The Ongoing Challenge of Antimicrobial Resistance

Editors

RICHARD R. WATKINS
ROBERT A. BONOMO

INFECTIOUS DISEASE CLINICS OF NORTH AMERICA

www.id.theclinics.com

Consulting Editor
HELEN W. BOUCHER

December 2020 • Volume 34 • Number 4

ELSEVIER

1600 John F. Kennedy Boulevard • Suite 1800 • Philadelphia, Pennsylvania, 19103-2899.

http://www.theclinics.com

INFECTIOUS DISEASE CLINICS OF NORTH AMERICA Volume 34, Number 4
December 2020 ISSN 0891–5520, ISBN-13: 978-0-323-75943-4

Editor: Kerry Holland
Developmental Editor: Donald Mumford

Infectious Disease Clinics of North America (ISSN 0891–5520) is published in March, June, September, and December by Elsevier Inc., 360 Park Avenue South, New York, NY 10010-1710. Periodicals postage paid at New York, NY and additional mailing offices. Subscription prices are $340.00 per year for US individuals, $703.00 per year for US institutions, $100.00 per year for US students, $396.00 per year for Canadian individuals, $878.00 per year for Canadian institutions, $432.00 per year for international individuals, $878.00 per year for international institutions, $100.00 per year for Canadian students, and $200.00 per year for international students. To receive student rate, orders must be accompanied by name of affiliated institution, date of term, and the *signature* of program/residency coordinator on institution letterhead. Orders will be billed at individual rate until proof of status is received. Foreign air speed delivery is included in all *Clinics* subscription prices. All prices are subject to change without notice. **POSTMASTER**: Send address changes to *Infectious Disease Clinics of North America*, Elsevier Health Sciences Division, Subcription Customer Service, 3251 Riverport Lane, Maryland Heights, MO 63043. **Customer Service: 1-800-654-2452 (US). From outside of the US and Canada, call 1-314-447-8871. Fax: 1-314-447-8029. E-mail: JournalsCustomerService-usa@elsevier.com (print support) or JournalsOnlineSupport-usa@elsevier.com (online support).**

Infectious Disease Clinics of North America is also published in Spanish by Editorial Inter-Médica, Junin 917, 1er A 1113, Buenos Aires, Argentina.

Reprints. For copies of 100 or more, of articles in this publication, please contact the Commercial Reprints Department, Elsevier Inc., 360 Park Avenue South, New York, New York 10010-1710. Tel. 212-633-3874, Fax: 212-633-3820, E-mail: reprints@elsevier.com.

Infectious Disease Clinics of North America is covered in *MEDLINE/PubMed (Index Medicus), Current Contents/ Clinical Medicine, Science Citation Alert, SCISEARCH,* and *Research Alert.*

Contributors

CONSULTING EDITOR

HELEN W. BOUCHER, MD, FIDSA, FACP
Director, Infectious Diseases Fellowship Program, Division of Geographic Medicine and Infectious Diseases, Tufts Medical Center, Associate Professor of Medicine, Tufts University School of Medicine, Boston, Massachusetts, USA

EDITORS

RICHARD R. WATKINS, MD, MS, FACP, FIDSA, FISAC
Professor of Internal Medicine, Northeast Ohio Medical University, Rootstown, Ohio; Staff Physician, Division of Infectious Diseases, Cleveland Clinic Akron General, Akron, Ohio, USA

ROBERT A. BONOMO, MD
Louis Stokes Cleveland Veterans Affairs Medical Center, Departments of Medicine, Biochemistry, Pharmacology, Molecular Biology, and Microbiology, Case Western Reserve University School of Medicine, Cleveland, Ohio, USA

AUTHORS

AMOS ADLER, MD
Clinical Microbiology Laboratory, Tel-Aviv Sourasky Medical Center, Sackler School of Medicine, Tel-Aviv University, Tel-Aviv, Israel

WILLIAM ALEGRIA, PharmD
Infectious Diseases Pharmacist, Stanford Health Care, Stanford, California, USA

YOSHICHIKA ARAKAWA, MD, PhD
Department of Bacteriology, Nagoya University Graduate School of Medicine, Nagoya, Aichi, Japan

CESAR A. ARIAS, MD, PhD
Professor of Medicine, Microbiology and Molecular Genetics, Herbert L. and Margaret W. DuPont Chair in Infectious Diseases, Laurel and Robert H. Graham Faculty Fellow at McGovern Medical School, Director, Center for Antimicrobial Resistance and Microbial Genomics, Director, Center for Infectious Diseases, School of Public Health, Houston, Texas, USA; Molecular Genetics and Antimicrobial Resistance Unit, International Center for Microbial Genomics, Universidad El Bosque, Bogota, Colombia

CHARLES M. BARK, MD
Division of Infectious Diseases, MetroHealth Medical Center, Cleveland, Ohio, USA

ROBERT A. BONOMO, MD
Louis Stokes Cleveland Veterans Affairs Medical Center, Departments of Medicine, Biochemistry, Pharmacology, Molecular Biology, and Microbiology, Case Western Reserve University School of Medicine, Cleveland, Ohio, USA

STAN DERESINSKI, MD
Division of Infectious Diseases and Geographic Medicine, Clinical Professor of Medicine, Stanford University School of Medicine, Stanford, California, USA

YOHEI DOI, MD, PhD
Division of Infectious Diseases, University of Pittsburgh School of Medicine, Pittsburgh, Pennsylvania, USA; Departments of Microbiology and Infectious Diseases, Fujita Health University School of Medicine, Toyoake, Japan

KHALID M. DOUSA, MD
Division of Infectious Diseases & HIV Medicine, University Hospitals Cleveland Medical Center, Case Western Reserve University, Cleveland, Ohio, USA

DONALD DUMFORD 3RD, MD, MPH
Assistant Professor, Department of Medicine, Northeast Ohio Medical University, Rootstown, Ohio, USA; Staff Physician, Division of Infectious Diseases, Cleveland Clinic Akron General, Akron, Ohio, USA

ANDREA ENDIMIANI, MD, PhD
Institute for Infectious Diseases, Faculty of Medicine, University of Bern, Bern, Switzerland

THOMAS M. FILE Jr, MD, MSc
Chair, Infectious Disease Division, Co-Director, Antimicrobial Stewardship Program, Summa Health, Akron, Ohio, USA; Professor, Internal Medicine, Master Teacher, Chair, Infectious Disease Section, Northeast Ohio Medical University (NEOMED), Rootstown, Ohio, USA

JENNIFER J. FURIN, MD, PhD
Division of Infectious Diseases & HIV Medicine, University Hospitals Cleveland Medical Center, Case Western Reserve University, Cleveland, Ohio, USA; Department of Global Health and Social Medicine, Harvard Medical School, Boston, Massachusetts, USA

MAHMOUD GHANNOUM, PhD
Professor, Center for Medical Mycology, Case Western Reserve University, University Hospitals Cleveland, Cleveland, Ohio, USA

DEBRA A. GOFF, PharmD, FCCP
Infectious Diseases Specialty Pharmacist, Department of Pharmacy, Associate Professor, College of Pharmacy, The Ohio State University Wexner Medical Center, Columbus, Ohio, USA

MARISA HOLUBAR, MD, MS
Division of Infectious Diseases and Geographic Medicine, Clinical Associate Professor of Medicine, Stanford University School of Medicine, Stanford, California, USA

MICHAEL R. JACOBS, MD, PhD
Department of Pathology, Case Western Reserve University and University Hospitals, Cleveland Medical Center, Cleveland, Ohio, USA

ROBIN L.P. JUMP, MD, PhD
Associate Professor, Department of Medicine, Case Western Reserve University, Geriatric Research, Education and Clinical Center (GRECC), VA Northeast Ohio Healthcare System, Cleveland, Ohio, USA

DAVID E. KATZ, MD, MPH
Division of Internal Medicine, Shaare Zedek Medical Center, Jerusalem, Israel

KEITH S. KAYE, MD, MPH
Department of Internal Medicine, University of Michigan Medical School, Ann Arbor, Michigan, USA

SEBASTIAN G. KURZ, MD, PhD
Mount Sinai National Jewish Health Respiratory Institute, New York City, New York, USA

JIAN LI, PhD
Laboratory of Antimicrobial Systems Pharmacology, Department of Microbiology, Monash University, Victoria, Australia

ZEKUN LI, BS
Department of Clinical Laboratory, Peking Union Medical College Hospital, Peking Union Medical College, Chinese Academy of Medical Sciences, Beijing, China

ANDREW R. MACK, BS
Research Service, Louis Stokes Cleveland Department of Veterans Affairs, Department of Molecular Biology and Microbiology, Case Western Reserve University, Cleveland, Ohio, USA

DROR MARCHAIM, MD
Sackler School of Medicine, Tel-Aviv University, Tel-Aviv, Israel; Unit of Infection Control, Shamir (Assaf Harofeh) Medical Center, Zerifin, Israel

LINA MENG, PharmD
Infectious Diseases Pharmacist, Stanford Health Care, Stanford, California, USA

WILLIAM R. MILLER, MD
Assistant Professor of Medicine, Department of Internal Medicine, Division of Infectious Diseases, University of Texas Health Science Center at Houston, McGovern Medical School, Center for Antimicrobial Resistance and Microbial Genomics (CARMiG), Houston, Texas, USA

BARBARA E. MURRAY, MD
J. Ralph Meadows Professor of Medicine, Department of Internal Medicine, Division of Infectious Diseases, University of Texas Health Science Center at Houston, McGovern Medical School, Center for Antimicrobial Resistance and Microbial Genomics (CARMiG), Professor, Department of Microbiology and Molecular Genetics, Houston, Texas, USA

ROGER L. NATION, PhD
Drug Delivery, Disposition and Dynamics, Monash Institute of Pharmaceutical Sciences, Faculty of Pharmacy and Pharmaceutical Sciences, Monash University, Victoria, Australia

KRISZTINA M. PAPP-WALLACE, PhD
Assistant Professor, Research Service, Louis Stokes Cleveland Department of Veterans Affairs, Departments of Medicine and Biochemistry, Case Western Reserve University, Cleveland, Ohio, USA

DAVID L. PATERSON, MD, PhD
University of Queensland Centre for Clinical Research, Royal Brisbane & Women's Hospital Campus, Herston, Queensland, Australia

JOHN R. PERFECT, MD
James B. Duke Professor, Duke University Medical Center, Durham, North Carolina, USA

JASON M. POGUE, PharmD
Department of Clinical Pharmacy, University of Michigan College of Pharmacy, Ann Arbor, Michigan, USA

ALBAN RAMETTE, PhD
Institute for Infectious Diseases, Faculty of Medicine, University of Bern, Bern, Switzerland

DANIEL D. RHOADS, MD
Pathology and Laboratory Medicine Institute and Department of Infectious Diseases, Cleveland Clinic, Cleveland, Ohio, USA

LOUIS B. RICE, MD
Joukowsky Family Professor of Medicine, Professor of Molecular Microbiology and Immunology, Chair of Medicine, Department of Internal Medicine, Brown University, Providence, Rhode Island, USA

MARION J. SKALWEIT, MD, PhD
Staff Physician, Infectious Diseases Section, VA Northeast Ohio Health System and Professor of Medicine, Case Western Reserve University, Cleveland, Ohio, USA

MAGDALENA A. TARACILA, MS
Research Service, Louis Stokes Cleveland Department of Veterans Affairs, Department of Medicine, Case Western Reserve University, Cleveland, Ohio, USA

DAVID VAN DUIN, MD, PhD
Division of Infectious Diseases, University of North Carolina, Chapel Hill, North Carolina, USA

JUN-ICHI WACHINO, PhD
Department of Bacteriology, Nagoya University Graduate School of Medicine, Nagoya, Aichi, Japan

RICHARD R. WATKINS, MD, MS, FACP, FIDSA, FISAC
Professor of Internal Medicine, Northeast Ohio Medical University, Rootstown, Ohio; Staff Physician, Division of Infectious Diseases, Cleveland Clinic Akron General, Akron, Ohio, USA

QIWEN YANG, MD
Department of Clinical Laboratory, Peking Union Medical College Hospital, Peking Union Medical College, Chinese Academy of Medical Sciences, Beijing, China

Contents

Preface: The Ongoing Threat of Antimicrobial Resistance xiii

Richard R. Watkins and Robert A. Bonomo

Overview: The Ongoing Threat of Antimicrobial Resistance 649

Richard R. Watkins and Robert A. Bonomo

The effectiveness of antibiotics continues to erode because of the relentless spread of antimicrobial resistance (AMR). Public and private foundations, professional organizations, and international health agencies recognize the threat posed by AMR and have issued calls for action. One of the main drivers of AMR is overprescription of antibiotics, both in human and in veterinary medicine. The One Health concept is a response from a broad group of stakeholders to counter the global health threat posed by AMR. In this article, we discuss current trends in AMR and suggest strategies to mitigate its ongoing dissemination.

The Evolving Role of the Clinical Microbiology Laboratory in Identifying Resistance in Gram-Negative Bacteria: An Update 659

Andrea Endimiani, Alban Ramette, Daniel D. Rhoads, and Michael R. Jacobs

The evolution of resistance to antimicrobial agents in gram-negatives has challenged the role of the clinical microbiology laboratory to implement new methods for their timely detection. Recent development has enabled the use of novel methods for more rapid pathogen identification, antimicrobial susceptibility testing, and detection of resistance markers. Commonly used methods improve the rapidity of resistance detection from both cultured bacteria and specimens. This review focuses on the commercially available systems available together with their technical performance and possible clinical impact.

The Continuing Plague of Extended-Spectrum β-Lactamase Producing Enterbacterales Infections: An Update 677

Amos Adler, David E. Katz, and Dror Marchaim

Antimicrobial resistance is a common iatrogenic complication of modern life and medical care. One of the most demonstrative examples is the exponential increase in the incidence of extended-spectrum β-lactamases (ESBLs) production among Enterobacteriaceae, that is, the most common human pathogens outside of the hospital setting. Infections resulting from ESBL-producing bacteria are associated with devastating outcomes, now affecting even previously healthy individuals. This poses an enormous burden and threat to public health. This article aims to narrate the evolving epidemiology of ESBL infections and highlights current challenges in terms of management and prevention of these common infections.

gram-negative bacterial infections. Plazomicin, a next-generation aminoglycoside, was introduced for the treatment of complicated urinary tract infections and acute pyelonephritis. In contrast, bacteria have resisted aminoglycosides, including plazomicin, by producing 16S ribosomal RNA (rRNA) methyltransferases (MTases) that confer high-level and broad-range aminoglycoside resistance. Aminoglycoside-resistant 16S rRNA MTase-producing gram-negative pathogens are widespread in various settings and are becoming a grave concern. This article provides up-to-date information with a focus on aminoglycoside-resistant 16S rRNA MTases.

The Role of Antibiotic Stewardship and Telemedicine in the Management of Multidrug-Resistant Infections **903**

Thomas M. File Jr, Robin L.P. Jump, and Debra A. Goff

This article summarizes the literature describing how antimicrobial stewardship and telemedicine interventions affect antimicrobial resistance. Discussion includes why we need stewardship, how to collaborate with team members, and the evidence of stewardship's and telemedicine's impact on resistance.

Emerging Issues in Antifungal Resistance **921**

John R. Perfect and Mahmoud Ghannoum

Invasive fungal diseases continue to cause substantial mortality in the enlarging immunocompromised population. It is fortunate that the field has moved past amphotericin B deoxycholate as the only available antifungal drug but despite new classes of antifungal agents, both primary and secondary drug resistance in molds and yeasts abound. From the rise of multiple-drug–resistant Candida auris to the agrochemical selection of environmental azole-resistant Aspergillus fumigatus, it is and will be critical to understand antifungal drug resistance and both prevent and treat it with new strategies and agents.

INFECTIOUS DISEASE CLINICS OF NORTH AMERICA

FORTHCOMING ISSUES

March 2021
Skin and Soft Tissue Infections
Henry Chambers, *Editor*

June 2021
Fungal Infections
Luis Ostrosky-Zeichner, *Editor*

September 2021
Infection Prevention and Control in Healthcare, Part I: Facility Planning
Keith S. Kaye and Sorabh Dhar, *Editors*

RECENT ISSUES

September 2020
Infectious Disease Complications of Opioid Use and Other Substance Use Disorders
Sandra A. Springer and Carlos Del Rio, *Editors*

June 2020
Infections Related to Biologics
Dora Y. Ho and Aruna K. Subramanian, *Editors*

March 2020
Collaborative Antimicrobial Stewardship
Elizabeth Dodds Ashley and Steven Schaeffer Spires, *Editors*

Preface

The Ongoing Threat of Antimicrobial Resistance

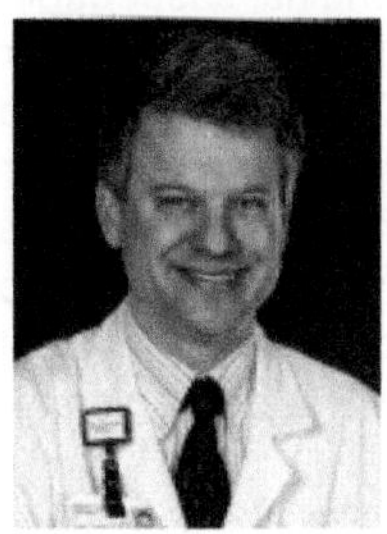

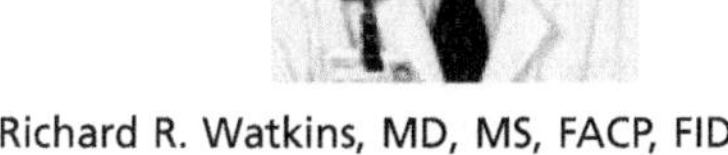

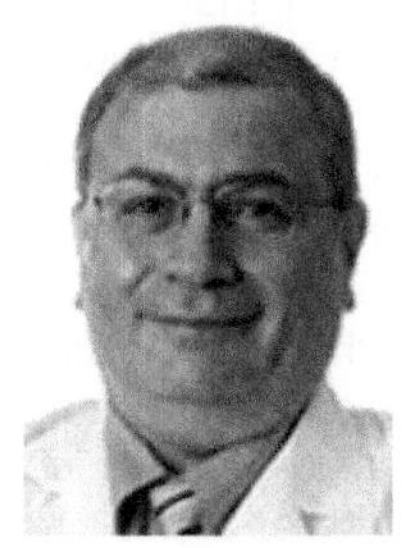

Richard R. Watkins, MD, MS, FACP, FIDSA, FISAC   Robert A. Bonomo, MD
Editors

The relentless spread of antimicrobial resistance (AMR) remains as salient a threat today as it was in 2016, when we last served as editors for this issue of *Infectious Disease Clinics of North America*. Since then, AMR continues to undermine progress in health care, economic development, food production, and life expectancy. Numerous governmental and nongovernmental organizations have called for action to curtail the unnecessary use of antibiotics and to strengthen antibiotic stewardship efforts. For example, the Centers for Disease Control and Prevention (CDC) issued "Antibiotic Resistance Threats in the United States, 2019" that estimated antibiotic-resistant bacteria and fungi cause 2,868,700 infections leading to 35,900 deaths in the United States each year. This document identified 5 pathogens as "urgent threats" that require aggressive action: (1) carbapenem-resistant *Acinetobacter*, (2) *Candida auris*, (3) *Clostridioides difficile*, (4) carbapenem-resistant Enterobacteriaceae (Enterobacterales), and (5) drug-resistant *Neisseria gonorrhoeae*. Our first article in this issue reviews how we got to this point, describes the factors that drive AMR, and suggests strategies to curtail its ongoing spread.

Another difficulty in this field is that diagnosing antibiotic-resistant bacteria remains challenging. This leads clinicians to prescribe empiric antibiotics that are often subsequently shown to be unnecessarily broad or sometimes too narrow. Despite progress from newer technologies (eg, matrix-assisted laser desorption/ionization time-of-flight mass spectrometry and whole-genome sequencing), making a microbiological diagnosis remains primarily culture-based, usually taking 12 to 24 hours from the time of culture collection to reach preliminary identification, then longer for antimicrobial susceptibilities. Indeed, many patients with infections end up with negative culture results. Rapid tests are available for some clinical scenarios, such as acute respiratory panels for viruses and group A streptococcal throat swabs, but they have limitations, such as the inability to report antimicrobial susceptibilities. What is truly needed is a rapid, inexpensive, point-of-care test that detects antibiotic-resistant bacteria in blood or other body fluids. Once available, this technology could be used to inform rational antibiotic

Infect Dis Clin N Am 34 (2020) xiii–xiv
https://doi.org/10.1016/j.idc.2020.09.001

prescribing, thus limiting toxicities and reducing health care costs. The second article discusses the changing role of the microbiology laboratory as it pertains to identifying AMR in gram-negative bacteria. These advances need to be evaluated critically in terms of impact on clinical decision making.

The mechanisms of AMR are diverse and complex. The exposure of susceptible bacterial populations to an antibiotic exerts selection pressure for genetic mutations. This results in resistant mutants that outcompete the original susceptible population. Another mechanism is the acquisition and sharing of highly mobile plasmids among bacteria of different species and genera. A notable example is the spread of the colistin-resistance gene *mcr-1*in *Escherichia coli*, which was first reported in 2016 from Shandong Province, China. Given that *E coli* is the most common cause of urinary tract infections (UTIs), the dissemination of *mcr-1* and other resistance genes raises the concern that UTIs could become untreatable with all currently available antibiotics. The next 2 articles further describe how AMR is spreading in gram-negative pathogens, including those in the community.

The remaining articles tackle a range of topics related to AMR, including how resistance develops to the major classes of antibiotic agents, principles of antimicrobial stewardship and telemedicine, and recent advances in understanding AMR in fungi. The authors are a distinguished group of experts whose articles provide the latest and most accurate information on AMR, with the primary goal to help clinicians make informed treatment decisions when confronted with infections from antibiotic-resistant pathogens. The issue should also help identify gaps in our current knowledge about AMR and suggest future directions for research. With the world in the midst of the COVID-19 pandemic, the possibility of coinfections with antibiotic-resistant bacteria is a real concern that requires further investigation. Ultimately, the goal of science and medicine is to preserve the existence of human life. Our ability to understand and mitigate the threat posed by AMR is crucial for human progress and to avoid a return to the preantibiotic era.

We would again like to thank Dr Helen Boucher for inviting us to develop this issue, along with the excellent editorial staff at Elsevier for their assistance, including Donald Mumford and Kerry Holland. Comments and feedback from the readers are welcome as we look forward to preparing future issues on the important topic of AMR.

Richard R. Watkins, MD, MS, FACP, FIDSA, FISAC
Division of Infectious Diseases
Cleveland Clinic Akron General
224 West Exchange Street, Suite 290
Akron, OH 44302, USA

Robert A. Bonomo, MD
Louis Stokes Cleveland Veterans Affairs
Medical Center
Departments of Medicine, Biochemistry, Pharmacology
Molecular Biology, and Microbiology
Case Western Reserve University
School of Medicine
10701 East Boulevard
Cleveland, OH 44106, USA

E-mail addresses:
WatkinR2@ccf.org (R.R. Watkins)
robert.bonomo@va.gov (R.A. Bonomo)

Overview

The Ongoing Threat of Antimicrobial Resistance

Richard R. Watkins, MD, MS[a,b,*], Robert A. Bonomo, MD[c,d]

KEYWORDS

- Antimicrobial resistance • Antibiotics • Public health

KEY POINTS

- The effectiveness of antibiotics continues to erode because of the relentless spread of antimicrobial resistance (AMR).
- Public and private foundations, professional organizations, and international health agencies recognize the threat posed by AMR and have issued calls for action.
- One of the main drivers of AMR is overprescription of antibiotics, both in human and in veterinary medicine.
- The One Health concept is a response from a broad group of stakeholders to counter the global health threat posed by AMR.

INTRODUCTION

The discovery and clinical implementation of antibiotics in the twentieth century is one of the greatest achievements in modern medicine. These "miracle drugs" treat infections ranging from minor to life threatening, enable surgeons to perform complex procedures in challenging anatomic locations, allow organ transplantation to be feasible, and empower oncologists to give higher doses of curative chemotherapy for cancer, thereby increasing the chance for remission. Unfortunately, the global dissemination of antimicrobial resistance (AMR) threatens to undo all these advances and lead us back to the "preantibiotic era." Moreover, the global economic cost of AMR is staggering and estimated to result in a loss of $3 trillion in gross domestic product annually.[1]

According to a recent Centers for Disease Control and Prevention (CDC) report, approximately 2.8 million infections from antibiotic-resistant bacteria occur annually

[a] Division of Infectious Diseases, Cleveland Clinic Akron General, Akron, OH, USA; [b] Department of Medicine, Northeast Ohio Medical University, Rootstown, OH, USA; [c] Medical Service, Louis Stokes Cleveland Department of Veterans Affairs Medical Center, Cleveland, OH, USA; [d] Case VA Center for Antimicrobial Resistance and Epidemiology (Case VA-CARES), Case Western Reserve University, Cleveland, OH, USA

* Corresponding author. Division of Infectious Diseases, Cleveland Clinic Akron General, Akron, OH.

E-mail address: WatkinR2@ccf.org

Infect Dis Clin N Am 34 (2020) 649–658
https://doi.org/10.1016/j.idc.2020.04.002
id.theclinics.com

in the United States, resulting in more than 35,000 deaths.[2] Moreover, these infections have a higher risk for hospitalization and complications.[3] AMR is an inevitable evolutionary outcome because all organisms develop genetic mutations to avoid lethal selective pressure. As long as antibiotics are used against human pathogens, these bacteria will continue to develop and use resistance mechanisms.[4] At present, more than 70% of pathogenic bacteria are resistant to at least 1 antibiotic.[5] Notably, a survey of infectious diseases physicians in the United States found that 60% had encountered a bacterial infection resistant to available drugs in the previous year.[6]

AMR is a complicated process that is driven by multiple factors (**Box 1**). Despite the global spread of AMR, regulatory approval of new antibiotics has declined 90% during the past 30 years in the United States.[7] In addition to the high cost of antibiotic research and development, the rapid evolution of AMR has meant diminished market returns for the pharmaceutical industry.[8] For example, the 4 antibiotics (ceftazidime-avibactam, meropenem-vaborbactam, plazomicin, and eravacycline) approved since 2015 that target carbapenem-resistant Enterobacteriales (CRE) compete against each other for market share, which has led to disappointing sales.[9] The present economic incentives in place to sustainably develop new antibiotics may be failing, and new models that incentivize long-term growth and development are needed.

After many years out of the mainstream, the serious threat posed by AMR has been increasingly recognized by the media and governmental organizations. In September 2014, the White House proposed the National Strategy for Combating Antibiotic-Resistant Bacteria, wherein President Obama charged Congress with designing a research agenda to combat AMR on multiple fronts.[10]

The CDC has prepared a list of AMR bacteria in the United States that are of most concern (**Box 2**). Of these threats, the widespread dissemination of AMR gram-negative bacilli (GNB) is arguably the most worrisome at present. Limited treatment options, the ease of plasmid-mediated transfer of resistance genes among GNB, the widespread distribution of Enterobacteriales (formally Enterobacteriaceae) as part of the human microbiome, the asymptomatic colonization present in certain individuals, and higher mortality associated with CRE compared with susceptible strains

Box 1
Factors that promote antimicrobial resistance

- Bacterial population density in health care facilities; allows transfer of bacteria within a community and enables resistance to emerge
- Inadequate adherence to best infection control practices
- Increase of high-risk patient populations (eg, chemotherapy, dialysis, and transplant patients and patients residing in long-term care facilities)
- Antibiotic overuse in agriculture
- Global travel and tourism (including medical tourism)
- Poor sanitation and contaminated water systems; can lead to the spread of resistant bacteria in sewage
- Improper antibiotic prescribing in human medicine (eg, for viral infections or for inappropriately long courses of therapy)
- Overprescription of broad-spectrum antibiotics; can exert selective pressure on commensal bacteria
- Paucity of rapid diagnostic tests to guide proper antibiotic prescribing
- Lack of approved vaccines for drug-resistant pathogens

Box 2
Antibiotic-resistant bacteria of concern in the United States

Urgent threat level
- Carbapenem-resistant Enterobacteriaceae
- *Candida auris*
- *Clostridioides difficile*
- Carbapenem-resistant *Acinetobacter*
- Drug-resistant *N gonorrhoeae*

Serious threat level
- Drug-resistant *Campylobacter*
- Drug-resistant *Candida*
- ESBL-producing Enterobacteriaceae
- Vancomycin-resistant *Enterococcus*
- Multidrug-resistant *P aeruginosa*
- Drug-resistant *Salmonella* serotype Typhi
- Drug-resistant nontyphoidal *Salmonella*
- Drug-resistant *Shigella*
- Methicillin-resistant *S aureus*
- Drug-resistant *Streptococcus pneumoniae*
- Drug-resistant tuberculosis

Concerning threat level
- Erythromycin-resistant group A *Streptococcus*
- Clindamycin-resistant group B *Streptococcus*

Watch list
- Azole-resistant *Aspergillus fumigatus*
- Drug-resistant *Mycoplasma genitalium*
- Drug-resistant *Bordetella pertussis*

Adapted from Centers for Disease Control and Prevention. Antibiotic resistance threats in the United States, 2019. Report available at https://www.cdc.gov/drugresistance/pdf/threats-report/2019-ar-threats-report-508.pdf. Accessed December 3, 2019.

can be insurmountable challenges.[11] Moreover, risk factors are increasingly identified for acquiring AMR-GNB and include recent antibiotic usage, residence in extended care facilities, admission to an intensive care unit (ICU), possessing an indwelling device or wounds, poor functional status, organ or stem cell transplantation, receipt of immunomodulatory therapies, and travel to an endemic area.[12]

Of the drug classes to which AMR can emerge, the most problematic is against the β-lactams. These drugs (penicillins, cephalosporins, monobactams, and carbapenems) are among the most time-honored, safest, and most potent of antibiotics. β-Lactam resistance in GNB is primarily mediated through β-lactamase genes (*bla*) that are frequently encoded on plasmids and other mobile genetic elements. β-Lactamases are classified into 4 main groups based on their amino acid sequences (classes A, B, C, and D).[13] Class A includes extended-spectrum β-lactamases (ESBLs) and *Klebsiella pneumoniae* carbapenemase enzymes; class B enzymes are the metallo-β-lactamases (of which New Delhi metallo-β-lactamase [NDM] is a prime example); class C enzymes are the chromosomal and plasmid encoded cephalosporinases; and class D enzymes are oxacillinases. Class D β-lactamases are among the most diverse and complex families possessing many carbapenem hydrolyzing variants (carbapenem hydrolyzing class D). It is notable that *Acinetobacter baumannii*, although at 1 time considered a "less-virulent" pathogen compared with *K pneumoniae* and *Pseudomonas aeruginosa*, plays a significant role in spreading broad-spectrum resistance genes and many *bla* variants of every major class to other gram-negative organisms.[14]

EVOLUTION OF ANTIBIOTIC RESISTANCE

The first effective antimicrobial agent, sulfonamide, was introduced into clinical practice in 1935. Within 2 years, sulfonamide resistance was reported, and the same AMR mechanisms are still present more than 80 years later.[15] One useful way to understand the basic mechanisms of AMR is through the "bullet-and-target" concept, whereby the sites of drug activity (the target) can be changed by enzymatic modification, transformed by genomic mutations, and bypassed metabolically (eg, sulfonamide resistance); the antibiotic (the bullet) can undergo enzymatic inactivation and degradation (eg, β-lactamases), reduced access into the cell (eg, porin loss), and increased removal from the cell (eg, efflux pumps).[16,17] Emerging evidence suggests that resistance mechanisms in *Mycobacterium tuberculosis* (MTb), one of the oldest and most widespread human pathogens, are induced by mutations caused by subinhibitory concentrations of antibiotics.[18] Indeed, the sole source of resistance to anti-MTb drugs is by mutation of the target genes. To illustrate, patients infected with MTb who previously received quinolone antibiotics developed resistance to this antibiotic class as well as to first-line anti-MTb drugs.[19] These data highlight the phenomenon of "collateral damage" by showing a strong and direct correlation between the use of antibiotics and resistance.

One important example of contemporary evolution in resistance phenotypes is *Salmonella typhi*. In the early twentieth century, the preantibiotic era, typhoid fever exacted a 20% mortality, which was significantly reduced with the introduction of effective therapy. Fluoroquinolones became the agents of choice in the 1990s, but 1 lineage of *Salmonella* with reduced susceptibility has widely disseminated.[20] Unfortunately, efforts to develop novel therapies against *S typhi* are minimal.[21] Thus, we are on the verge of widespread resistance with few effective alternatives for typhoid fever, raising the possibility of a return to the preantibiotic era for this disease.[22] Two other notable examples are (i) the evolution of penicillin resistance in *Neisseria gonorrhea* whereby alterations in penicillin-binding proteins accelerated the development of resistance to penicillin; and (ii) the discovery of ESBLs whereby single point mutations in β-lactamase genes undermined the impact of expanded-spectrum cephalosporins (eg, ceftazidime).

Although AMR has traditionally been identified as a hospital-acquired problem, the impact from the environment is increasingly recognized. Certain environmental compartments (eg, municipal wastewater systems, pharmaceutical manufacturing effluents, and agricultural waste products) are characterized by extremely high concentrations of bacteria coupled with subtherapeutic concentrations of antibiotics, leading to the discharge of AMR bacteria and AMR genes into the wider environment.[23] For example, river sediment downstream from a waste water treatment plant had 10 novel combinations of cephalosporin-resistance genes as well as an imipenem-resistant *Escherichia coli*.[24] Uncertainty exists as to whether AMR genes that are acquired by both clinically relevant bacteria and nonpathogenic ones in the environment originate from the same sources. Furthermore, the role of environmental bacteria in spreading AMR genes to nosocomial pathogens is unknown. Investigating these conundrums should be a priority because of the global scale of AMR.

ANTIBIOTICS AND AGRICULTURE

The use of antibiotics in agriculture is becoming increasingly scrutinized. More than 13 million kilograms of antibiotics are used annually in agriculture in the United States, approximately 80% of the antibiotics consumed in the country.[25] Most of this usage is not for treating disease in animals (livestock), but for growth promotion and disease prevention, usually at subtherapeutic concentrations. Chang and colleagues[26] have suggested the following 3 mechanisms by which AMR in agriculture could threaten human health:

1. A human is infected by a resistant pathogen through contact with livestock or through ingestion of bacteria from contaminated food or water;
2. A human becomes colonized by resistant bacteria through one of these means and then spreads it to another person who subsequently becomes ill;
3. Resistance genes arising in agriculture are spread to humans through horizontal gene transfer, and the resulting resistant strains are selected by antibiotic use in people.

Evidence suggests several strains of pathogens that infect humans have originated from animals, including stains of AMR *Campylobacter* spp,[27] *Salmonella* spp,[28] methicillin-resistant *Staphylococcus aureus* (MRSA),[29] vancomycin-resistant *Enterococcus* (VRE),[30] ESBL-producing Enterobacteriales,[31] and CRE.[32] The transfer of resistance determinants from animals to humans, however, is difficult to trace, and the role of these animal reservoirs in clinical AMR remains enigmatic.

Given the link between AMR and antibiotic use in farm animals, a possible solution is to ban antibiotics except when livestock are ill. The European Union banned all nontherapeutic antibiotics in animals in 2006, and the Food and Drug Administration issued a policy in 2012 asking farmers to voluntarily decrease their use of antibiotics. Theoretically, antibiotic selection pressure should be reduced by a ban, leading to less-resistant organisms in the environment. Avoparcin, a vancomycin analogue, was banned as a feed additive in Taiwan in 2000, and a nationwide surveillance study found the frequency of VRE in chicken farms decreased in association with this legislation.[33] Despite a paucity of definitive data, a better argument for restricting antibiotics in agriculture may be to reduce the prevalence of resistant pathogens and, thereby, lower the chances for horizontal transfer of resistance genes.

Significant challenges exist for banning antibiotics in agriculture in the United States. Given the wide geographic distribution of farms, regulatory oversight would likely be difficult to enforce. Also, it would be problematic to clearly know what the antibiotics were being used for, such as treating sick animals versus prophylaxis against infections. One proposal is to implement an antibiotic user fee. According to Hollis and Ahmed,[25] a user fee would be easier to administer because it could be collected at the manufacturing stage, would discourage low-value uses of antibiotics, would generate revenues that could help pay for new antibiotic development by the pharmaceutical industry or support antimicrobial stewardship efforts, and could encourage governments to collaborate, such as signing treaties to collect revenue generated by the user fees. Finally, a "One Health" approach has been advocated as a way to engage multiple sectors and stakeholders (eg, human health, animal health, agriculture, and the environment) to address AMR on multiple fronts.[34]

SOCIETAL BURDEN OF ANTIBIOTIC RESISTANCE

The economic impact of AMR is enormous. Overall, AMR is estimated to cost $55 billion in the United States annually.[35] Furthermore, an infection by an ESBL-producing *E coli* or *Klebsiella* spp can increase hospitalization costs by $16,450 and add an additional 9.7 days to the length of stay.[36]

Novel AMR genes disproportionately originate in lower-income countries, with downstream impact on the originating country and in those outside the region.[20] For example, NDM-1 was first identified in a strain of *K pneumoniae* from a patient in Sweden who had returned from India.[37] Regarding the health impact of AMR, the World Health Organization (WHO) reported a significant increase in all-cause mortality and 30-day mortality from infections caused by third-generation cephalosporin-resistant (including ESBL) and fluoroquinolone-resistant *E coli* as well as expanded-spectrum cephalosporin (eg, ceftazidime and cefepime) -resistant and carbapenem-resistant *K pneumoniae*.[38] MRSA infections lead to significant increases in all-cause mortality, bacterium-attributable mortality, ICU mortality, septic shock, length of stay, and a 2-fold risk increase for discharge to long-term care compared with methicillin-sensitive *S aureus*.[39] Thus, the management of MRSA imposes important economic costs to health care organizations, although there is a scarcity of definitive evidence available to allow for a comprehensive evaluation of the economic burden.

WHAT CAN BE DONE TO AVOID A POSTANTIBIOTIC ERA?

Although identifying and developing new drugs or vaccines are an important solution to the AMR problem, the development of therapeutics is a costly and complicated endeavor. In addition to novel antibiotics in development, early preliminary data obtained by using phage cocktails against *Acinetobacter* spp seem promising.[40] A phage-derived enzyme with highly potent lytic activity has been shown to improve therapy against MRSA.[41] Monoclonal vaccines have also been tested, but their clinical applications are still in the early stages (eg, *P aeruginosa* monoclonal vaccine under development by Medimmune). Therefore, alternative strategies are necessary, particularly in low-income countries.

An important and effective way to limit the spread of AMR is to reduce the consumption of antibiotics. In 2004, Bergman and colleagues[42] showed that regional macrolide use was closely associated with erythromycin resistance in *Streptococcus pyogenes*. Reducing antibiotics use is one of the central tenets of antibiotic stewardship, now universally recognized as beneficial.[43] For example, a stewardship program from a Swedish university hospital decreased antibiotic usage by 27% without any negative impact on patient outcomes, primarily by limiting broad-spectrum agents.[44] On a wider scale, antibiotic prescribing nationally in the United States has improved, with a 5% decrease from 2011 to 2016.[45] However, reducing antibiotic consumption alone is not a panacea for stopping AMR, which requires a multifaceted approach.

The World Alliance Against Antibiotic Resistance has put forward a declaration that includes 10 proposals for tackling AMR.[46] Several of them (eg, more rapid diagnostic tests, antibiotic stewardship, and surveillance networks) are not new ideas, but nonetheless are widely recognized as beneficial. Therefore, the value of the declaration is that it convincingly and authoritatively conveys the recommendations through a global perspective. One important concept in the document that deserves emphasis is the pressing need for an improved national surveillance mechanism in the United States. Currently there are several public databases and global surveillance projects, including Antimicrobial Resistance: Global Report on Surveillance, from the WHO; the European Antimicrobial Resistance Interactive Database; the Surveillance Network database in the United States and Australia; and the Global Study for Monitoring Antimicrobial Resistance Trends. In 2002, this last study began to monitor in vitro resistance of GNB in intraabdominal infections and more recently has focused on resistance to carbapenems and ESBLs.[47] Efforts to improve and coordinate microbiological information with clinical outcomes among these various programs are truly necessary.

Despite increasing media attention, the general public largely remains unaware of the threat posed by AMR. Of concern, a recent global survey conducted by the

WHO found that even in countries where national antibiotic awareness programs had been conducted, there was still widespread belief that antibiotics were effective against viral illnesses.[48] Certainly better educational efforts are needed.

Another disconcerting finding from the report was the widespread practice of antibiotics available without a prescription.[48] This ill-informed practice undoubtedly leads to overconsumption, especially among commonly used drugs in low-income settings (eg, fluoroquinolones to treat viral illnesses where typhoid fever is endemic). Changing antibiotics to prescription status will require strong government action, which is also necessary to make improvements in infrastructure and to provide better access to health care providers and laboratory facilities.

The role of the microbiome in the spread and control of AMR is increasingly recognized. Many commensal bacterial species, which were previously considered relatively harmless residents of the human gut, are now seen as disease-causing organisms.[49] Indeed, the microbiome is host to a vast reservoir of antibiotic resistance genes (ARG), which vary because of a multitude of factors, including diet, antibiotic use, country of residence, and occupation. For example, Yang and colleagues[50] showed residents of China have a higher relative abundance of ARG in the gut, followed by Americans and Europeans. Although antibiotics clearly affect the microbiome, the confounding effects of illness and aging make investigating their role a challenge.[51]

Finally, fecal microbiota transplant (FMT) has been shown to decrease ARG and potential pathogens, along with changing the function and composition of the microbiome.[52] Although promising, the potential benefits of FMT must be carefully weighed against the risks, which can include bacteremia or death, as described in a recent report.[53]

SUMMARY

AMR can only be tackled through a comprehensive approach that includes drug discovery and development, sustainable antibiotic usage policies, and disease-prevention strategies, like improving sanitation in low-income countries, infection-control practices in hospitals, and better diagnostic testing. Whether novel vaccines or phage therapy can be used to treat specific AMR bacteria remains to be seen, although there appears to be some promise in the use of phages against *A baumanii, P aeruginosa*, and *Mycobacteria*. Most of the political will and necessary resources must come from high-income countries. AMR is a complicated existential threat to humanity that requires a coordinated effort across a multitude of organizations and political boundaries.

REFERENCES

1. Naylor NR, Atun R, Zhu N, et al. Estimating the burden of antimicrobial resistance: a systematic literature review. Antimicrob Resist Infect Control 2018;7:58.
2. CDC. Antibiotic resistance threats in the United States, 2019. Atlanta (GA): U.S. Department of Health and Human Services, CDC; 2019. Available at: https://www.cdc.gov/drugresistance/Biggest-Threats.html. Accessed December 3, 2019.
3. Livermore D. Current epidemiology and growing resistance of gram-negative pathogens. Korean J Intern Med 2012;27:128–42.
4. National Institute of Allergy and Infectious Diseases. NIAID's antibacterial resistance program: current status and future directions. 2014. Available at: http://

www.niaid.nih.gov/topics/antimicrobialResistance/documents/arstrategicplan2014.pdf. Accessed December 3, 2019.
5. Katz ML, Mueller LV, Polyakov M, et al. Where have all the antibiotic patents gone? Nat Biotechnol 2006;24:1529–31.
6. Hersh AL, Newland JG, Beekmann SE, et al. Unmet medical need in infectious diseases. Clin Infect Dis 2012;54:1677–8.
7. Shlaes DM, Sahm D, Opiela C, et al. The FDA reboot of antibiotic development. Antimicrob Agents Chemother 2013;57:4605–7.
8. Payne DJ, Gwynn MD, Holmes DJ, et al. Drugs for bad bugs: confronting the challenges of antibiotic discovery. Nat Rev Drug Discov 2007;6:29–40.
9. Nielsen TB, Brass EP, Gilbert DN, et al. Sustainable discovery and development of antibiotics–is a nonprofit approach the future? N Engl J Med 2019;38:503–5.
10. Obama B. National strategy for combating antibiotic-resistant bacteria. Washington, DC: White House; 2014. p. 1–33.
11. Vasoo S, Barreto JN, Tosh PK. Emerging issues in gram-negative bacterial resistance: an update for the practicing clinician. Mayo Clin Proc 2015;90:395–403.
12. Tzouvelekis LS, Markogiannakis A, Psichogiou M, et al. Carbapenemases in *Klebsiella pneumoniae* and other Enterobacteriaceae: an evolving crisis of global dimensions. Clin Microbiol Rev 2012;25:682–707.
13. Hall BG, Barlow M. Revised Ambler classification of beta-lactamases. J Antimicrob Chemother 2005;55:1050–1.
14. Potron A, Poirel L, Nordmann P. Emerging broad-spectrum resistance to *Pseudomonas aeruginosa* and *Acinetobacter baumannii*: mechanisms and epidemiology. Int J Antimicrob Agents 2015;45(6):568–85.
15. Davies J, Davies D. Origins and evolution of antibiotic resistance. Microbiol Mol Biol Rev 2010;77:417–33.
16. Aminov RI. A brief history of the antibiotic era: lessons learned and challenges for the future. Front Microbiol 2010;1:134.
17. Tang SS, Apisarnthanarak A, Hsu LY. Mechanisms of b-lactam antimicrobial resistance and epidemiology of major community- and healthcare-associated multidrug-resistant bacteria. Adv Drug Deliv Rev 2014;78:3–13.
18. Fonseca JD, Knight GM, McHugh TD. The complex evolution of antibiotic resistance in *Mycobacterium tuberculosis*. Int J Infect Dis 2015;32:94–100.
19. Deutschendorf C, Goldani LZ, Santos RP. Previous use of quinolones: a surrogate marker for first line anti-tuberculosis drugs resistance in HIV-infected patients? Braz J Infect Dis 2012;16:142–5.
20. Kariuki S, Revathi G, Kiiru J, et al. Typhoid in Kenya is associated with a dominant multidrug-resistant *Salmonella enterica* serovar Typhi haplotype that is also widespread in Southeast Asia. J Clin Microbiol 2010;48:2171–6.
21. Baker S. A return to the pre-antimicrobial era? Science 2015;347:1064–6.
22. Koirala KD, Thanh DP, Thapa SD, et al. Highly resistant *Salmonella enterica* serovar Typhi with a novel gyrA mutation raises questions about the long-term efficacy of older fluoroquinolones for treating typhoid fever. Antimicrob Agents Chemother 2012;56:2761–2.
23. Berendonk TU, Manaia CM, Merlin C, et al. Tackling antibiotic resistance: the environmental framework. Nat Rev Microbiol 2015;13:310–7.
24. Amos GCA, Hawkey PM, Gaze WH, et al. Waste water effluent contributes to the dissemination of CTX-M-15 in the natural environment. J Antimicrob Chemother 2014;69:1785–91.
25. Hollis A, Ahmed Z. Preserving antibiotics, rationally. N Engl J Med 2013;369: 2474–6.

26. Chang Q, Wang W, Regev-Yochay G, et al. Antibiotics in agriculture and the risk to human health: how worried should we be? Evol Appl 2015;8:240–7.
27. Travers K, Barza M. Morbidity of infections caused by antimicrobial-resistant bacteria. Clin Infect Dis 2002;34(Suppl 3):S131–4.
28. Brunelle BW, Bearson BL, Bearson SM. Chloramphenicol and tetracycline decrease motility and increase invasion and attachment gene expression in specific isolates of multi-drug resistant *Salmonella enterica* serovar Typhimurium. Front Microbiol 2015;5:801.
29. Van der Mee-Marquet N, Francois P, Domelier-Valentin AS, et al. Emergence of unusual bloodstream infections associated with pig-borne-like *Staphylococcus aureus* ST398 in France. Clin Infect Dis 2011;52:152–3.
30. Lebreton F, van Schaik W, McGuire AM, et al. Emergence of epidemic multi-drug-resistant *Enterococcus faecium* from animal and commensal strains. MBio 2013;4 [pii:e00534-13].
31. Reich F, Atanassova V, Klein G. Extended-spectrum b-lactamase- and AmpC-producing enterobacteria in healthy broiler chickens, Germany. Emerg Infect Dis 2013;19:1253–9.
32. Wang Y, Wu C, Zhang Q, et al. Identification of New Delhi metallo-b-lactamase 1 in *Acinetobacter lwoffii* of food animal origin. PLoS One 2012;7:e37152.
33. Lauderdale TL1, Shiau YR, Wang HY, et al. Effect of banning vancomycin analogue avoparcin on vancomycin-resistant enterococci in chicken farms in Taiwan. Environ Microbiol 2007;9:819–23.
34. Cabrera-Pardo JR, Lood R, Udekwu K, et al. A One Health–One World initiative to control antibiotic resistance: a Chile-Sweden collaboration. One Health 2019; 14(8):100100.
35. Smith R, Coast J. The true cost of antimicrobial resistance. BMJ 2013;346:f1493.
36. Lee SY, Kotapati S, Kuti JL, et al. Impact of extended-spectrum beta-lactamase-producing *Escherichia coli* and *Klebsiella* species on clinical outcomes and hospital costs: a matched cohort study. Infect Control Hosp Epidemiol 2006;27: 1226–32.
37. Walsh TR, Weeks J, Livermore DM, et al. Dissemination of NDM-1 positive bacteria in the New Delhi environment and its implications for human health: an environmental point prevalence study. Lancet Infect Dis 2011;11:355–62.
38. World Health Organization. Antimicrobial resistance: global report on surveillance. Geneva (Switzerland): WHO; 2014.
39. Antonanzas F, Lozano C, Torres C. Economic features of antibiotic resistance: the case of methicillin-resistant *Staphylococcus aureus*. Pharmacoeconomics 2015; 33:285–325.
40. LaVergne S, Hamilton T, Biswas B, et al. Phage therapy for a multidrug-resistant *Acinetobacter baumannii* craniectomy site infection. Open Forum Infect Dis 2018; 5:ofy064.
41. Fujiki J, Nakamura T, Furusawa T, et al. Characterization of the lytic capability of a LysK-like endolysin, Lys-phiSA012, derived from a polyvalent *Staphylococcus aureus* bacteriophage. Pharmaceuticals (Basel) 2018;11(1) [pii:E25].
42. Bergman M, Huikko S, Pihlajamäki M, et al. Effect of macrolide consumption on erythromycin resistance in *Streptococcus pyogenes* in Finland in 1997-2001. Clin Infect Dis 2004;38:1251–6.
43. Livermore DM. Of stewardship, motherhood and apple pie. Int J Antimicrob Agents 2014;43:319–22.
44. Nilholm H, Holmstrand L, Ahl J, et al. An audit-based, infectious disease specialist-guided antimicrobial stewardship program profoundly reduced

antibiotic use without negatively affecting patient outcomes. Open Forum Infect Dis 2015;2(2):ofv042.
45. CDC. Antibiotic use in the United States, 2018 update; progress and opportunities. Atlanta (GA): US Department of Health and Human Services, CDC; 2019.
46. Claret J. The World Alliance Against Antibiotic Resistance: consensus for a declaration. Clin Infect Dis 2015;60(12):1837–41.
47. Morrissey I, Hackel M, Badal R, et al. A review of ten years of study for monitoring antimicrobial resistance trends (SMART) from 2002 to 2011. Pharmaceuticals (Basel) 2013;6:1335–46.
48. World Health Organization. Worldwide country situation analysis: response to antimicrobial resistance. Geneva (Switzerland): WHO; 2015.
49. Sommer MOA, Dantas G, Church GM. Functional characterization of the antibiotic resistance reservoir in the human microflora. Science 2009;325:1128–31.
50. Yang Z, Guo Z, Qiu C, et al. Preliminary analysis showed country-specific gut resistome based on 1,267 feces samples. Gene 2016;581:178–82.
51. Relman DA, Lipsitch M. Microbiome as a tool and a target in the effort to address antimicrobial resistance. Proc Natl Acad Sci U S A 2018;115:12902–10.
52. Hourigan SK, Ahn M, Gibson KM, et al. Fecal transplant in children with *Clostridioides difficile* gives sustained reduction in antimicrobial resistance and potential pathogen burden. Open Forum Infect Dis 2019;6:ofz379.
53. DeFilipp Z, Bloom PP, Torres Soto M, et al. Drug-resistant *E. coli* bacteremia transmitted by fecal microbiota transplant. N Engl J Med 2019;381:2043–50.

The Evolving Role of the Clinical Microbiology Laboratory in Identifying Resistance in Gram-Negative Bacteria: An Update

Andrea Endimiani, MD, PhD[a,*], Alban Ramette, PhD[a], Daniel D. Rhoads, MD[b], Michael R. Jacobs, MD, PhD[c]

KEYWORDS

• AST • PCR • LAMP • MALDI-TOF • Sequencing • Rapid • Blood • T2MR

KEY POINTS

- Extensively drug resistant and pan–drug-resistant gram-negatives represent a global public health challenge.
- Rapid commercial phenotypic antimicrobial susceptibility tests now are available for laboratory use.
- Detection of resistance genes can be rapidly accomplished in cultures by immunoassays and nucleic acid amplification testing–based methods.
- Whole-genome sequencing directly on specimens is being developed for clinical applications.
- Advances have been made with direct detection of resistance genes from specimens.

INTRODUCTION

The clinical microbiology laboratory is challenged with detecting and characterizing antimicrobial resistance (AMR) in gram-negatives. Examples of recent and emerging resistance include the detection of extensively/pan–drug-resistant Enterobacterales, *Pseudomonas aeruginosa*, and *Acinetobacter* spp producing carbapenemases (eg, KPC, NDM, and OXA types) together with other traits, such as 16S rRNA methylases

[a] Institute for Infectious Diseases, Faculty of Medicine, University of Bern, Bern, Switzerland; [b] Pathology and Laboratory Medicine Institute and Department of Infectious Diseases, Cleveland Clinic, Cleveland, OH, USA; [c] Department of Pathology, Case Western Reserve University and University Hospitals Cleveland Medical Center, Cleveland, OH, USA

* Corresponding author. Institute for Infectious Diseases, University of Bern, Friedbühlstrasse 51, Bern CH-3001, Switzerland.

E-mail addresses: andrea.endimiani@ifik.unibe.ch; aendimiani@gmail.com

Infect Dis Clin N Am 34 (2020) 659–676

https://doi.org/10.1016/j.idc.2020.08.001 **id.theclinics.com** and mobilized colistin resistance (MCR), conferring resistance to aminoglycosides and polymyxins, respectively.[1–3]

More rapid identification of AMR is a perpetual goal. Increased emphasis on rapid detection of resistance has focused on infections with the highest morbidity and mortality, in particular sepsis associated with bloodstream infections (BSIs). A mean decrease in survival of 7.6% for each hour after onset of infection until effective antibiotics are administered has been reported in sepsis.[4] Recent studies also have documented the value of more rapid resistance detection by the laboratory, which needs to be paired with more extralaboratory intervention. Rapid resistance detection has been shown to improve patient outcomes, with lower mortality, decreased hospital length of stay, lower superinfection and adverse drug reaction rates, and decreased costs.[5]

Although the rapid detection of bacteria and their resistance mechanisms directly from blood specimens is still a challenging target, this has been achieved on growing blood cultures (BCs), which typically become positive after 12 hours to 16 hours of incubation.[6] Many systems for rapid bacterial identification from positive BCs have been developed and, more recently, rapid automated antimicrobial susceptibility tests (ASTs) have been made available. Many of these systems also can detect AMR genes (ARGs).

AVAILABLE METHODS

Standard Antimicrobial Susceptibility Test Methods

Conventional AST procedures have been in use for many decades and follow methods and interpretations of various organizations, such as European Committee on Antimicrobial Susceptibility Testing and Clinical and Laboratory Standards Institute (CLSI)[7,8] as well as regulatory agencies such as US Food and Drug Administration (FDA) and European Agency for the Evaluation of Medicinal Products. These organizations have established reference AST methods based on minimum inhibitory concentration determination by microdilution and agar dilution, with incubation times ranging from 18 hours to 48 hours. Disk diffusion methods also have been standardized.

Many commercial methods for AST are available and are based on using these methods directly or by methods providing comparable results. Commercial systems using reference microdilution methods include, for instance, MicroScan WalkAway (Beckman) and Sensititre (Thermo Fisher Scientific). Methods providing results comparable to reference testing include gradient diffusion minimum inhibitory concentration determination (Etest [bioMérieux] and MTS [Liofilchem]), and automated systems, such as Vitek (bioMérieux), Phoenix (BD Diagnostic Systems), and the rapid versions of MicroScan and Sensititre. Several of the methods have faster turnaround time (TAT) than reference methods, and those automated are coupled with machine-generated results. Instruments that record and interpret disk diffusion zone also are available (eg, ADAGIO [Bio-Rad]; Scan 1200 [Interscience]; and SIRscan [i2a]). Faster TAT also is available for disk diffusion testing using standard and enhanced media.[9,10]

Antimicrobial Susceptibility Test Methods to Detect Resistance Mechanisms

These reference AST methods include methods for determination of resistance mechanisms, such as (1) the presence of extended-spectrum β-lactamases (ESBLs) using cefotaxime and ceftazidime alone and combined with clavulanate and (2) the presence of carbapenemases using lowered carbapenem breakpoints, the modified carbapenem inactivation method, and enzyme inhibitors (eg, boronic and dipicolinic acids).[7,11] These approaches are incorporated in many commercially available systems, such as those automated (eg, the Phoenix system)[12] or those based on disk diffusion (eg, the disk diffusion Neo-Rapid CARB kit [Rosco]).[13]

Rapid Antimicrobial Susceptibility Tests

The rapid AST systems include those based on flow cytometry; microfluidic; real-time high-resolution video imager; ATP bioluminescence; cell lysis; nanoechanical, electro-echanical, and optomechanical; and other techniques (reviewed by Endimiani and Jacobs[14] and by Behera and colleagues[15]). Only a few, so far, however, are available commercially.

The Accelerate Pheno system (Accelerate Diagnostics) combines species identification (ID) through fluorescence in situ hybridization probes with rapid ASTs based on time-lapse automated morphokinetic cell microscopic analysis. Both ID and AST are performed automatically on positive BCs, with results provided in maximum 1.5 hours and 7 hours, respectively (at least 24 hours before those provided with routine approaches).[16] In a recent study, the system accurately identified the pathogens with a sensitivity ranging from 94.6% to 100%, whereas for the AST results, the categorical agreement was 97.9%.[17] Overall, the Accelerate Pheno system may significantly anticipate the definitive antibiotic therapy, improving the outcome of BSI patients.[18]

The Alfred 60 (Alifax) is another automatic AST system implemented for positive BCs that provides results in approximately 6 hours. It analyzes the turbidity of bacteria that grow in broth and has demonstrated a 93% categorical agreement with the standard ASTs.[19]

Rapid Biochemical Tests to Detect Extended-Spectrum β-Lactamase and Carbapenemase Producers

The ESBL Nordmann/Dortet/Poirel (NDP) test is a rapid (15 minutes to 2 hours) and cost-effective biochemical test used to detect ESBL producers. ESBL production is evidenced by a color change (red to yellow) of the pH indicator phenol red due to acid formation resulting from cefotaxime hydrolysis that is reversed by adding tazobactam, with reported 93% sensitivity and 100% specificity for detecting ESBL-producing Enterobacterales (ESBL-PE). The test has been evaluated on BC and urine samples, showing excellent sensitivity and specificity (>98% and >99%, respectively). This homemade test has been upgraded to a commercially available kit named Rapid ESBL NP test.[20]

The Carba Nordmann/Poirel (NP) test is an in-house assay designed to detect carbapenemase producers. It detects a change in pH due to the hydrolysis of imipenem in presence of carbapenemases in less than 2 hours. β-Lactamases are extracted rapidly from bacterial cells and then incubated with imipenem and phenol red. This test demonstrated an excellent ability to detect carbapenemases in Enterobacterales and *Pseudomonas* spp, as well as in *Acinetobacter* spp, in an improved version (CarbAcineto NP test),[20,21] although there are concerns regarding the low sensitivity for OXA-48–like producers. The test also was implemented directly on positive BCs with carbapenemase-producing Enterobacterales (CPE) and *Pseudomonas* spp, demonstrating greater than 98% sensitivity and 100% specificity.[22,23] Notably, the Carba NP test is recommended for the confirmation of carbapenemase production in gram-negatives by the CLSI.[7] This test now is available commercially in an easy-to-use rapid kit (RAPIDEC Carba NP test [bioMérieux]). Another version of the original Carba NP test (Carba NP II test) includes additional wells with clavulanic acid and EDTA, making the assay able to distinguish the different classes of carbapenemases.[24] This test, however, is not commercially available.[20]

The Blue-Carba test is another in-house biochemical assay for carbapenemases detection, but it uses a different indicator (bromothymol blue) and a simplified protocol compared with the Carba NP test. The main advantage of the Blue-Carba is its faster TAT, because there is no need to extract the β-lactamase(s) from colonies. Overall, the test shows comparable performance to the in-house Carba NP, with reported better sensitivity for the detection of OXA-type carbapenemases.[25] In a recent study with CPE, Carba NP had higher specificity than Blue-Carba (98.9% vs 91.7%, respectively), whereas both tests had 100% sensitivity.[26] A commercially available version of Blue-Carba test (Neo-CARB kit, formerly Rapid CARB Screen) has shown similar sensitivity (97% vs 98%, respectively) but superior specificity (100% vs 83%) compared with the Carba NP test.[27] In contrast, in another evaluation, the Carba NP had sensitivities of 91% for Enterobacterales and 100% for *P aeruginosa*, whereas those for the Rapid CARB Screen kit were 73% and 67%, respectively; the specificity of both tests was 100%.[28]

β LACTA and β CARBA tests (Bio-Rad) are commercially available tests used for the detection of ESBL-PE and CPE, respectively. They rely on the use of chromogenic β-lactams that yield a different color when they are hydrolyzed by the β-lactamase (from yellow to red). Both tests are easy to perform and the results are obtained within 1 hour.[29] The β LACTA test has been evaluated not only with colonies but also directly from blood, urine, and bronchial samples. These samples yielded both specificity and sensitivity of 100%.[30] The β CARBA test showed high sensitivity (98%) and high specificity (100%) in detecting CPE, including those producing OXA-48–like enzymes, from cultures.[31] Recently, it has been used directly on the pellet of positive spiked BCs: all CPE were detected and no false-positive results were recorded. Sensitivity and specificity were 100% and 94%, respectively, with TATs ranging between 20 minutes and 45 minutes.[32]

Biochemical Tests to Detect Other Resistance Phenotypes

The Rapid Polymyxin NP test (ELITechGroup) is a commercial assay that quickly detects polymyxin resistance. This test is based on the detection of glucose metabolism related to bacterial growth (when resistant to polymyxins) in the presence of a defined concentration of colistin. The formation of acid metabolites is evidenced by a color change of the pH indicator red phenol in less than 2 hours. The assay showed greater than 98% sensitivity and greater than 94% specificity.[33,34] It was also evaluated for detection of colistin-resistant *Enterobacterales* directly from BCs, exhibiting excellent discrimination between colistin-resistant and susceptible isolates.[35]

Based on the same principle used in the Rapid Polymyxin NP, further rapid phenotypic tests to detect aminoglycoside-resistant and fosfomycin-resistant Enterobacterales have been developed.[36,37] Because *Acinetobacter baumannii* and *P aeruginosa* do not metabolize glucose, a new assay (Rapid ResaPolymyxin *Acinetobacter/Pseudomonas* NP test) based on the utilization of resazurin (alamarBlue) has been developed. Metabolically active cells (polymyxin-resistant) reduce blue resazurin to the pink product resorufin. In less than 4 hours, the test showed 100% sensitivity and 95% specificity.[38]

Immunochromatographic Tests

Antigen detection can be used to detect enzymes or cell components of bacteria that are associated with AMR. The immunochromatographic tests often are lateral flow assays (LFAs) where antigen detection is identified by visualization of a line (as in pregnancy tests). These LFAs are useful because of their rapidity (results within

15 minutes), low cost, and accuracy that typically are comparable to nucleic acid amplification testing.[39]

The LFAs designed to detect β-lactamases started being commercialized during 2015-2016. Although at the beginning they were targeting only one enzyme (eg, OXA-48),[40] nowadays multiplex LFAs are available. For instance, the RESIST-4 O.K.N.V. kit (Coris BioConcept) detects OXA-48–like, KPC, NDM, and VIM carbapenemases, with greater than 99% sensitivity and 100% specificity in culture strains belonging to Enterobacterales and *Pseudomonas* spp.[41] The NG-Test CARBA 5 (NG Biotech) detects the 5 most common carbapenemases: KPC, OXA-48–like, VIM, IMP, and NDM. Having shown 99.3% sensitivity and 99.8% specificity for cultured colonies,[42] this LFA now is FDA-cleared. Remarkably, CARBA 5 also has demonstrated high accuracy when testing positive BCs for detecting CPE (sensitivity and specificity of >97.7% and >96.1%, respectively).[43,44] An LFA to detect the colistin resistance trait MCR-1 also has been developed.[45]

Matrix-Assisted Laser Desorption Ionization–Time of Flight Mass Spectroscopy

The matrix-assisted laser desorption ionization–time of flight (MALDI-TOF) mass spectroscopy (MS) nowadays is used routinely to identify bacterial species from growth on agar plates as well as organisms present in positive BCs. Overall, the main advantages of MALDI-TOF MS are its speed, relatively low costs, and consistency.[46]

Numerous studies also have assessed the utility of MALDI-TOF MS for the identification of β-lactam degradation products in the presence of hydrolyzing β-lactamases, including directly from positive BCs and urine. In particular, many investigators have evaluated the identification of carbapenemase producers where antibiotics (imipenem, meropenem, and ertapenem) are incubated with the organism and then analyzed for degradation products of the antibiotics with the MS; the time required to do this assay is approximately 1 hour to 4 hours.[47] Bruker Daltonics also produces the MBT STAR-Carba IVD commercial kit to rapidly detect carbapenemase producers. The assay showed high sensitivity (100%) and specificity (>98%) for CPE but not for OXA-23/-24–producing *A baumannii.*[48,49] All of these MALDI-TOF MS approaches, however, can detect only the presence of β-lactam hydrolysis as a generic resistance mechanism and not the specific enzyme (eg, distinguishing NDM from KPC); this identical information can be obtained easily by implementing rapid and cost-effective biochemical tests (discussed previously) or polymerase chain reaction (PCR)-based methods. Interestingly, the MALDI-TOF MS is able to detect the specific KPC-2 peak (28′544 m/z) in Enterobacterales and *P aeruginosa* with both sensitivity and specificity of 100%.[50]

Single and Multiplex Endpoint Polymerase Chain Reaction

A single PCR frequently is sufficient for detection of a unique ARG of interest. Subsequent DNA sequencing, however, may be necessary (eg, to distinguish SHVs with ESBL from those with non-ESBL spectrum). Results of PCR amplification can be obtained in less than 3 hours to 4 hours for simple amplification to greater than or equal to 24 hours if DNA sequencing is required. Making use of multiple primer sets, multiplex endpoint PCRs have the advantage of simultaneously amplifying many different targets. In the past, numerous single and multiplex PCRs have been designed to detect ARGs, including ESBL, carbapenemase, aminoglycoside-modifying enzyme, and outer membrane porin genes associated with carbapenem resistance (reviewed by Endimiani and Jacobs[14] and Lupo and colleagues[51]).

Single and Multiplex Real-Time Polymerase Chain Reaction

Real-time PCR consists of an amplification reaction of the target gene coupled with the detection of the exponentially amplified DNA product by various methods, such as monitoring fluorescence emission with SYBR Green or TaqMan probes. Real-time PCR avoids time consuming steps, such as running gels; is sensitive, reliable, and cost-effective; and usually does not require DNA sequencing. Modern apparatuses also can perform a high-resolution melting analysis of DNA products, giving information on single-nucleotide polymorphisms in the sequence.[52]

Many in-house single or multiplex platforms for detecting plasmid-mediated AmpC (pAmpC), ESBL, carbapenemase, and other ARGs have been designed (see, Endimiani and Jacobs[14] and Lupo and colleagues[51]), and many commercially available kits now are available. For example, Check-Points Health B.V. provides quantitative multiplex real-time PCR kits to detect ESBL and carbapenemase genes directly from rectal swabs. Results are available within 2 hours to 3 hours, along with genotypic differentiation of the *bla* types based on probes labeled with different fluorescent dyes. Kits can be adapted to the BD MAX system (Becton-Dickinson), a diagnostic platform that operates as an open real-time PCR, allowing automated sample lysis, extraction, amplification, and detection processes. The Check-Direct ESBL screening kit detects CTX-M and SHV ESBL genes. For rectal swabs, it displayed sensitivity of 88% to 95% and specificity of 96% to 99%.[53,54] The Check-Direct CPE assay identifies bla_{KPC}, bla_{NDM}, bla_{VIM}, and $bla_{OXA\text{-}48\text{-}like}$, with reported sensitivity of 100% and specificity of 88% to 100%, respectively. Moreover, compared with standard approaches, this molecular system reduced TAT from 18 hours to 24 hours (using direct culture) or 48 hours (using broth enrichment) to only 3 hours.[55–58] For both Check-Direct kits, false-positive results (negative by culture) can arise from the presence of DNA residual of dead bacteria, or detection of bacteria harboring, but not expressing, *bla* genes.[53,54,56,58]

GeneXpert (Cepheid) is another real-time PCR system that performs fully automated nucleic acid detection and analysis directly from clinical samples. To minimize contamination, it is a cartridge-based, closed, self-contained platform. The company provides many cartridges for detection of different pathogens and ARGs. Among them, the Xpert Carba-R (v2) cartridge is designed to detect bla_{KPC}, bla_{NDM}, bla_{IMP}, bla_{VIM}, and $bla_{OXA\text{-}48\text{-}like}$, requiring 2 minutes of hands-on time and less than 48 minute to achieve results.[59] For rectal swabs, this kit demonstrated overall sensitivity of 97% to 100% and specificity of 99%. As for Check-Direct, the Xpert Carba-R assay reported the presence of carbapenemase genes in culture-negative samples.[60,61] In another study, Xpert Carba-R was implemented for rapid screening for colonization with carbapenemase-producing species, coupled with implementation of infection prevention strategies. Isolation of positive patients led to a reduction in both colonization (from 28.6% to 5.6%; $P<.05$) and infection (from 35.7% to 2.8%; $P<.05$) rates during the study period.[62]

Other companies have developed further real-time PCR-based platforms to detect carbapenemases, *mcr-1/-2* associated with polymyxins resistance and other ARGs. Examples include PANA RealTyper CRE kit (PANAGENE)[63]; Tandem-Plex CRE EU kit (AusDiagnostics)[64]; Acuitas AMR Gene Panel (OpGen)[65]; and GenePOC Carba/ Revogene Carba C assay (Meridian Bioscience).[66] Their analytical performance directly on clinical samples, however, has not yet been extensively evaluated.

BioFire FilmArray

The BioFire FilmArray (bioMérieux) is a closed, very rapid (1-hour), fully automated system (only 2 minutes hands-on-time) that combines DNA extraction from samples, nested multiplex PCRs, post-PCR amplicon high-resolution melting analysis, and automated interpretation of results.[67] This method initially was developed for the detection of respiratory pathogens,[68] but later additional assays have been developed. The FilmArray Blood Culture Identification (BCID) kit has been approved by FDA for direct implementation on positive BCs. It identifies 27 targets, including gram-positives, gram-negatives, 6 *Candida* spp, and the ARGs *mecA*, *vanA/B*, and bla_{KPC}. Similarly, the FilmArray Pneumonia Panel *plus* has 34 targets, including 27 major respiratory pathogens and several ARGs (*mecA/C*, bla_{KPC}, bla_{NDM}, bla_{VIM}, bla_{IMP}, $bla_{OXA\text{-}48\text{-}like}$, $bla_{CTX\text{-}M}$, and bla_{KPC}).

The FilmArray BCID has been evaluated in numerous recent studies. In a large multicenter trial (2207 samples), the system showed an identification sensitivity greater than 96%. Moreover, sensitivity and specificity for *mecA* were both 98%, whereas those for *vanA/B* and bla_{KPC} were both 100%.[69] In another study, it was shown that the use of the BCID system reduced the time to optimal antimicrobial treatment in intensive care unit (ICU) patients by an average of 10 hours (from 15 hours to 5 hours; $P<.05$).[70] Although focusing on bacteremia due to gram-positives, another analysis showed that the implementation of the BCID panel resulted in shorter postculture length of stay and saved approximately $30,000 per 100 patients tested.[71] A new BC panel (BCID2), able to detect further species and ARGs (including major carbapenemases and *mcr-1*), will be released shortly.

Loop-Mediated Isothermal Amplification

The loop-mediated isothermal amplification (LAMP) method allows amplification and fluorescent detection of the target DNA at a constant temperature, avoiding the need for a thermocycler. Genomic extraction from samples is not required as the activity of the *Bst* DNA polymerase is not hampered by serum or heparin.[72] Recently, many investigators have designed in-house LAMP platforms to detect different ARGs. Overall, for clinical samples the LAMP was very rapid (<1-hour), more sensitive, and with a lower limit of detection than PCR-based approaches.[14,73,74]

The commercially available eazyplex LAMP system (Amplex Diagnostics) consists of a series of freeze-dried and ready-to-use kits coupled by real-time photometric detection of amplified targets using the transportable Genie II instrument (OptiGene). One of the kits was designed to detect KPC, NDM, OXA-48, VIM, OXA-23, OXA-24/40, and OXA-58 carbapenemase genes. Its first evaluation was performed on *Acinetobacter* spp and all isolates were characterized correctly in less than 30 minutes.[75] In another study focusing on Enterobacterales, an advanced kit (eazyplex SuperBug CRE kit) was assessed to detect KPC, VIM, NDM, OXA-48–like, and CTX-M-1/-9–like genes: all carbapenemase and/or CTX-M producers were identified correctly within 15 minutes.[76]

The same kit also was used directly on 50 urine samples, 30 of which contained ESBL producers; the assay showed sensitivity of 100% and specificity of 97.9%, with results obtained in less than 20 minutes.[77] Recently, it was shown that implementation of the eazyplex SuperBug CRE kit on positive BCs significantly improved the clinical outcome of BSIs due to CTX-M- and/or KPC/VIM-producing *Escherichia coli* and *Klebsiella pneumoniae*. In particular, after notification of SuperBug CRE results (on average 20 hours after sample collection), the proportion of appropriate treatment increased from 6% to 71% and from 30% to 92% for BSIs caused by KPC/VIM and CTX-M producers, respectively.[78] Extended kit versions able to further detect pAmpCs (eazyplex AmpC), OXA-23–like, OXA-24/40–like, OXA-58–like, and OXA-181–like (eazyplex SuperBug complete A/B/C and Acineto), IMI, GES, GIM (eazyplex SuperBug expert), and the *mcr-1* (eazyplex SuperBug mcr-1) genes also are available.

Microarrays

Microarrays possess great diagnostic capacity because they can simultaneously detect and analyze a large number of target genes.[79] In the past, numerous in-house assays have been designed to characterize ARGs, but their implementation was difficult because of problems related to standardization of the procedures. Recently, commercially available microarrays have become available. These platforms are easy to perform and can be updated readily, although the TAT is rather long (6–8 hours) and commercial kits are relatively expensive.[51]

Check-Points Health B.V. has developed an automated DNA microarray platform to detect the major *bla* genes. Over the past 10 years, several kits have been released, including Check KPC/ESBL, Check-MDR CT101, CT102, CT103, and CT103XL. Overall, these assays showed high accuracy in detecting ESBL, pAmpC, and carbapenemase genes in cultured strains.[80–82] Moreover, one of these kits (Check-KPC/ESBL) was used to detect ESBL and KPC genes directly from positive BCs, reducing the reporting time of these resistance traits by 18 hours to 20 hours.[83] The latest microarray kit made available by the company (New Check-MDR CT103XL) can detect the most epidemiologically important ESBL, pAmpC, and carbapenemase, along with the *mcr-1* and *mcr-2* genes. In a recent evaluation against a collection of Enterobacterales, all *bla* and *mcr-1/2* genes were correctly identified.[84]

Verigene System

Verigene (Luminex Corporation) is an automated multiplex microarray-based system that uses small aliquots of positive BC broths to identify a panel of major bacterial pathogens and ARGs. Results are available within 2.5 hours from Gram stain result on positive BCs. The test uses a disposable kit and cartridge, the latter inserted in a processor (5-minute hands-on-time) that carries out extraction of nucleic acid and microarray reactions. Final results are obtained by inserting the cartridge into a dedicated reader. Assays for gram-positives and gram-negatives are available. The Verigene gram-negative BC nucleic acid (BC-GN) test can identify *E coli*, *K pneumoniae*, *K oxytoca*, *P aeruginosa*, *S marcescens*, *Acinetobacter* spp, *Proteus* spp, *Citrobacter* spp, *Enterobacter* spp, and the ARGs bla_{KPC}, bla_{NDM}, $bla_{CTX\text{-}M}$, bla_{VIM}, bla_{IMP}, and bla_{OXA}. In a large study (1847 BCs), agreement of the BC-GN assay with the reference method for monomicrobial cultures was *E coli*, 100%; *K pneumoniae*, 92.9%; *P aeruginosa*, 98.9%; and *Acinetobacter* spp, 98.4%. Agreement for identification of ARGs was $bla_{CTX\text{-}M}$, 98.9%; $bla_{KPC/VIM/IMP}$, 100%; bla_{NDM}, 96.2%; and bla_{OXA}, 94.3%.[85]

Numerous studies also have demonstrated that implementation of Verigene BC-GN has a significant positive clinical impact. For instance, it was shown that ID (mean 10.9 hours vs 37.9 hours, respectively; $P<.001$) and time to effective therapy for BSI due to ESBL producers were achieved more quickly (mean 7.3 hours vs 41.4 hours, respectively; $P = .04$); moreover, length of ICU stay (12.0 days vs 16.2 days, respectively) and 30-day mortality (8.1% vs 19.2%, respectively) were significantly lowered.[86]

T2 Magnetic Resonance

The T2 magnetic resonance (T2MR) (T2 Biosystems) is a recently marketed system that combines PCR amplification, hybridization with nanoparticles and T2MR in a closed apparatus to detect diverse targets directly from complex matrices, such as blood.[87] With a limit of detection of 1 colony-forming unit/mL, the system can identify 5 *Candida* spp (T2Candida Panel) or *E faecium*, *Staphylococcus aureus*, *K pneumoniae*, *P aeruginosa*, and *E coli* (T2Bacteria Panel) from 2 mL of whole blood.[88] In ICU patients, T2Bacteria Panel showed sensitivity of 83.3% and specificity of 97.6% in detecting bacterial targets that were present in BCs. Sensitivity increased to 89.5% when patients with clinical indication of infection, regardless of BC results, were considered. A considerable number of patients, especially those receiving antimicrobials, had T2Bacteria-positive/BC-negative results. Mean times to detection of species or negative results were 5.5 hours and 6.1 hours, respectively; in comparison, those for conventional BCs were 25.2 hours and 120 hours, respectively.[89] Recently, the company has developed a panel (T2Resistance) to rapidly detect 13 ARGs (bla_{KPC}, $bla_{NDM/IMP/VIM}$, bla_{OXA-48}, $bla_{CTX-M-14/15}$, $bla_{CMY/DHA}$, *vanA/B*, and *mecA/C*).

Next-Generation Sequencing

In the clinical setting, whole-genome sequencing of bacteria increasingly is used to inform on the emergence and spread of AMR, with the final objective to better tailor antimicrobial prescription.[90,91] Pathogen genomic sequencing provides the most complete ARG and species identification currently available directly from BCs. or provide a full picture of the susceptibility profile as well as insights about novelty, transmission, and virulence of associated genetic elements. Genomic workflows typically involve several steps, from raw sequence data production to the further processing of the generated data into interpretable nucleic acid sequences using bioinformatic tools.

Over the past 15 years, the low-throughput, costly, yet accurate, Sanger sequencing has been replaced by high-throughput sequencing technologies, such as 454 pyrosequencing (discontinued in 2013) and Illumina sequencing. Currently, clinical genomic applications are based mostly on Illumina sequencing technology, which allows for the sequencing of entire genomes in mixed samples or the detection of sequence variants with enough coverage and with satisfactory base accuracy.[92] Although successfully used to profile human-associated antibiotic resistomes (eg, Forsberg and colleagues[93] and Gonzalez-Escalona and collaegues[94]), the short reads (few hundreds of bases) produced by the Illumina technology may lead to downstream sequence processing difficulties (eg, for contig assembly), especially when multiple copies of the same genes, high guanine-cytosine (GC), or homopolymeric regions are present in the target genome.[95]

High-quality de novo microbial genome assemblies can alternatively be obtained via Pacific Biosciences Single-molecule real-time (SMRT) sequencing, which may produce sequences efficiently, even when long repeat regions are present.[96] The Pacific Biosciences technology introduced in 2011, however, needs significant capital investment, dedicated personnel, and laboratory space, which may explain why only few applications have been reported in the clinical setting.[92] Consequently, clinically applicable workflows that provide straightforward, affordable, and comprehensive resistome characterization still are lacking, and technologies addressing those needs are highly desirable.

Oxford Nanopore Technologies introduced its first product, MinION, consisting of a single-molecule sensing system embedded in a cheap, light-weight (100-g) sequencer.[97] Nanopore sequencing works by threading individual DNA or RNA molecules through nanoscopic pores fixed to a membrane on which an ionic current is applied. As the molecule passes through the pore, the current is altered as a function of the identity of the base and of its residues. This signal then is recorded and converted into a nucleotide sequence by a suite of bioinformatic tools, while further processing of the data is done using software scripts provided by the company and by the user community. The strategy of Oxford Nanopore Technologies was to let a limited number of laboratories assess the sequencing performance of the device, acknowledging the developing nature of the technology. This early access to this technology has helped rapidly develop wet laboratory protocols, software scripts to optimize the sequencing process and also downstream analyses by a large group of users. It also lets users explore potential applications, thus contributing to publicize the new technology across a large array of scientific fields in a record amount of time. Nanopore reads are long, often reaching lengths greater than 100 kb,[98] and typically capture entire genomic fragments, which facilitates downstream analysis of the genomic context when ARGs are identified.[99] This is significant particularly for clinical applications that aim at reducing TAT, particularly when a culture-independent, direct processing method to detect mixed microbial populations in samples is needed. In that respect, Cao and colleagues[100] demonstrated that bacterial species and strain information could be obtained within 30 minutes of nanopore sequencing based on approximately 500 reads, whereas initial drug-resistance profiles could be established in less than 2 hours, and complete resistance profiles could be available within 10 hours.

Whole-genome sequencing–based AMR predictions and antibiotic-resistance phenotypes often are concordant, with high sensitivity and specificity (>95%) reported for many phenotypes across several pathogen species,[101] although some notable exceptions were found, such as with levofloxacin resistance in *P aeruginosa*, where sensitivity and specificity may be below 95%.[102] Successful genomic applications in the context of bacterial drug-resistance characterization include the analysis of the structure and insertion site of an antibiotic resistance island in *Salmonella* Typhi[103] and the characterization of carbapenemase and ESBL genes in gram-negatives.[104,105] A functional metagenomics approach combined with nanopore sequencing was reported by van der Helm and colleagues[99] to characterize the resistome of clinical samples: clones from metagenomic expression libraries, derived from fecal samples obtained from an ICU patient, which could grow on each of a panel of 7 antibiotics, were selected, pooled, and barcoded with custom adapters and sequenced with the MinION nanopore sequencer. Resistome profiling identified a variety of ARGs with annotation accuracies of greater than 97% mean sequence identity, such as $bla_{\text{CTX-M}}$ and bla_{TEM}, genes coding for aminoglycoside-modifying enzymes, and diverse genes encoding ribosomal and efflux mediated resistance to tetracycline antibiotics.

Despite successful applications for strain identification and resistome profiling, emerging sequencing technologies that offer real-time, long-read, single-molecule sequencing of DNA or RNA molecules need further development in terms of (1) sensitivity, especially when applied to mixed samples, for which high-sequence yields providing sufficient genome coverage are required[100]; (2) sequencing accuracy to overcome the high error rate of the current nanopore sequencing technology (currently at approximately 4% per raw read), so that AMR-associated with mutations in chromosomal genes also can be identified[104] or multilocus sequencing typing schemes that attempt to identify bacterial strains from nanopore data be obtained reliably[92,100]; meanwhile, several postsequencing algorithms may be used to produce error-corrected reads with accuracy greater than 99%; those algorithms include several rounds of mapping the raw reads to a consensus sequence in order to improve the overall consensus sequence quality[99,106]; (3) costs of flow cell and associated consumables[107]; and (4) easy-to-use bioinformatic tools and interfaces that facilitate the interpretation of the sequencing results by clinicians and that would enable a broader adoption of the technology in clinical settings in different countries.[108]

Overall, single-molecule, real-time sequencing technologies, which may help better identify and characterize the genomic makeup of drug-resistant bacteria, have been shown not only to be technically feasible but also time- and cost-effective. Moreover, portable technology and rapid TAT provide actionable results with respect to infection control, implementation of personalized antibiotic treatment in high-risk patients, and on-site monitoring of resistome in both clinical and environmental settings. It is hoped that diagnostic laboratories soon will be able to implement routine genome sequencing as part of their surveillance programs for drug-resistant bacteria.

DISCUSSION

The spread of extensively drug-resistant and pan–drug-resistant gram-negatives has challenged the clinical microbiology laboratory to recognize the presence of responsible resistance mechanisms, appreciate their clinical significance, and develop techniques to rapidly detect their existence. This overall challenge is significant and, in many instances, difficult to address when conventional AST fails to recognize the presence of clinically important resistance mechanisms, such as ESBLs and carbapenemases. A further challenge is to rapidly detect these resistance traits in established cultures as well as directly from specimens. This review shows the impressive advances that have been made in rapid detection of resistance in cultures (eg, positive BCs). Moreover, direct detection of ARGs from screening specimens (eg, rectal swabs) is a reality, whereas that from other primary samples (eg, whole blood) in the routine clinical context still is on the horizon.

There also is the inherent conflict between choosing between phenotypic and genotypic methods. Genotypic methods are rapid and can be used to test cultures as well as specimens but are limited by the complexity of the genetic targets and the continuing emergence of new resistance mechanisms. Phenotypic methods are slow and best suited for use on cultures, but speed has been improved significantly using rapid AST systems. It is likely that these challenges will continue as new resistance mechanisms emerge and that phenotypic and genotypic methods will continue to be needed and used in parallel.

DISCLOSURE

A. Endimiani is a consultant for (Merck Sharp and Dohme AG). M.R. Jacobs and D.D. Rhoads received grant support from bioMérieux and OpGen. A. Ramette received travel grants from Oxford Nanopore Technologies to attend scientific conferences. The sponsor had no role in the design, execution, interpretation, or writing of the study. A. Endimiani and A. Ramette are supported by the Swiss National Science Foundation (SNF), NRP72 National Research Programme, Antimicrobial Resistance (SNF grant no. 177378). A. Endimiani also is supported by SNF grant no. 170063.

REFERENCES

1. Bonomo RA, Burd EM, Conly J, et al. Carbapenemase-producing organisms: a global scourge. Clin Infect Dis 2018;66(8):1290–7.
2. Poirel L, Jayol A, Nordmann P. Polymyxins: antibacterial activity, susceptibility testing, and resistance mechanisms encoded by plasmids or chromosomes. Clin Microbiol Rev 2017;30(2):557–96.
3. Potron A, Poirel L, Nordmann P. Emerging broad-spectrum resistance in *Pseudomonas aeruginosa* and *Acinetobacter baumannii*: Mechanisms and epidemiology. Int J Antimicrob Agents 2015;45(6):568–85.

4. Kothari A, Morgan M, Haake DA. Emerging technologies for rapid identification of bloodstream pathogens. Clin Infect Dis 2014;59(2):272–8.
5. Timbrook TT, Morton JB, McConeghy KW, et al. The effect of molecular rapid diagnostic testing on clinical outcomes in bloodstream infections: a systematic review and meta-analysis. Clin Infect Dis 2017;64(1):15–23.
6. Altun O, Almuhayawi M, Luthje P, et al. Controlled evaluation of the new BacT/alert virtuo blood culture system for detection and time to detection of bacteria and yeasts. J Clin Microbiol 2016;54(4):1148–51.
7. CLSI. Performance standards for antimicrobial susceptibility testing: 29th informational supplement. Wayne (PA): Clinical and Laboratory Standard Institute; 2019. CLSI document M100-S29.
8. EUCAST. European Committee on Antimicrobial Susceptibility Testing Breakpoint Tables for interpretation of MICs and zone diameters Version 90, valid from 2019-01-01. 2019.
9. Humphries RM, Kircher S, Ferrell A, et al. The continued value of disk diffusion for assessing antimicrobial susceptibility in clinical laboratories: report from the Clinical and Laboratory Standards Institute Methods Development and Standardization Working Group. J Clin Microbiol 2018;56(8). e00437–18.
10. Perillaud C, Pilmis B, Diep J, et al. Prospective evaluation of rapid antimicrobial susceptibility testing by disk diffusion on Mueller-Hinton rapid-SIR directly on blood cultures. Diagn Microbiol Infect Dis 2019;93(1):14–21.
11. European Committee on Antimicrobial Susceptibility Testing (EUCAST). EUCAST guidelines for detection of resistance mechanisms and specific resistances of clinical and/or epidemiological importance. Version 2.0. July 2017.
12. Ong CH, Ratnayake L, Ang MLT, et al. Diagnostic Accuracy of BD Phoenix CPO detect for carbapenemase production in 190 enterobacteriaceae isolates. J Clin Microbiol 2018;56(12):e01043-18.
13. Noel A, Huang TD, Berhin C, et al. Comparative evaluation of four phenotypic tests for detection of carbapenemase-producing gram-negative bacteria. J Clin Microbiol 2017;55(2):510–8.
14. Endimiani A, Jacobs MR. The changing role of the clinical microbiology laboratory in defining resistance in gram-negatives. Infect Dis Clin North Am 2016; 30(2):323–45.
15. Behera B, Anil Vishnu GK, Chatterjee S, et al. Emerging technologies for antibiotic susceptibility testing. Biosens Bioelectron 2019;142:111552.
16. Charnot-Katsikas A, Tesic V, Love N, et al. Use of the accelerate pheno system for identification and antimicrobial susceptibility testing of pathogens in positive blood cultures and impact on time to results and workflow. J Clin Microbiol 2018; 56(1). e01166-17.
17. Pancholi P, Carroll KC, Buchan BW, et al. Multicenter Evaluation of the Accelerate PhenoTest BC kit for rapid identification and phenotypic antimicrobial susceptibility testing using morphokinetic cellular analysis. J Clin Microbiol 2018; 56(4). e01329-17.
18. Henig O, Cooper CC, Kaye KS, et al. The hypothetical impact of Accelerate Pheno system on time to effective therapy and time to definitive therapy in an institution with an established antimicrobial stewardship programme currently utilizing rapid genotypic organism/resistance marker identification. J Antimicrob Chemother 2019;74(Supplement_1):i32–9.
19. Van den Poel B, Meersseman P, Debaveye Y, et al. Performance and potential clinical impact of Alfred60(AST) (Alifax(R)) for direct antimicrobial susceptibility

testing on positive blood culture bottles. Eur J Clin Microbiol Infect Dis 2020; 39(1):53–63.
20. Decousser JW, Poirel L, Nordmann P. Recent advances in biochemical and molecular diagnostics for the rapid detection of antibiotic-resistant Enterobacteriaceae: a focus on β-lactam resistance. Expert Rev Mol Diagn 2017;17(4): 327–50.
21. Dortet L, Poirel L, Errera C, et al. CarbAcineto NP test for rapid detection of carbapenemase-producing *Acinetobacter* spp. J Clin Microbiol 2014;52(7): 2359–64.
22. Dortet L, Brechard L, Poirel L, et al. Rapid detection of carbapenemase-producing *Enterobacteriaceae* from blood cultures. Clin Microbiol Infect 2014; 20(4):340–4.
23. Dortet L, Boulanger A, Poirel L, et al. Bloodstream infections caused by *Pseudomonas* spp.: how to detect carbapenemase producers directly from blood cultures. J Clin Microbiol 2014;52(4):1269–73.
24. Dortet L, Poirel L, Nordmann P. Rapid identification of carbapenemase types in Enterobacteriaceae and Pseudomonas spp. by using a biochemical test. Antimicrob Agents Chemother 2012;56(12):6437–40.
25. Pires J, Novais A, Peixe L. Blue-carba, an easy biochemical test for detection of diverse carbapenemase producers directly from bacterial cultures. J Clin Microbiol 2013;51(12):4281–3.
26. Pires J, Tinguely R, Thomas B, et al. Comparison of the in-house made Carba-NP and Blue-Carba tests: Considerations for better detection of carbapenemase-producing Enterobacteriaceae. J Microbiol Methods 2016; 122:33–7.
27. Huang TD, Berhin C, Bogaerts P, et al. Comparative evaluation of two chromogenic tests for rapid detection of carbapenemase in *Enterobacteriaceae* and in *Pseudomonas aeruginosa* isolates. J Clin Microbiol 2014;52(8):3060–3.
28. Yusuf E, Van Der Meeren S, Schallier A, et al. Comparison of the Carba NP test with the Rapid CARB Screen Kit for the detection of carbapenemase-producing *Enterobacteriaceae* and *Pseudomonas aeruginosa*. Eur J Clin Microbiol Infect Dis 2014;33(12):2237–40.
29. Renvoise A, Decre D, Amarsy-Guerle R, et al. Evaluation of the betaLacta test, a rapid test detecting resistance to third-generation cephalosporins in clinical strains of Enterobacteriaceae. J Clin Microbiol 2013;51(12):4012–7.
30. Gallah S, Benzerara Y, Tankovic J, et al. beta LACTA test performance for detection of extended-spectrum β-lactamase-producing Gram-negative bacilli directly on bronchial aspirates samples: a validation study. Clin Microbiol Infect 2018;24(4):402–8.
31. Bayraktar B, Baris A, Malkocoglu G, et al. Comparison of Carba NP-Direct, Carbapenem Inactivation Method, and beta-CARBA tests for detection of carbapenemase production in enterobacteriaceae. Microb Drug Resist 2019;25(1): 97–102.
32. Meier M, Hamprecht A. Rapid detection of carbapenemases directly from positive blood cultures by the beta-CARBA test. Eur J Clin Microbiol Infect Dis 2019; 38(2):259–64.
33. Nordmann P, Jayol A, Poirel L. Rapid detection of polymyxin resistance in enterobacteriaceae. Emerg Infect Dis 2016;22(6):1038–43.
34. Jayol A, Kieffer N, Poirel L, et al. Evaluation of the Rapid Polymyxin NP test and its industrial version for the detection of polymyxin-resistant Enterobacteriaceae. Diagn Microbiol Infect Dis 2018;92(2):90–4.

35. Jayol A, Dubois V, Poirel L, et al. Rapid detection of polymyxin-resistant enterobacteriaceae from blood cultures. J Clin Microbiol 2016;54(9):2273–7.
36. Nordmann P, Poirel L, Mueller L. Rapid detection of fosfomycin resistance in *Escherichia coli.* J Clin Microbiol 2019;57(1). e01531-18.
37. Nordmann P, Jayol A, Dobias J, et al. Rapid Aminoglycoside NP test for rapid detection of multiple aminoglycoside resistance in enterobacteriaceae. J Clin Microbiol 2017;55(4):1074–9.
38. Lescat M, Poirel L, Tinguely C, et al. A resazurin reduction-based assay for rapid detection of polymyxin resistance in *Acinetobacter baumannii* and *Pseudomonas aeruginosa.* J Clin Microbiol 2019;57(3). e01563-18.
39. Bishop JD, Hsieh HV, Gasperino DJ, et al. Sensitivity enhancement in lateral flow assays: a systems perspective. Lab Chip 2019;19(15):2486–99.
40. Wareham DW, Shah R, Betts JW, et al. Evaluation of an Immunochromatographic Lateral Flow Assay (OXA-48 K-SeT) for Rapid Detection of OXA-48-like carbapenemases in enterobacteriaceae. J Clin Microbiol 2016;54(2):471–3.
41. Glupczynski Y, Evrard S, Huang TD, et al. Evaluation of the RESIST-4 K-SeT assay, a multiplex immunochromatographic assay for the rapid detection of OXA-48-like, KPC, VIM and NDM carbapenemases. J Antimicrob Chemother 2019;74(5):1284–7.
42. Hopkins KL, Meunier D, Naas T, et al. Evaluation of the NG-Test CARBA 5 multiplex immunochromatographic assay for the detection of KPC, OXA-48-like, NDM, VIM and IMP carbapenemases. J Antimicrob Chemother 2018;73(12): 3523–6.
43. Takissian J, Bonnin RA, Naas T, et al. NG-Test Carba 5 for rapid detection of carbapenemase-producing enterobacterales from positive blood cultures. Antimicrob Agents Chemother 2019;63(5). e00011-19.
44. Giordano L, Fiori B, D'Inzeo T, et al. Simplified testing method for direct detection of carbapenemase-producing organisms from positive blood cultures using the NG-Test Carba 5 Assay. Antimicrob Agents Chemother 2019;63(7). e00550-19.
45. Volland H, Dortet L, Bernabeu S, et al. Development and multicentric validation of a lateral flow immunoassay for rapid detection of MCR-1-Producing Enterobacteriaceae. J Clin Microbiol 2019;57(5). e01454-18.
46. Bryson AL, Hill EM, Doern CD. Matrix-assisted laser desorption/ionization time-of-flight: the revolution in progress. Clin Lab Med 2019;39(3):391–404.
47. Neonakis IK, Spandidos DA. Detection of carbapenemase producers by matrix-assisted laser desorption-ionization time-of-flight mass spectrometry (MALDI-TOF MS). Eur J Clin Microbiol Infect Dis 2019;38(10):1795–801.
48. Rapp E, Samuelsen O, Sundqvist M. Detection of carbapenemases with a newly developed commercial assay using Matrix Assisted Laser Desorption Ionization-Time of Flight. J Microbiol Methods 2018;146:37–9.
49. Dortet L, Tande D, de Briel D, et al. MALDI-TOF for the rapid detection of carbapenemase-producing Enterobacteriaceae: comparison of the commercialized MBT STAR(R)-Carba IVD Kit with two in-house MALDI-TOF techniques and the RAPIDEC(R) CARBA NP. J Antimicrob Chemother 2018;73(9):2352–9.
50. Figueroa-Espinosa R, Costa A, Cejas D, et al. MALDI-TOF MS based procedure to detect KPC-2 directly from positive blood culture bottles and colonies. J Microbiol Methods 2019;159:120–7.
51. Lupo A, Papp-Wallace KM, Sendi P, et al. Non-phenotypic tests to detect and characterize antibiotic resistance mechanisms in Enterobacteriaceae. Diagn Microbiol Infect Dis 2013;77(3):179–94.

52. Navarro E, Serrano-Heras G, Castano MJ, et al. Real-time PCR detection chemistry. Clin Chim Acta 2015;439:231–50.
53. Souverein D, Euser SM, van der Reijden WA, et al. Clinical sensitivity and specificity of the Check-Points Check-Direct ESBL Screen for BD MAX, a real-time PCR for direct ESBL detection from rectal swabs. J Antimicrob Chemother 2017;72(9):2512–8.
54. Engel T, Slotboom BJ, van Maarseveen N, et al. A multi-centre prospective evaluation of the Check-Direct ESBL Screen for BD MAX as a rapid molecular screening method for extended-spectrum beta-lactamase-producing Enterobacteriaceae rectal carriage. J Hosp Infect 2017;97(3):247–53.
55. Nijhuis R, Samuelsen O, Savelkoul P, et al. Evaluation of a new real-time PCR assay (Check-Direct CPE) for rapid detection of KPC, OXA-48, VIM, and NDM carbapenemases using spiked rectal swabs. Diagn Microbiol Infect Dis 2013; 77(4):316–20.
56. Huang TD, Bogaerts P, Ghilani E, et al. Multicentre evaluation of the Check-Direct CPE(R) assay for direct screening of carbapenemase-producing *Enterobacteriaceae* from rectal swabs. J Antimicrob Chemother 2015;70(6):1669–73.
57. Lau AF, Fahle GA, Kemp MA, et al. Clinical Performance of Check-Direct CPE, a Multiplex PCR for Direct Detection of bla(KPC), bla(NDM) and/or bla(VIM), and bla(OXA)-48 from Perirectal Swabs. J Clin Microbiol 2015;53(12):3729–37.
58. Antonelli A, Arena F, Giani T, et al. Performance of the BD MAX instrument with Check-Direct CPE real-time PCR for the detection of carbapenemase genes from rectal swabs, in a setting with endemic dissemination of carbapenemase-producing Enterobacteriaceae. Diagn Microbiol Infect Dis 2016;86(1):30–4.
59. Dortet L, Fusaro M, Naas T. Improvement of the Xpert Carba-R Kit for the detection of carbapenemase-producing enterobacteriaceae. Antimicrob Agents Chemother 2016;60(6):3832–7.
60. Tato M, Ruiz-Garbajosa P, Traczewski M, et al. Multisite evaluation of cepheid Xpert Carba-R assay for detection of carbapenemase-producing organisms in rectal swabs. J Clin Microbiol 2016;54(7):1814–9.
61. Hoyos-Mallecot Y, Ouzani S, Dortet L, et al. Performance of the Xpert((R)) Carba-R v2 in the daily workflow of a hygiene unit in a country with a low prevalence of carbapenemase-producing Enterobacteriaceae. Int J Antimicrob Agents 2017;49(6):774–7.
62. Zhou M, Kudinha T, Du B, et al. Active Surveillance of Carbapenemase-Producing Organisms (CPO) Colonization With Xpert Carba-R assay plus positive patient isolation proves to be effective in CPO containment. Front Cell Infect Microbiol 2019;9:162.
63. Jeong S, Kim JO, Jeong SH, et al. Evaluation of peptide nucleic acid-mediated multiplex real-time PCR kits for rapid detection of carbapenemase genes in gram-negative clinical isolates. J Microbiol Methods 2015;113:4–9.
64. Meunier D, Woodford N, Hopkins KL. Evaluation of the AusDiagnostics MT CRE EU assay for the detection of carbapenemase genes and transferable colistin resistance determinants mcr-1/-2 in MDR Gram-negative bacteria. J Antimicrob Chemother 2018;73(12):3355–8.
65. Evans SR, Tran TTT, Hujer AM, et al. Rapid molecular diagnostics to inform empiric use of ceftazidime/avibactam and ceftolozane/tazobactam against Pseudomonas aeruginosa: PRIMERS IV. Clin Infect Dis 2019;68(11):1823–30.
66. Lucena Baeza L, Pfennigwerth N, Hamprecht A. Rapid and easy detection of carbapenemases in enterobacterales in the routine laboratory using the new

GenePOC Carba/Revogene Carba C Assay. J Clin Microbiol 2019;57(9). e00597-19.
67. Poritz MA, Blaschke AJ, Byington CL, et al. FilmArray, an automated nested multiplex PCR system for multi-pathogen detection: development and application to respiratory tract infection. PLoS One 2011;6(10):e26047.
68. Babady NE. The FilmArray respiratory panel: an automated, broadly multiplexed molecular test for the rapid and accurate detection of respiratory pathogens. Expert Rev Mol Diagn 2013;13(8):779–88.
69. Salimnia H, Fairfax MR, Lephart PR, et al. Evaluation of the filmarray blood culture identification panel: results of a multicenter controlled trial. J Clin Microbiol 2016;54(3):687–98.
70. Verroken A, Despas N, Rodriguez-Villalobos H, et al. The impact of a rapid molecular identification test on positive blood cultures from critically ill with bacteremia: A pre-post intervention study. PLoS One 2019;14(9):e0223122.
71. Pardo J, Klinker KP, Borgert SJ, et al. Clinical and economic impact of antimicrobial stewardship interventions with the FilmArray blood culture identification panel. Diagn Microbiol Infect Dis 2016;84(2):159–64.
72. Mori Y, Notomi T. Loop-mediated isothermal amplification (LAMP): Expansion of its practical application as a tool to achieve universal health coverage. J Infect Chemother 2020;26(1):13–7.
73. Liu W, Zou D, Li Y, et al. Sensitive and rapid detection of the new Delhi metallo-β-lactamase gene by loop-mediated isothermal amplification. J Clin Microbiol 2012;50(5):1580–5.
74. Nakano R, Nakano A, Ishii Y, et al. Rapid detection of the Klebsiella pneumoniae carbapenemase (KPC) gene by loop-mediated isothermal amplification (LAMP). J Infect Chemother 2015;21(3):202–6.
75. Vergara A, Zboromyrska Y, Mosqueda N, et al. Evaluation of a loop-mediated isothermal amplification-based methodology to detect carbapenemase carriage in *Acinetobacter* clinical isolates. Antimicrob Agents Chemother 2014;58(12): 7538–40.
76. Garcia-Fernandez S, Morosini MI, Marco F, et al. Evaluation of the eazyplex(R) SuperBug CRE system for rapid detection of carbapenemases and ESBLs in clinical *Enterobacteriaceae* isolates recovered at two Spanish hospitals. J Antimicrob Chemother 2015;70(4):1047–50.
77. Hinic V, Ziegler J, Straub C, et al. Extended-spectrum beta-lactamase (ESBL) detection directly from urine samples with the rapid isothermal amplification-based eazyplex(R) SuperBug CRE assay: Proof of concept. J Microbiol Methods 2015;119:203–5.
78. Fiori B, D'Inzeo T, Posteraro B, et al. Direct use of eazyplex((R)) SuperBug CRE assay from positive blood cultures in conjunction with inpatient infectious disease consulting for timely appropriate antimicrobial therapy in *Escherichia coli* and *Klebsiella pneumoniae* bloodstream infections. Infect Drug Resist 2019; 12:1055–62.
79. Miller MB, Tang YW. Basic concepts of microarrays and potential applications in clinical microbiology. Clin Microbiol Rev 2009;22(4):611–33.
80. Endimiani A, Hujer AM, Hujer KM, et al. Evaluation of a commercial microarray system for detection of SHV-, TEM-, CTX-M-, and KPC-type β-lactamase genes in Gram-negative isolates. J Clin Microbiol 2010;48(7):2618–22.
81. Bogaerts P, Hujer AM, Naas T, et al. Multicenter evaluation of a new DNA microarray for rapid detection of clinically relevant *bla* genes from β-lactam-resistant gram-negative bacteria. Antimicrob Agents Chemother 2011;55(9):4457–60.

82. Cunningham SA, Vasoo S, Patel R. Evaluation of the check-points check MDR CT103 and CT103 XL microarray kits by use of preparatory rapid cell lysis. J Clin Microbiol 2016;54(5):1368–71.
83. Fishbain JT, Sinyavskiy O, Riederer K, et al. Detection of extended-spectrum β-lactamase and *Klebsiella pneumoniae* Carbapenemase genes directly from blood cultures by use of a nucleic acid microarray. J Clin Microbiol 2012; 50(9):2901–4.
84. Bernasconi OJ, Principe L, Tinguely R, et al. Evaluation of a New Commercial Microarray Platform for the Simultaneous Detection of beta-Lactamase and mcr-1 and mcr-2 Genes in Enterobacteriaceae. J Clin Microbiol 2017;55(10): 3138–41.
85. Ledeboer NA, Lopansri BK, Dhiman N, et al. Identification of gram-negative bacteria and genetic resistance determinants from positive blood culture broths by use of the verigene gram-negative blood culture multiplex microarray-based molecular assay. J Clin Microbiol 2015;53(8):2460–72.
86. Walker T, Dumadag S, Lee CJ, et al. Clinical impact of laboratory implementation of Verigene BC-GN microarray-based assay for detection of gram-negative bacteria in positive blood cultures. J Clin Microbiol 2016;54(7): 1789–96.
87. Neely LA, Audeh M, Phung NA, et al. T2 magnetic resonance enables nanoparticle-mediated rapid detection of candidemia in whole blood. Sci Transl Med 2013;5(182):182ra154.
88. Clancy CJ, Nguyen MH. T2 magnetic resonance for the diagnosis of bloodstream infections: charting a path forward. J Antimicrob Chemother 2018; 73(suppl_4):iv2–5.
89. De Angelis G, Posteraro B, De Carolis E, et al. T2Bacteria magnetic resonance assay for the rapid detection of ESKAPEc pathogens directly in whole blood. J Antimicrob Chemother 2018;73(suppl_4):iv20–6.
90. Eichenberger EM, Thaden JT. Epidemiology and mechanisms of resistance of extensively drug resistant gram-negative bacteria. Antibiotics (Basel) 2019; 8(2):37.
91. Hendriksen RS, Bortolaia V, Tate H, et al. Using genomics to track global antimicrobial resistance. Front Public Health 2019;7:242.
92. Schurch AC, van Schaik W. Challenges and opportunities for whole-genome sequencing-based surveillance of antibiotic resistance. Ann N Y Acad Sci 2017;1388(1):108–20.
93. Forsberg KJ, Reyes A, Wang B, et al. The shared antibiotic resistome of soil bacteria and human pathogens. Science 2012;337(6098):1107–11.
94. Gonzalez-Escalona N, Allard MA, Brown EW, et al. Nanopore sequencing for fast determination of plasmids, phages, virulence markers, and antimicrobial resistance genes in Shiga toxin-producing Escherichia coli. PLoS One 2019; 14(7):e0220494.
95. Salzberg SL, Phillippy AM, Zimin A, et al. GAGE: A critical evaluation of genome assemblies and assembly algorithms. Genome Res 2012;22(3):557–67.
96. Chin CS, Alexander DH, Marks P, et al. Nonhybrid, finished microbial genome assemblies from long-read SMRT sequencing data. Nat Methods 2013;10(6): 563–9.
97. Quick J, Quinlan AR, Loman NJ. A reference bacterial genome dataset generated on the MinION portable single-molecule nanopore sequencer. Gigascience 2014;3:22.

98. Ma ZS, Li L, Ye C, et al. Hybrid assembly of ultra-long Nanopore reads augmented with 10x-Genomics contigs: Demonstrated with a human genome. Genomics 2019;111(6):1896–901.
99. van der Helm E, Imamovic L, Hashim Ellabaan MM, et al. Rapid resistome mapping using nanopore sequencing. Nucleic Acids Res 2017;45(8):e61.
100. Cao MD, Ganesamoorthy D, Elliott AG, et al. Streaming algorithms for identification of pathogens and antibiotic resistance potential from real-time MinION(TM) sequencing. Gigascience 2016;5(1):32.
101. Su M, Satola SW, Read TD. Genome-based prediction of bacterial antibiotic resistance. J Clin Microbiol 2019;57(3). e01405-18.
102. Kos VN, Deraspe M, McLaughlin RE, et al. The resistome of Pseudomonas aeruginosa in relationship to phenotypic susceptibility. Antimicrob Agents Chemother 2015;59(1):427–36.
103. Ashton PM, Nair S, Dallman T, et al. MinION nanopore sequencing identifies the position and structure of a bacterial antibiotic resistance island. Nat Biotechnol 2015;33(3):296–300.
104. Judge K, Harris SR, Reuter S, et al. Early insights into the potential of the Oxford Nanopore MinION for the detection of antimicrobial resistance genes. J Antimicrob Chemother 2015;70(10):2775–8.
105. Turton JF, Doumith M, Hopkins KL, et al. Clonal expansion of Escherichia coli ST38 carrying a chromosomally integrated OXA-48 carbapenemase gene. J Med Microbiol 2016;65(6):538–46.
106. Loman NJ, Quick J, Simpson JT. A complete bacterial genome assembled de novo using only nanopore sequencing data. Nat Methods 2015;12(8):733–5.
107. Votintseva AA, Bradley P, Pankhurst L, et al. Same-day diagnostic and surveillance data for tuberculosis via whole-genome sequencing of direct respiratory samples. J Clin Microbiol 2017;55(5):1285–98.
108. Bradley P, Gordon NC, Walker TM, et al. Rapid antibiotic-resistance predictions from genome sequence data for Staphylococcus aureus and Mycobacterium tuberculosis. Nat Commun 2015;6:10063.

The Continuing Plague of Extended-Spectrum β-Lactamase Producing Enterbacterales Infections

An Update

Amos Adler, MD[a,b], David E. Katz, MD, MPH[c], Dror Marchaim, MD[b,d,*]

KEYWORDS

• Gram-negative • MDRO • *Escherichia coli* • *Klebsiella pneumoniae* • *Proteus mirabilis*

KEY POINTS

- The continued spread of extended-spectrum β-lactamase (ESBL) infections is highly correlated with the shift in modern continuums of medical care, whereby patients with severe and complex medical conditions are now frequently managed in suboptimal conditions outside of hospital settings.
- Emergence of a new class of ESBL enzymes, the $bla_{CTX\text{-}M}$, contributed to the epidemiologic evolution of human ESBL infections in community settings.
- Appropriate antimicrobial therapy is frequently delayed in patients with ESBL infections, which leads to worse outcomes. Rapid diagnostics and reliable clinical predicting tools could aid in reducing delays to initiation of appropriate antimicrobials and might improve patient outcomes.
- Carbapenems should still be perceived as the mainstay of therapy for severe ESBL infections.

Portions of this article were previously published in Adler A, Katz DE, Marchaim D. The Continuing Plague of Extended-spectrum β-lactamase–producing Enterobacteriaceae Infections. Infect Dis Clin North Am 2016; 30(2): 347-375.

[a] Clinical Microbiology Laboratory, Tel-Aviv Sourasky Medical Center, 6 Weizmann Street, Tel-Aviv 6423906 Israel; [b] Sackler School of Medicine, Tel-Aviv University, Tel-Aviv, Israel; [c] Division of Internal Medicine, Shaare Zedek Medical Center, 12 Shmuel Bait Street, Jerusalem 9103102, Israel; [d] Unit of Infection Control, Shamir (Assaf Harofeh) Medical Center, Zerifin, Israel

* Corresponding author. Unit of Infection Control, Shamir (Assaf Harofeh) Medical Center, Zerifin 7030000, Israel.

E-mail address: drormarchaim@gmail.com

Infect Dis Clin N Am 34 (2020) 677–708
https://doi.org/10.1016/j.idc.2020.06.003 id.theclinics.com
0891-5520/20/

INTRODUCTION

The incidence of infections caused by multidrug-resistant (MDR) gram-negative bacilli (GNB) pathogens, affecting humans in hospitals, outpatient health care facilities, and community settings, is continually growing worldwide.[1–3] The Infectious Diseases Society of America defined the "ESKAPE" pathogens as the pathogens that currently cause most of hospital infections and can effectively "escape" the effects of available therapeutics.[1] The World Health Organization further reinforced this statement and named some of the same pathogens as imposing one of the biggest challenges and threats in modern medicine.[4] Among the ESKAPE pathogens are common Enterobacteriaceae (eg, *Klebsiella pneumoniae*, *Enterobacter* species, and *Escherichia coli*).[1] *Proteus mirabilis* is another enteric pathogen in which the rate of resistance to multiple antimicrobials is increasing, more commonly outside of the United States.[5,6] Emergence of resistance to a wide range of antibiotics among the most common human pathogens,[7] that is, the Enterobacteriaceae, is hazardous, and it poses a huge burden on individual patients and the general public.[1,8,9]

THE EMERGENCE OF EXTENDED-SPECTRUM β-LACTAMASES

The incremental growth in resistance to β-lactam agents (eg, penicillins and cephalosporins) among Enterobacteriaceae is frightful. β-Lactams are among safest therapeutics.[10,11] Given susceptible isolates, they are potent bactericidal agents.[12] In addition, well-controlled data on their clinical efficacy against Enterobacteriaceae are readily available because of their extended years of usage.[1,13] Because of their safety, tolerability, potency, and (usually) low price, β-lactams are the most commonly prescribed drugs worldwide.[14] β-Lactams are used as first-line agents for many infectious clinical syndromes resulting from Enterobacteriaceae infections.[15,16]

The first report of a naturally occurring β-lactam hydrolyzing enzyme in *E coli* was published even before penicillin was marketed for use.[17] In 1960, the plasmid mediated β-lactamase bla_{TEM} was first reported from Greece.[18] Later on, additional transmissible types of β-lactamases were identified, for example, $bla_{SHV\text{-}1}$.[13] These β-lactamases confer resistance to penicillins and narrow-spectrum cephalosporins, but not to extended-spectrum penicillins or cephalosporins.[13] Soon thereafter, new broader-spectrum β-lactam agents became widely used (eg, cephalosporins with oxymino side chain, cephamycins, carbapenems, and monobactam). Subsequently, new families of β-lactamases soon started to emerge.[19,20] One of the most epidemiologically "successful" groups of such enzymes is the extended-spectrum β-lactamases (ESBLs).

The ESBLs are serine β-lactamases, characterized according to their biochemically functional Ambler classification as class A, and are inhibited by β-lactamase inactivators, such as clavulanate or tazobactam.[11] This feature constitutes the basis for the phenotypic diagnosis of ESBL-producing bacteria in many laboratories, measuring the zone of inhibition of the isolates in the presence and absence of a β-lactamase inhibitor (BLI; ie, the "ESBL test").[11] According to the functional Bush-Jacoby-Medeiros classification, ESBLs are classified under group 2be.[21,22]

ESBLs confer resistance to most β-lactam antibiotics, including expanded-spectrum cephalosporins and monobactams, but not to carbapenems and cephamycins.[16,18,23] Even though ESBL-producing Enterobacteriaceae hydrolyze penicillins, cephalosporins (excluding cephamycins), and monobactam, their degree of hydrolytic activity can vary greatly. This variable degree of hydrolytic activity results in both diagnostic challenges and controversies pertaining to treatment efficacy of agents for which isolates are supposedly "susceptible."[24] It took several years before clinicians realized that treatment with β-lactams for an ESBL-producing strain, even when the strain is supposedly "susceptible" (per older criteria[25]), could fail in various infectious syndromes and settings.[23,24,26,27] Moreover, ESBL-producing Enterobacteriaceae are often coresistant to other classes of antibiotics, such as fluoroquinolones, aminoglycosides, and trimethoprim/sulfamethoxazol (TMP/SMX),[28,29] further limiting available therapeutic options and increasing the epidemiologic significance posed by these offending human strains.[24,30,31]

ESBLs have been discovered in *K pneumoniae*, *E coli*, and *P mirabilis*, as well as in other enteric bacteria (eg, *Klebsiella oxytoca*, *Citrobacter*, *Enterobacter*, *Salmonella*, *Serratia*), and in nonfermenting nosocomial pathogens (eg, *Acinetobacter baumannii*, *Pseudomonas aeruginosa*).[20] Some Enterobacteriaceae (eg, *Enterobacter*, *Citrobacter*, *Providencia*, *Morganella*, and *Serratia*) inherently possess chromosomal genes (bla_{AmpC}), which confer resistance to the same extended-spectrum cephalosporins and penicillins through an Ambler C hydrolyzing bla_{AmpC} β-lactamases.[20,22] This review focuses solely on Ambler A ESBL-producing *K pneumoniae*, *E coli*, and *P mirabilis* infections, because this has proved to be a somewhat distinct epidemiologic clinical entity.

WORLDWIDE PREVALENCE OF EXTENDED-SPECTRUM β-LACTAMASES

Overall, the rates and types of ESBL-producing Enterobacteriaceae infections increased dramatically in the past 30 years; however, distinct geographic patterns and institutional variation exist.[18,32] Huge surveillance programs are periodically reporting the prevalence of ESBLs among offending pathogens from all over the world.[33,34] For example, database from 2004 to 2006 reported that the rates of ESBL production in Latin America was 44% among *K pneumoniae* and 13.5% among *E coli* isolations.[33] In Europe, the rates of ESBL production reported during the same years were 13.3% of *K pneumoniae* and 7.6% of *E coli*; in Asia/Pacific Rim 22.4% of *K pneumoniae* and 12% of *E coli*, and in North America, 7.5% of *K pneumoniae* and 2.2% among *E coli*.[33,35–37] Presently, the rates reported from many facilities are much higher, that is, up to 45% among *K pneumoniae* and up to 35% among *E coli*.[38–40]

THE HISTORIC EVOLUTION OF bla_{TEM}- AND bla_{SHV}-TYPES EXTENDED-SPECTRUM β-LACTAMASES–PRODUCING ENTEROBACTERIACEAE INFECTIONS

Expanded-spectrum cephalosporins were introduced to clinical practice in the early 1980s.[41,42] In many institutions, they were prescribed in high volumes and with very little regulation.[43] These agents were safe, potent, accessible, relatively cheap, and extremely effective against a wide array of human pathogens.[44,45] In many facilities, they became the backbone of empiric regimens for various indications.[46] Frequently, administration of these broad-spectrum agents was continued, even following the isolation of a more susceptible causative pathogen.[43]

Soon thereafter, plasmid-encoded β-lactamases, which hydrolyze expanded-spectrum cephalosporins, started to be reported in Western Europe (Germany, 1983), Asia, and the Americas.[18] The first ESBLs reported were developed via point mutations in the narrow-spectrum β-lactamases bla_{SHV-1}, bla_{TEM-1}, and bla_{TEM-2}.[47] These substitutions in amino acids changed the active site of the β-lactamase and consequently resulted in resistance also to the extended-spectrum cephalosporins, to all penicillins, and monobactam.[48] As new alleles of the bla_{SHV} and bla_{TEM} families of enzymes were discovered, they were named in chronologic order (ie, bla_{SHV-2}, bla_{SHV-3}, and so on, and bla_{TEM-3}, bla_{TEM-4}, and so on, respectively),[20,22,48] but not necessarily according to their antimicrobial spectrum. For instance, the bla_{SHV-9} is categorized as a type 2be (ie, ESBL) enzyme, whereas the bla_{SHV-11} is a type 2b (narrow spectrum) enzyme (http://www.lahey.org/Studies/).

Initially, ESBL-producing pathogens were primarily isolated in tertiary facilities, particularly from very sick patients hospitalized in intensive care units (ICUs).[18,49–51] These patients were exposed to broad-spectrum antibiotics and had multiple invasive devices and exposure to instrumentation.[52,53] After establishing endemicity in certain facilities, reports of nosocomial outbreaks of Enterobacteriaceae-producing bla_{SHV} or bla_{TEM} ESBLs were starting to emerge, consisting mostly of ESBL-producing *K pneumoniae*.[52,54–56] In the mid to late 1990s, case reports and case series suggested that ESBL-producing Enterobacteriaceae had started to spread to outpatient settings as well.[57–64] This phenomenon was extremely worrisome at that time and was defined by experts as a global sentinel event that should be closely monitored and controlled.[52,65]

One hypothesis explaining this spread of ESBL producers to community settings stems from the dramatic global change related to the continuum of medical care that gradually took place during those years. Medically complex patients, who previously were exclusively managed in acute care settings (eg, the severely ill, patients with chronic invasive foreign devices, central lines, urinary catheter, and even ventilated patients), were now being managed for prolonged periods in specified long-term care facilities (LTCF).[66] The motivation for this gradual change was primarily fiscal.[66] These LTCFs are in many instances "for-profit" facilities and were initially reluctant to invest in infection control and antimicrobial stewardship measures.[66,67] Therefore, LTCFs soon became an important pathway between the hospital and the community settings, contributing to the exponential increase in the prevalence of multidrug-resistant organisms (MDROs),[68] including ESBL-producing Enterobacteriaceae.[69,70] These patients with complicated medical conditions were continually transmitted back and forth between acute and chronic health care facilities, serving as "Trojan horses" of MDROs.[69,71] Multiple case-control analyses conducted in various locations worldwide showed that an LTCF stay was an independent predictor for acquisition of various MDROs, including ESBLs.[31,72–75] Misuse of antimicrobials, which facilitate the predominance of resistant strains and emergence of resistance among susceptible strains, coupled with nonimplementation of infection control measures, further facilitating patient-to-patient transmission, and poor patients' basic characteristics, were all common in certain LTCFs.[8,66,69,70] This evolution of the continuum of medical care probably aided the spread of formerly "pure nosocomial ESBLs," for example, bla_{SHV} and bla_{TEM}, into nonhospital settings.[75]

The epidemiology of ESBL-producing strains further evolved soon thereafter. Approximately 15 years ago, ESBL-producing Enterobacteriaceae began to appear in the community among patients with no prior documented contact with LTCFs, no recent antibiotic exposure, and no other known risk factors for ESBL acquisition and carriage.[31,72,73,76,77] This lack of common known predictors for ESBL infections created an additional clinical challenge, because apart from being resistant to extended-spectrum β-lactam agents, resistances to commonly prescribed oral agents, frequently prescribed in community settings, became prevalent as well.[28,72] The plasmid harboring the ESBL gene (ie, the "resistome"[78]) was carrying additional genes conferring resistance to commonly prescribed oral antimicrobials, such as fluoroquinolones and TMP/SMX,[72,73,75,79–81] resulting in delays in instituting appropriate therapy in the community setting and worse outcomes for relatively "simple" infections among previously healthy and young individuals.[23,31,80,82]

THE bla_{CTX-M}-PRODUCING *E COLI* OUTBREAK IN NONHOSPITAL SETTINGS

Following the reports of increased incidence of ESBL infections in nonhospital settings among patients with none of the known "traditional" risk factors (ie, associated with health care exposures), molecular investigations revealed that a change in ESBL types might be related to this epidemiologic shift.[29,49,70,72,74,76,77,83–91] As previously mentioned, *K pneumoniae* was initially the main isolate harboring ESBL genes (most often bla_{TEM} and bla_{SHV} types) during the 1990s.[11] However, a decade later, *E coli*–producing ESBLs became prevalent in various regions, producing a different class of ESBLs, that is, the $bla_{CTX\text{-}M}$.[76,77,91] The $bla_{CTX\text{-}M}$ were discovered more than a decade before, but were initially not prevalent among ESBL producing human offending pathogens (with the exception of few alleles, ie, $bla_{CTX\text{-}M\text{-}93}$[92]).[13,21,93]

In recent years, the $bla_{CTX\text{-}M}$ families have seen a tremendous diversification. This family is divided into 5 main groups,[94] with different enzymes prevalent in different locations worldwide.[95,96] In comparison to the "old epidemiology," whereby *K pneumoniae* ESBL infections (ie, mainly bla_{SHV} and bla_{TEM}) were associated with various infectious clinical syndromes (eg, pneumonia, intraabdominal infections, urinary tract infections [UTI], and skin and soft tissue infections), most $bla_{CTX\text{-}M}$-producing *E coli* infections from the community were UTIs.[28,77,79]

The risk factors for $bla_{CTX\text{-}M}$-producing *E coli* infections were assessed in multiple analyses.[72,97–101] One of the unique features of this endemic strain is the tight statistical correlation to prior usage of fluoroquinolones and recent invasive urologic procedures.[28,72,77] The common practice of many urologists is to prescribe "prophylactic" regimens of antimicrobials, mostly consisting of fluoroquinolones, for several days preinvasive and postinvasive urologic procedure. This practice is not supported by professional guidelines[102,103] or based on solid scientific clinical data.[104–106] Regardless, this practice is still common with urologists and primary practitioners worldwide.[102,103] The increase in the number of such ambulatory urologic procedures in the modern era might have also contributed to the spread of $bla_{CTX\text{-}M}$-producing *E coli* infections in some community settings.[72] Some risk factor analyses even pointed to the fact that being a middle-aged man became an independent risk factor for $bla_{CTX\text{-}M}$-producing *E coli* infection, despite the fact that UTIs are usually more common among women in this age group. Sex might have served as a possible confounder for urologic invasive procedures in some of these studies.[28,73]

Additional contributing factors to the epidemic of ESBL infections in the community in general, and of $bla_{CTX\text{-}M}$-producing *E coli* infections in particular, may be related to the agriculture and food industries.[107–110] Unfortunately, misuse of antibiotics in these industries is common and not tightly regulated.[111–113] Many community outbreaks of $bla_{CTX\text{-}M}$-producing *E coli* infections, originating from agriculture and food products and industries, were reported.[86,107–110,114–122] In 2011, a huge outbreak in Europe of a $bla_{CTX\text{-}M}$-producing *E coli* strain, associated with hemolytic uremic syndrome, resulted in several deaths among previously healthy and young individuals, mainly from Germany and France.[123,124] It was suggested that the outbreak resulted from contaminated food products that were distributed in various countries.[122] CTX-Ms have also been isolated from wild birds, poultry, urban rats, companion animals, and retail meat from supermarkets in various states in the United States.[86,90,116,125–133] These findings led several investigators to suggest that $bla_{CTX\text{-}M}$ enzymes could potentially spread from the community to the health care environment and not universally vice versa.[28,55] Despite the appeal of this concept, the importance of this connection beyond isolated outbreaks (as mentioned above) is questionable. Although ESBLs are certainly not uncommon in livestock, there are important differences in the prevalence of specific genes and clones in animals versus humans.[133] This difference in ESBLs found in animals vs humans is in contrast with other organisms, for example, *Staphylococcus aureus*, whereby specific clones have been shown to be transferred from livestock to humans.[134] More importantly, considering the production process of food products from livestock, the transmission mechanism of living organisms from food to human is not clear.

International travel to certain locations (eg, India, the Middle East, and Africa) used to be an additional factor that had facilitated the spread of bla_{CTX-M}-producing strains in the community, specifically in certain countries (particularly in North America).[135] A detailed Canadian risk factor analysis found that the distribution of bla_{CTX-M} enzymes among travelers was highly correlated with the predominant bla_{CTX-M} that were reported from the respective travel destination.[135] However, these enzymes had already established endemicity in most regions. As of 2013, bla_{CTX-M} were considered the most common ESBLs in Latin America, Canada, South America, and in many parts of Europe and the United States.[55,76,95,136,137] Thus, unlike carbapenemases that are still rare in the community of many parts of the world, ESBL's endemicity is much wider, and thus, the contribution of international travel to current spread is probably minor.

THE CLONAL EXPANSION OF A SPECIFIC *bla*$_{CTX-M}$-PRODUCING *E COLI* STRAIN IN THE COMMUNITY

Following the recognition that *bla*$_{CTX-M}$ might be related in part to the epidemiologic shift in ESBL human infections and its dissemination into community settings, advanced investigational molecular techniques soon revealed the predominance of a specific *E coli* clone, producing mainly *bla*$_{CTX-M15}$ enzymes in at least 3 continents.[138,139] This successful clone was classified as (1) sequence type (ST) 131 per multilocus sequence typing (MLST)[72,76,138,140–144]; (2) phylogenetic group B2 (classified according to major *E coli* phylogenetic groups [A, B1, B2, D])[145]; and (3) serotype O25:H4.[146] This clone, referred to as ST-131 for the rest of this review, is a pandemic clone that has disseminated exponentially since 2003.[147] Although other lineages, such as the ST-405 or ST-38, have also played an important role in the dissemination of *bla*$_{CTX-M}$-producing *E coli* in certain countries,[139] they have been less predominant compared with the ST-131 clone. This clone is primarily associated with community-associated ESBL UTIs, which are frequently accompanied by bloodstream infections (BSI).[148] Most ST-131 isolates are also resistant to fluoroquinolones.[149]

Until recently, the reasons that made this specific clone so successful were obscure. It was isolated from companion animals, seagulls, rats, poultry, and even retail chicken, with all of these sources suggested as possible reservoirs.[148] In a recent trial conducted in Seville, Spain, a case-control and cohort investigation of the risk factors and clinical outcomes, respectively, were compared between 110 patients with ST-131 *E coli* ESBL infections versus 288 patients with non-ST-131 ESBL *E coli* infections.[150] Previous use of antibiotics was the main modifiable risk factor for infections caused by ST-131 strains. The severity of sepsis, rates of bacteremia, and mortality were similar among ST-131 and non-ST-131 groups.[150] These same findings were later reported from a US site[77] and from Nepal.[151] These analyses suggest that misuse of antimicrobials, particularly in the community, plays an important role in the acquisition and spread of this clone. Other common modes of MDRO acquisition, that is, patient-to-patient transmission, probably play a lesser role in the dissemination of this clone in the community.[8] This understanding led to the initiation of extensive systematic efforts to reduce the misuse of antibiotics in the "community": that is, in ambulatory clinical settings and in the agriculture and food industries,[152] which also contributes to the on-going debate whether patients with ESBL carriage should be subjected to contact isolation precautions when they are admitted to the hospital.[153]

WHAT ARE THE PREDICTORS FOR EXTENDED-SPECTRUM β-LACTAMASES–PRODUCING ENTEROBACTERIACEAE INFECTIONS ACQUIRED OUTSIDE OF THE HOSPITAL SETTINGS?

Many risk factor analyses pertaining to ESBLs acquired outside the hospital settings have been published from diverse geographic settings using various definitions.[63,64,135,154–160] The debate on how best to define "community-onset infections" is beyond the scope of this article and is reviewed in detail elsewhere.[9] The risk factors analyses, which were published up until 2008, were nicely summarized by Pitout and Laupland.[29] However, this was before the magnitude of the bla_{CTX-Ms}-producing ST-131 *E coli* pandemic was fully acknowledged.[73] Their review highlighted the different predictors of hospital-onset and community-onset infections. In the hospital setting, ESBL infections were significantly linked to ICU stay, prolonged "time at risk" (ie, time from admission to culture), presence of foreign medical devices (eg, central lines, nasogastric tubes, urinary catheters, endotracheal tubes), recent prior invasive procedures, and recent prior administration of antimicrobials (especially third-generation cephalosporins).[11,18,161–163] In community-onset infections, or infections "upon admission" to hospitals, admission from an LTCF was the major risk factor for ESBL infection.[11,28,72] Other risk factors for community-onset ESBL infections were recurrent UTIs coupled with underlying renal pathologic condition, recent exposure to fluoroquinolones, previous hospitalization, advanced age, diabetes mellitus, and underlying liver disease.[29] Later, in 2008, Rodriguez-Bano and colleagues[73] published a detailed prospective analysis of risk factors for "community-acquired" ESBL-producing *E coli* infections in 11 Spanish hospitals. The independent predictors per the multivariable model were age older than 60 years, female sex, diabetes mellitus, recurrent UTIs, previous urologic invasive procedures, follow-up visits to outpatient clinics, and previous recent receipt of antibiotics (in particular, β-lactams or fluoroquinolones).[73] Many of these independent predictors simply reflected health care exposures.[164] The misuse of antibiotics before and following minimally invasive urologic procedures (by urologist and primary care physicians), frequently with no established indication,[165] may have contributed to the emergence and spread of ESBLs in nonhospital settings.[73]

This former "epidemiologic era" of community-onset ESBL infections is also well summarized by a multinational metasynthesis investigation conducted by Ben-Ami and colleagues[72] and published in 2009. This study included a synthesis of data collected from 6 centers in Europe, Asia, and North America. A total of 983 patient-specific isolates were reviewed (91% were *E coli*, 7% were *Klebsiella* species, and 2% were *P mirabilis*). CTX-M types were already the most frequent ESBLs (65%).

Independent predictors for community-onset ESBL infections included recent antibiotic use, residence in an LTCF, recent hospitalization, age older than 65 years, and male sex (in contrast to female predominance reported from Seville[73]). This comprehensive analysis illustrates again the resemblance of independent predictors for ESBL infections acquired outside of a hospital, and the complexities associated with the definition of health care-associated infections set by Friedman and colleagues.[164] It highlights that ESBL infections upon admission to acute-care hospitals should be suspected when "health care exposure" is documented.[40,166]

A multicenter prospective case-control study, conducted in 10 Israeli hospitals (2007–2009), was published in 2010[31]; this was already after bla_{CTX-M}-producing strains had established endemicity in most of Israel.[7,28] Overall, 447 patients with bacteremia owing to Enterobacteriaceae were enrolled: 205 cases with ESBLs and 242 controls with susceptible strains. Independent predictors of ESBL were increased age, multiple comorbid conditions, poor functional status, recent contact with health care settings, invasive procedures, and prior receipt of antimicrobial therapy. An interesting, previously unreported finding of this prospective trial was that patients presenting with septic shock or multiorgan failure were more likely to have an ESBL infection (ie, as opposed to infection resulting from susceptible Enterobacteriaceae). This finding may be indirectly related to the increased virulence properties of these ESBL-producing strains. It is very common in epidemiologic analyses that patients affected by the resistant strain suffer worse outcomes compared with its susceptible counterpart strain.[167–171] However, when controlling for various confounders, particularly for delays in initiation of appropriate antimicrobial therapy (DAAT), antimicrobial resistance alone has not always been shown to be independently associated with worse clinical outcomes[172]; many times, the opposite was actually evident.[172,173] Among ESBL-containing strains though, this might be different, and it is postulated by some that virulence properties are coupled with resistance genes on some of the transmissible "resistomes" in some of the circulating ESBL strains.[174,175] This aspect, however, is beyond the scope of this review. An additional finding of this multicenter Israeli trial was that patients infected with ESBL strains suffered more frequently from DAAT (odds ratio = 4.7), again highlighting the importance of early pathogen detection and identification (ie, by rapid diagnostics), the standardization of appropriate empirical regimens, and the development of reliable prediction tools. These measures could shorten the time to initiation of appropriate therapy, thereby improving patient outcomes,[82] while adhering to stewardship guidelines and recommendations.[31,40]

The spread of human ESBL infections caused by $bla_{\text{CTX-M}}$-producing *E coli* strains was introduced to the United States a few years after earlier reports from other locations.[77,84,176–180] A prospective observational study to examine the epidemiology of "community-associated" (both community-acquired and health care-associated) infections owing specifically to ESBL-producing *E coli* at 5 centers in the United States was published in 2013.[76] Of the 291 patients infected or colonized with ESBL-producing *E coli* who were enrolled either as outpatients or within 48 hours of hospitalization, 107 (36.8%) had "community-acquired" infections (with none of the health care-associated exposures as set by Freidman and colleagues[164]), and in 81.5% of them, the infectious syndrome was UTI.[76] Independent risk factors for health care-associated infection (with $\geq$1 health care exposures as per the Friedman criteria[164]) were the presence of cardiovascular disease, chronic renal failure, dementia, solid organ malignancy, and hospitalization within the previous 12 months. Of the "community-acquired" infections (ie, with no health care exposures[164]), 54.2% were caused by the globally epidemic ST131 strain, and 91.3% of the isolates produced $bla_{\text{CTX-M}}$-type ESBL.[76]

A case-case-control study of risk factors for $bla_{\text{CTX-M}}$-producing *E coli* was conducted later in Detroit.[77] Overall, 575 patients with community-onset ESBL-producing *E coli* were enrolled, and 491 (85.4%) of the isolates contained a $bla_{\text{CTX-M}}$ ESBL gene. Independent risk factors for $bla_{\text{CTX-M}}$ *E coli* isolation compared with non-$bla_{\text{CTX-M}}$ *E coli* included male gender, impaired consciousness, H2 blocker use, immunosuppression, and exposure to penicillins or TMP/SMX. Compared with uninfected controls, independent risk factors for isolation of $bla_{\text{CTX-M}}$ *E coli* included presence of a urinary catheter, previous UTI, exposure to oxyimino-cephalosporins, dependent functional status, non–home residence, and multiple baseline comorbidities. In addition, $bla_{\text{CTX-M}}$ strains were more resistant to multiple antibiotics than non-$bla_{\text{CTX-M}}$ ESBL-producing strains.[77]

To summarize this section, independent predictors for ESBL infections acquired in the community resemble some of the criteria as set by Friedman and colleagues[164] for defining health care-associated exposures. These criteria include LTCF stay, recent hospitalization in acute-care facilities, exposure to antibiotics, recent invasive procedures (specifically urologic), presence of foreign devices, and certain baseline complex comorbidities.

WHAT IS THE ISOLATED IMPACT OF EXTENDED-SPECTRUM β-LACTAMASES ACQUISITION ON PATIENTS' CLINICAL OUTCOMES?

In a matched case-case-control investigation, patients with ESBL infections have been shown to suffer worse clinical outcomes compared with patients with susceptible Enterobacteriaceae and compared with uninfected controls.[73,80,82,181–183] In a metaanalysis looking at the impact of ESBL production on mortality, comprising 16 studies conducted from 1996 to 2003, there was a significant increase in mortality among patients with ESBL-associated BSI (relative risk [RR] 1.85, $P<.001$). Moreover, patients with ESBL infections had significant DAAT (RR 5.56, $P<.001$).[82] Because DAAT is the strongest modifiable independent predictor for mortality in sepsis,[184] and because every hour of DAAT in septic shock reduces survival rates by approximately 7.6%,[185] this might be one of the main reasons for worse outcomes among these patients.[82]

There are various methods for reducing DAAT, including implementation of rapid diagnostic techniques and developing genuine prediction tools for early identification of ESBL infections, all to aid in reducing DAAT and avoiding the inappropriate administration of wide-spectrum antibiotics for patients with susceptible organisms.[186] In an attempt to reduce DAAT, several approaches to hasten the diagnosis of ESBLs have been explored, including the detection of bla_{ESBL} genes by microarray[187] or by using matrix-assisted laser desorption/ionization-time of flight to detect cefotaxime-hydrolyzing Gram negatives from positive blood cultures.[188] Unfortunately, these methods are both expensive and require significant amount of work and expertise. In addition, unlike other important resistance traits, such as methicillin resistance in *S aureus* that are conferred by a single molecular mechanism, cephalosporin resistance may be caused by a multitude of genetic mechanisms that are difficult to detect by a single test. Thus, such methods are unlikely to be implemented on a routine basis in most clinical microbiology laboratories. There were also attempts to develop prediction tools for ESBL infection upon admission to hospitals, with the aim of reducing DAAT, and avoiding misuse of broad-spectrum antimicrobials in patients without ESBL infection.[186] However, these tools have not yet been validated or implemented in many centers.[189] Difficulty in developing these tools arises from the fact that MDRO infections upon admission are not limited only to Enterobacteriaceae.[40,166,190]

TREATMENT OPTIONS FOR EXTENDED-SPECTRUM β-LACTAMASES–PRODUCING ENTEROBACTERIACEAE INFECTIONS IN HOSPITAL SETTINGS

Despite being prevalent pathogens, in both hospital and community settings, a limited number of prospective randomized controlled trials have been conducted addressing the most efficacious therapy for ESBL-producing Enterobacteriaceae infections (except the MERINO trial, discussed later).[191] The efficacy of some of the antimicrobial classes is reviewed in the following sections.

Carbapenems

This class is considered by many first-line agents, particularly for serious invasive ESBL infections.[15] Carbapenems have favorable pharmacokinetic/pharmacodynamic

(PK/PD) properties, are relatively safe, and have the most established clinical track record in this field.[15,16,192] A multicenter prospective observational trial demonstrated a significant association between carbapenems and lower mortalities in *K pneumoniae* BSIs, compared with other supposedly appropriate agents.[192] Notably, this was at a time when the prevalent ESBLs were bla_{TEM} and bla_{SHV}, not like current epidemiology. Other relative older trials, summarized in a review in 2008,[29] were small and retrospective, with multiple methodological flaws.[29] A few years later, a metaanalysis comparing carbapenems to alternative antibiotics demonstrated superiority of carbapenems over other therapeutic regimens.[193]

It should be noted that both group 1 (eg, ertapenem) and group 2 (eg, imipenem, meropenem, and doripenem) carbapenems cannot be hydrolyzed by ESBLs. Group 1 has a potential advantage in terms of reducing selective pressure among non-glucose-fermenting GNB pathogens (eg, *A baumannii*, *P aeruginosa*).[194] However, group 1 carbapenems were not thoroughly tested against serious invasive ESBL infections (eg, BSIs), and therefore, initial expert reviews recommended group 2 carbapenems for serious ESBL infections.[15] A retrospective analysis of 261 patients with ESBL BSIs from Detroit, Michigan, showed that the outcomes of infections were equivalent between patients treated with ertapenem versus those treated with group 2 carbapenems.[16] The investigators stratified the analysis based on the SIRS (systemic inflammatory response syndrome[195]) level, and group 1 was equivalent to group 2 even in patients with severe sepsis, septic shock, or multiorgan failure.[16]

Despite being the agents of choice for microbiologically confirmed ESBL infections, the empiric usage of carbapenems should be limited, because of the emergence and spread of carbapenem-resistant Enterobacteriaceae (CRE).[8,196,197] A direct correlation between carbapenem usage and CRE acquisition, on an ecological level (not patient level), is still a matter of debate.[8,194] However, the strongest independent predictor for CRE acquisition, on a patient level, is exposure to antimicrobials in general.[167]

β-Lactam-β-Lactamase Inhibitors Combinations

Although ESBLs (as Ambler A enzymes) are inhibited by BLI, such as clavulanic acid and tazobactam, data and expert opinions pertaining to the efficacy of β-lactam-β-lactamase inhibitors (BLBLI) for treating ESBL infections are conflicting.[11,12,16] The efficacy of BLBLI is doubtful because of the mostly theoretic "inoculum effect" phenomenon, hypothesizing that with certain infected tissues (eg, lungs), the bacteria inoculum is high compared with the concentration of the BLI concentration reaching that tissue.[198,199] The clinical impact of this phenomenon is not supported by strong scientific data, although worse outcomes were consistently reported, mainly in "high inoculum infectious syndromes," such as in endovascular infections and endocarditis.[200] Because of these reports, the common practice among most experts in the field was to consider BLBLI as an inappropriate alternative for ESBL infections.[15] Many microbiologic laboratories converted the susceptibility results to BLBLI of ESBL-producing strains to "resistant" so that prescribers would not consider BLBLI for ESBL infections.[24]

In 2012, a post hoc analysis of 6 prospective studies from Spain was published, comparing the efficacy of BLBLI with carbapenems in BSIs caused by ESBL-producing *E coli*.[201] A total of 192 patients were included in the final analysis consisting of 2 distinct cohorts: one for empiric therapy and the other for definitive therapy. The investigators did not find significant correlations between any of the regimens to any of the measured outcomes. However, outcomes in general were better among the group of patients who received BLBLI, and in the definitive treatment arm this difference nearly reached statistical significance for some of the outcomes.[201] The investigators concluded that BLBLIs should be perceived as legitimate alternatives to carbapenems for *E coli* ESBL BSIs.[201] However, as displayed in the editorial that accompanied this publication,[202] it is problematic to extrapolate these results to all ESBL-producing Enterobacteriaceae (not solely to *E coli*) and to all clinical infectious syndromes, for the following reasons: First, nearly 70% of BSIs originated from the urinary (or biliary) tract. β-Lactamase inhibitors, the only "active" ingredient in the BLBLI combination, are excreted almost exclusively unchanged in urine (or bile).[203] Because UTIs are relatively "low inoculum infections,"[204] a somewhat "reverse inoculum effect" might be expected in ESBL UTIs. Second, nearly 90% of ESBL *E coli* BSIs were due to $bla_{CTX\text{-}M}$-producing pathogens, and these enzymes are known to be hydrolyzed more efficiently by tazobactam compared with other ESBLs (eg, bla_{TEM}, bla_{SHV}) more prevalent among other Enterobacteriaceae (eg,*K pneumoniae* and *P mirabilis*). Third, the investigators found an obvious and significant correlation between the piperacillin-tazobactam MIC and the clinical outcome: that is, mortality increased when the minimal inhibitory concentration was greater than 4 mg/L.[201,205] Many ESBL isolates in multiple locations worldwide exhibit much higher MICs to piperacillin-tazobactam.[24] Fourth, bla_{CMY}-producing *E coli* strains, which are not inhibited by tazobactam, are as common as ESBL-producing strains in certain areas.[202] Fifth, the recent spread of the ST-131 *E coli* clone, which is the prevalent strain in this Spanish region,[46] is known to have lower MICs to BLBLIs.[206] Despite all these issues, this was a meticulously executed analysis, which questioned a concept that was already well accepted in many regions worldwide, despite the fact it was based on poor scientific and clinical data. Interestingly, the investigators pointed out that the sickest patients in their cohort were treated with carbapenems,[201] perhaps implying that carbapenems are still more trusted. In order to test whether BLBLI are equal to carbapenems in treating ESBL-producing BSIs (all ESBL-producing Enterobacteriaceae), a study focusing on BSIs arising from a nonurinary, high inoculum source (eg, pneumonia) was warranted.

The MERINO trial was designed as a prospective randomized clinical trial and included hospitalized patients who were enrolled from 26 sites in 9 countries. Adult patients were eligible if they had at least 1 positive blood culture with *E coli* or *Klebsiella* spp testing nonsusceptible to ceftriaxone but susceptible to piperacillin-tazobactam. It was designed to determine whether definitive therapy with piperacillin-tazobactam is noninferior to meropenem in patients with ESBL BSI (from various sources). The study included 391 patients, and the 30-day mortality for patients treated with piperacillin-tazobactam compared with meropenem was 12.3% versus 3.7%, respectively. The difference did not meet the noninferiority margin of 5%, that is, implying that piperacillin-tazobactam was inferior to meropenem for this indication.[191] The main critiques to this trial relate to few methodological issues, that is, claiming the investigators had not strictly controlled for potential clustering effect (by site) and possible allocation/selection biases, to the fact it was open-label, and that it may have underestimated the "true" or "actual" rates of nonsusceptibility to piperacillin-tazobactam among the arm assigned to this agent.[207] However, it is the only large and very well-designed prospective randomized controlled trial in the field of ESBL infections.

An additional study that was published in this debatable field, that is, comparing the efficacy of carbapenems versus BLBLIs for all ESBL infections (not restricted to *E coli*), and specifically focusing on patients with BSIs arising from a nonurinary, high inoculum source (eg, pneumonia), was retrospective, and conducted at a US and an Israeli center.[208] Despite the fact that both centers were endemic for ESBLs, only 10 patients were enrolled to the piperacillin-tazobactam arm (ie, this was a retrospective noninterventional study, and in most patients, the treatment with BLBLI was discontinued after obtaining results of a confirmed ESBL). Nonetheless, despite the very low sample size, the mortality risk with piperacillin-tazobactam was significantly and independently higher compared with carbapenems (adjusted odds ratio = 7.9, P = .03).[208]

Because it is difficult to enroll patients with ESBL BSIs to a BLBLI consolidative regimen for a prospective controlled trial, specifically following the publication of the MERINO results, it is relevant to mention the study that was published before the MERINO publication, from a US group, who reported the isolated impact of the empiric regimen (only), on the clinical outcomes of patients with ESBL BSI.[209] The adjusted 14-day mortality risk was 1.92 times higher for 103 patients who received empiric piperacillin-tazobactam, compared with 110 patients who received empiric carbapenems (95% CI, 1.07–3.45).[209] This difference might suggest that carbapenems should be perceived as superior in terms of empiric regimen as well (on top of its advantages for definitive treatment, as depicted in the MERINO trial), in order to reduce DAAT for later confirmed ESBL BSIs.[193]

To summarize, current data are inconclusive as to the use of BLBLIs as definitive (or empiric) treatment of ESBL infections. It is probably inferior to carbapenems. However, further research is needed in order to better understand the role that BLBLI might play in the treatment of milder ESBL infections; specifically, those originating from various infectious syndromes caused by various ESBL-producing bacteria (but consisting mainly of *bla*$_{CTX\text{-}M}$-producing *E coli*) in the community setting (where oral BLBLI are still available), and targeting isolates with lower MICs to the relevant BLBLI agent. *bla*$_{CTX\text{-}M}$ -producing *E coli* lower inoculum infections might still be a niche where BLBLI, being safe and bacteriocidic, might still be considered a treatment option for ESBL infections.

The "Newer" β-Lactam-β-Lactamase Inhibitors Combinations

In the last decade, there has been a resurgence in the pharmaceutical research of novel BLI, particularly aiming to expand the armamentarium toward nosocomial carbapenem-resistant Gram negatives, not toward ESBLs. These BLIs are divided into "non-β-lactam" BLI, boronic-acid BLI, and cyclobutanone BLI.[210] From this plethora of new compounds, 4 new agents have been approved and marketed thus far: (1) ceftazidime-avibactam, (2) ceftolozane-tazobactam, (3) meropenem-vaborbactam, and (4) imipenem-relebactam.[211] Because the focus of this review is ESBLs, already susceptible to meropenem and imipenem, the discussion in this section is limited to the first 2 agents.

Ceftazidime-avibactam

Avibactam is a reversible non-β-lactam BLI that showed lower 50% inhibitory concentrations for class A (including ESBLs) and C β-lactamases, compared with older BLIs, such as clavulanic acid, sulbactam, and tazobactam.[210] In combination with ceftazidime, the activity of this drug was tested against ESBL isolates from a multitude of studies conducted globally. In a study from the United States, ceftazidime-avibactam was almost universally active against ESBL-producing Enterobacteriaceae of both the *bla*$_{CTX\text{-}M}$ and the *bla*$_{SHV}$ types.[212] A follow-up study from the same group reported 100% susceptibility rate among a different set of isolates.[213] A global surveillance program (INFORM) of strains collected from all around the world (2012–2014) had also reported almost universal in vitro activity of ceftazidime-avibactam against ESBLs.[214]

Because the knowledge pertaining to resistances to ceftazidime-avibactam by mechanisms other than carbapenemases has low clinical relevance, data pertaining to naturally occurring resistant isolates are lacking. In 1 study that evaluated various

ESBL-cloned isolates, the only ESBL gene that conferred resistance to ceftazidime-avibactam was PER-1, which is naturally found only in *P aeruginosa*, not in Enterobacteriaceae.[215] An additional study characterized the resistance mechanisms in in vitro selected mutants.[216] The resistant strains mostly had genetic modifications outside the β-lactamase gene, commonly affecting uptake, efflux, or β-lactamase quantity.[216] Although the results of these studies are encouraging by suggesting that the ESBL β-lactamases are unlikely to become stable to ceftazidime-avibactam,[215,216] this hypothesis is yet to be determined in future reports.

Ceftolozane + tazobactam

This drug consists of the fifth-generation cephalosporin ceftolozane and the β-lactam BLI tazobactam. Ceftolozane was developed in order to provide improved potency against bla_{AmpC}-producing *P aeruginosa*. The tazobactam component was added in order to provide activity against Ambler A β-lactamases (eg, ESBLs, bla_{KPC}).[211] Hence, the question that is relevant for this review is whether this new combination has provided extended activity against ESBLs compared with piperacillin-tazobactam (ie, the added value of ceftolozane vs piperacillin). In 1 study of Gram negatives from hospitalized patients with pneumonia from United States and Europe, the susceptibility rates for ceftolozane-tazobactam were higher compared with piperacillin-tazobactam: that is, 57.6% versus 33.8% and 93.4% versus 67.1% among ESBL-producing *K pneumoniae* and *E coli*, respectively.[217] In studies of urinary tract and intraabdominal infections, again conducted in both United States and Europe, susceptibility rate differences between the 2 agents were lower: that is, 81.8% versus 73% in the United States, and 82.8% versus 70.8% in Europe, for ceftolozane-tazobactam versus piperacillin-tazobactam, respectively.[218,219] In a study conducted on isolates from the Asia-Pacific region, the susceptibility rates were 79.1% versus 70.8% for ceftolozane-tazobactam versus piperacillin-tazobactam, respectively.[220] Comparative clinical data are still lacking.

To conclude, data suggest that the activity of ceftolozane-tazobactam is probably somewhat higher against ESBLs, as of now, compared with piperacillin-tazobactam. However, compared with ceftazidime-avibactam, susceptibility rates are expected to be lower. Nonetheless, none of these newer BLBLIs should be used to treat a monomicrobial ESBL infection, because they should be preserved as one of very few remaining options available to treat carbapenem-resistant gram-negative human offending strains. Moreover, the newer BLBLIs have no established advantage over carbapenems as anti-ESBL therapeutics.

Cephalosporins

Despite the fact that most cephalosporins are effectively inhibited by ESBLs, certain cephalosporins may retain in vitro activity (per older higher CLSI [Clinical and Laboratory Standards Institute] breakpoints[25]) against specific ESBL-producing isolates (eg, ceftazidime for $bla_{\mathrm{CTX\text{-}M}}$-producing strains).[221] However, studies (usually small retrospective observational case-series analyses) have shown that clinical outcomes are often unsatisfactory even when the drug is administered to a seemingly susceptible isolate[23,222,223]; this also pertains to cefepime, for which CLSI breakpoints were not reduced.[23] Other more conclusive studies found significant correlations between cephalosporin use and increased mortality among patients with ESBL infection.[224] As of 2010, the American CLSI has joined the European EUCAST in recommending that ESBL testing should not be used for breakpoints determination (it might still be done for epidemiologic purposes). This recommendation was combined with the recommendation to lower the MIC breakpoints for most cephalosporins.[225] These recommendations are still debated, because some experts are advocating that resistance mechanisms, including ESBL, are of importance to clinical decision making.[226] The implications of these changes in diagnostic policies have yet to be determined.[24]

Cephamycins

By definition, this group of β-lactams (eg, cefoxitin, cefotetan, and cefmetazole) is stable to hydrolysis by ESBL-producing Enterobacteriaceae.[11] A small retrospective study from Taiwan found flomoxef was as effective at treating ESBL-producing *K pneumoniae* infections as carbapenems[227]; however, these compounds have unfavorable PK/PD properties and are no longer distributed and marketed in many countries. In addition, there are reports of emerging coresistances to these molecules as a result of either decreased expression of external membrane porins or cocarriage of bla_{AmpC} enzyme conveying cephamycin resistance in some ESBL-producing strains.[49]

Fluoroquinolones

Some older data suggested that fluoroquinolones could be as effective as carbapenems for treatment of infections caused by ESBLs.[228] Kang and colleagues[224] found similar 30-day mortalities with ciprofloxacin and carbapenem therapy for patients with BSIs caused by ESBL-producing *E coli* and *K pneumoniae*. However, because of exponential increases in resistance to fluoroquinolones (in both community and health care settings), and mainly the spread of certain $bla_{\mathrm{CTX\text{-}M}}$, this therapeutic option became nearly irrelevant in many locations, with more than 90% of offending ESBL isolates becoming resistant to all fluoroquinolones.[81,229] Moreover, few reports have identified fluoroquinolone exposure as a strong independent predictor for ESBL emergence and acquisition.[229,230]

Aminoglycosides

The susceptibility rates of certain aminoglycosides (eg, gentamicin, amikacin, and tobramycin) to common ESBL-producing offending Enterobacteriaceae isolates might still be relatively high in some locales.[231–233] Despite its well-known elevated toxicity rates and unfavorable PK/PD properties,[234] aminoglycosides might still have a role for treatment of ESBL infections in hospital settings, particularly in mild to moderate (but not severe or life-threatening) UTIs, in patients without underlying renal or auditory compromise.[235] Aminoglycoside usage may be advantageous in terms of antimicrobial stewardship efforts on a population level, particularly as carbapenem-sparing substitutions.[236] However, there is lack of well-controlled clinical data pertaining to aminoglycosides' efficacy for the treatment of mild to moderate UTIs.[235] For non-UTI infectious syndromes, aminoglycosides should serve only as adjuncts and should not be trusted as the single effective agent.[234,237]

Tigecycline and polymyxins

ESBL-producing *E coli* and, to a lesser extent, *K pneumoniae* have shown high susceptibility rates to these compounds.[49,238] Tigecycline is a drug with unfavorable pharmacodynamic properties for BSI, and there was a Food and Drug Administration warning pertaining to its usage.[239] Colistin, the polymyxin used most often, is toxic, and its PK/PD properties have not been thoroughly determined after its recently revived usage.[240] However, as mentioned for the new BLBLIs as well, the main reason to avoid these agents for treating ESBL infections is that these are frequently the only remaining therapeutic options for CRE and other extensively drug resistant gram-negative MDROs (eg, *A baumannii* and *P aeruginosa*).[9] Therefore, it is of paramount importance to avoid these therapeutics while additional options are available.[15,241]

TREATING EXTENDED-SPECTRUM β-LACTAMASE INFECTIONS IN AMBULATORY SETTINGS

ESBLs have become prevalent in "the community" of many regions worldwide, particularly since the spread of the ESBL-producing *E coli* ST131 strain.[140,150,177] In ambulatory settings, DAAT is probably even more common than in acute-care hospitals[9] and impacts patient outcomes, although controlled data are lacking.[9] Some mild to moderate ESBL infections could probably be managed outside the hospital settings[30,235]; however, oral therapeutics that possess potential activity against ESBLs are limited, and controlled data pertaining to their efficacy are lacking as well.[9]

Fluoroquinolones and TMP/SMX can be used as definitive therapy against susceptible isolates.[26,228,242–245] Susceptibility rates from recent years, however, have been shown to be consistently low.[11,61,245–247] In a prospective multicenter observational study of community-associated infections caused by ESBL-producing *E coli* from the United States, only 11% and 32% of the isolates were susceptible to fluoroquinolones and TMP-SMX, respectively, and 64% were resistant to both agents.[76]

Nitrofurantoin and fosfomycin are 2 additional oral therapeutic options in ambulatory settings for mild/moderate ESBL UTIs. In vitro susceptibility to nitrofurantoin was shown to be 71.3% in a microbiological survey from Spain, conducted in 2006,[248] and 90% in 2013 in 1 US center.[76] Susceptibility rates to fosfomycin among Enterobacteriaceae (mostly CRE) recovered from a single US center was more than 90%.[30] Fosfomycin is approved in many countries for mild ESBL UTIs.[249] In a retrospective study from Spain, the cure rate of patients with cystitis was 93% with fosfomycin therapy, and all ESBL-producing offending strains were susceptible to fosfomycin.

Another potential option to manage ESBL infections in the community is oral BLBLI (eg, amoxicillin-clavulanate). A large Spanish multicenter publication demonstrated the significant association between BLBLI MIC and clinical outcome. Cure rates were up to 93% for susceptible isolates (MIC $\leq$8 μg/mL) but only 56% for intermediate or resistant isolates (MIC $\geq$16 μg/mL).[73] Susceptibility rates to oral BLBLI vary greatly, with some areas reporting more than 70% resistance rates.[250] For UTIs, the inherent broad-spectrum activity of BLBLI (covering many prevalent Gram positives, Gram negatives, and anaerobes) might pose an additional disadvantage, in terms of antimicrobial stewardship, when additional oral alternatives are available.

FUTURE PERSPECTIVE

Antimicrobial resistance is a worldwide prevalent iatrogenic complication of modern medical care. ESBL-producing Enterobacteriaceae are one of the most common markers for this complication. These infections are prevalent both in health care settings and in the community. Appropriate therapy is frequently delayed in these patients, who suffer as a result from worse clinical outcomes. Moreover, with the exception of 1 recent open-label study, no additional prospective randomized controlled trials have ever been conducted in this field, and there are still several debates and controversies pertaining to the most efficacious management of these common infections. There are few investigational efforts, which the authors think could lend significant aid to this research front in the future:

1. Studies that propose, develop, and validate a reliable bedside score that predict ESBL infections upon admission to acute care hospitals, in order to reduce DAAT among patients with severe invasive ESBL infections.
2. Improvement in the availability and applicability of rapid diagnostics tools, both for invasive ESBL infections (from blood cultures) and for ESBL asymptomatic carriage (from rectal samplings).
3. Investment in efforts and more studies conducted that will aid in the control and regulation of ESBL carriage, and of antimicrobial usage in general, in the food and agriculture industries.
4. Investment in efforts and more studies conducted of innovations in the field of antimicrobial stewardship in ambulatory settings and its impact on "emergence" and spread of ESBLs in the community settings.
5. Study of the role of oral agents (eg, fluoroquinolones, TMP/SMX, fosfomycin, nitrofurantoin, and amoxicillin-clavulonate) for treating mild to moderate ESBL infections, which are managed in ambulatory settings.
6. Implications of the changes in breakpoint reporting according to the current CLSI and EUCAST recommendations on both the epidemiology and the diagnosis of ESBL-producing bacteria have to be monitored and studied.

FUNDING

This review was not supported financially by any external source.

ACKNOWLEDGMENTS

D. Marchaim had in the past received payments for lectures and a research grant from Merck (all not related to this article). All other authors have no acknowledgments.

CONFLICTS OF INTEREST

No potential conflicts of interest.

REFERENCES

1. Boucher HW, Talbot GH, Bradley JS, et al. Bad bugs, no drugs: no eskape! An update from the Infectious Diseases Society of America. Clin Infect Dis 2009; 48(1):1–12.
2. Livermore DM. Has the era of untreatable infections arrived? J Antimicrob Chemother 2009;64(Suppl 1):i29–36.
3. Marchaim D, Perez F, Lee J, et al. Swimming in resistance": co-colonization with carbapenem-resistant enterobacteriaceae and Acinetobacter baumannii or Pseudomonas aeruginosa. Am J Infect Control 2012;40(9):830–5.
4. WHO. Global priority list of antibiotic-resistant bacteria to guide research, discovery, and development of new antibiotics. 2017.
5. Cohen-Nahum K, Saidel-Odes L, Riesenberg K, et al. Urinary tract infections caused by multi-drug resistant Proteus mirabilis: risk factors and clinical outcomes. Infection 2010;38(1):41–6.
6. Endimiani A, Luzzaro F, Brigante G, et al. Proteus mirabilis bloodstream infections: risk factors and treatment outcome related to the expression of extended-spectrum beta-lactamases. Antimicrob Agents Chemother 2005; 49(7):2598–605.

7. Marchaim D, Zaidenstein R, Lazarovitch T, et al. Epidemiology of bacteremia episodes in a single center: increase in gram-negative isolates, antibiotics resistance, and patient age. Eur J Clin Microbiol Infect Dis 2008;27(11):1045–51.
8. Bogan C, Marchaim D. The role of antimicrobial stewardship in curbing carbapenem resistance. Future Microbiol 2013;8(8):979–91.
9. Tal Jasper R, Coyle JR, Katz DE, et al. The complex epidemiology of extended-spectrum beta-lactamase-producing enterobacteriaceae. Future Microbiol 2015;10:819–39.
10. Bonomo RA, Rossolini GM. Importance of antibiotic resistance and resistance mechanisms. Expert Rev Anti Infect Ther 2008;6(5):549–50.
11. Paterson DL, Bonomo RA. Extended-spectrum beta-lactamases: a clinical update. Clin Microbiol Rev 2005;18(4):657–86.
12. Peterson LR. Antibiotic policy and prescribing strategies for therapy of extended-spectrum beta-lactamase-producing enterobacteriaceae: the role of piperacillin-tazobactam. Clin Microbiol Infect 2008;14(Suppl 1):181–4.
13. Bush K, Fisher JF. Epidemiological expansion, structural studies, and clinical challenges of new beta-lactamases from gram-negative bacteria. Annu Rev Microbiol 2011;65:455–78.
14. Gerber JS, Kronman MP, Ross RK, et al. Identifying targets for antimicrobial stewardship in children's hospitals. Infect Control Hosp Epidemiol 2013; 34(12):1252–8.
15. Peleg AY, Hooper DC. Hospital-acquired infections due to gram-negative bacteria. N Engl J Med 2010;362(19):1804–13.
16. Collins VL, Marchaim D, Pogue JM, et al. Efficacy of ertapenem for treatment of bloodstream infections caused by extended-spectrum-beta-lactamase-producing enterobacteriaceae. Antimicrob Agents Chemother 2012;56(4): 2173–7.
17. Abraham EP, Chain E. An enzyme from bacteria able to destroy penicillin. 1940. Rev Infect Dis 1988;10(4):677–8.
18. Bradford PA. Extended-spectrum beta-lactamases in the 21st century: characterization, epidemiology, and detection of this important resistance threat. Clin Microbiol Rev 2001;14(4):933–51 [table of contents].
19. Medeiros AA. Evolution and dissemination of beta-lactamases accelerated by generations of beta-lactam antibiotics. Clin Infect Dis 1997;24(Suppl 1):S19–45.
20. Jacoby GA, Munoz-Price LS. The new beta-lactamases. N Engl J Med 2005; 352(4):380–91.
21. Bush K, Jacoby GA, Medeiros AA. A functional classification scheme for beta-lactamases and its correlation with molecular structure. Antimicrob Agents Chemother 1995;39(6):1211–33.
22. Jacoby GA, Bush K. Beta-lactamase nomenclature. J Clin Microbiol 2005; 43(12):6220.
23. Chopra T, Marchaim D, Veltman J, et al. Impact of cefepime therapy on mortality among patients with bloodstream infections caused by extended-spectrum-beta-lactamase-producing Klebsiella pneumoniae and Escherichia coli. Antimicrob Agents Chemother 2012;56(7):3936–42.
24. Marchaim D, Sunkara B, Lephart PR, et al. Extended-spectrum beta-lactamase producers reported as susceptible to piperacillin-tazobactam, cefepime, and cefuroxime in the era of lowered breakpoints and no confirmatory tests. Infect Control Hosp Epidemiol 2012;33(8):853–5.

25. Institute CaLS, editor. CLSI. Performance standards for antimicrobial susceptibility testing. Nineteenth informational supplement. Approved standard m100-s19. Wayne (PA): CLSI; 2009.
26. Endimiani A, Paterson DL. Optimizing therapy for infections caused by enterobacteriaceae producing extended-spectrum beta-lactamases. Semin Respir Crit Care Med 2007;28(6):646–55.
27. Marchaim D, Lazarovitch Z, Efrati S, et al. Serious consequences to the use of cephalosporins as the first line of antimicrobial therapy administered in hemodialysis units. Nephron Clin Pract 2005;101(2):c58–64.
28. Ben-Ami R, Schwaber MJ, Navon-Venezia S, et al. Influx of extended-spectrum beta-lactamase-producing enterobacteriaceae into the hospital. Clin Infect Dis 2006;42(7):925–34.
29. Pitout JD, Laupland KB. Extended-spectrum beta-lactamase-producing enterobacteriaceae: an emerging public-health concern. Lancet Infect Dis 2008;8(3): 159–66.
30. Pogue JM, Marchaim D, Abreu-Lanfranco O, et al. Fosfomycin activity versus carbapenem-resistant enterobacteriaceae and vancomycin-resistant enterococcus, Detroit, 2008-10. J Antibiot (Tokyo) 2013;66(10):625–7.
31. Marchaim D, Gottesman T, Schwartz O, et al. National multicenter study of predictors and outcomes of bacteremia upon hospital admission caused by enterobacteriaceae producing extended-spectrum beta-lactamases. Antimicrob Agents Chemother 2010;54(12):5099–104.
32. Reinert RR, Low DE, Rossi F, et al. Antimicrobial susceptibility among organisms from the Asia/Pacific Rim, Europe and Latin and North America collected as part of test and the in vitro activity of tigecycline. J Antimicrob Chemother 2007; 60(5):1018–29.
33. Nagy E, Dowzicky MJ. In vitro activity of tigecycline and comparators against a European compilation of anaerobes collected as part of the Tigecycline Evaluation and Surveillance Trial (TEST). Scand J Infect Dis 2010;42(1):33–8.
34. Jones RN, Biedenbach DJ, Gales AC. Sustained activity and spectrum of selected extended-spectrum beta-lactams (carbapenems and cefepime) against enterobacter spp. and ESBL-producing Klebsiella spp.: report from the SENTRY antimicrobial surveillance program (USA, 1997-2000). Int J Antimicrob Agents 2003;21(1):1–7.
35. Bouchillon SK, Iredell JR, Barkham T, et al. Comparative in vitro activity of tigecycline and other antimicrobials against gram-negative and gram-positive organisms collected from the Asia-Pacific Rim as part of the Tigecycline Evaluation and Surveillance Trial (TEST). Int J Antimicrob Agents 2009;33(2): 130–6.
36. Rodloff AC, Leclercq R, Debbia EA, et al. Comparative analysis of antimicrobial susceptibility among organisms from France, Germany, Italy, Spain and the UK as part of the tigecycline evaluation and surveillance trial. Clin Microbiol Infect 2008;14(4):307–14.
37. Hoban DJ, Bouchillon SK, Johnson BM, et al. In vitro activity of tigecycline against 6792 gram-negative and gram-positive clinical isolates from the global Tigecycline Evaluation and Surveillance Trial (TEST program, 2004). Diagn Microbiol Infect Dis 2005;52(3):215–27.
38. Badura A, Feierl G, Pregartner G, et al. Antibiotic resistance patterns of more than 120 000 clinical Escherichia coli isolates in southeast Austria, 1998-2013. Clin Microbiol Infect 2015;21(6):569 e1–7.

39. Calbo E, Garau J. The changing epidemiology of hospital outbreaks due to ESBL-producing Klebsiella pneumoniae: the CTX-M-15 type consolidation. Future Microbiol 2015;10:1063–75.
40. Leibman V, Martin ET, Tal-Jasper R, et al. Simple bedside score to optimize the time and the decision to initiate appropriate therapy for carbapenem-resistant enterobacteriaceae. Ann Clin Microbiol Antimicrob 2015;14:31.
41. Livermore DM. Current epidemiology and growing resistance of gram-negative pathogens. Korean J Intern Med 2012;27(2):128–42.
42. Livermore DM. Defining an extended-spectrum beta-lactamase. Clin Microbiol Infect 2008;14(Suppl 1):3–10.
43. Dellit TH, Owens RC, McGowan JE Jr, et al. Infectious Diseases Society of America and the Society for Healthcare Epidemiology of America guidelines for developing an institutional program to enhance antimicrobial stewardship. Clin Infect Dis 2007;44(2):159–77.
44. del Rio MA, Chrane D, Shelton S, et al. Ceftriaxone versus ampicillin and chloramphenicol for treatment of bacterial meningitis in children. Lancet 1983; 1(8336):1241–4.
45. Bernstein Hahn L, Barclay CA, Iribarren MA, et al. Ceftriaxone, a new parenteral cephalosporin, in the treatment of urinary tract infections. Chemotherapy 1981; 27(Suppl 1):75–9.
46. Efficacy and toxicity of single daily doses of amikacin and ceftriaxone versus multiple daily doses of amikacin and ceftazidime for infection in patients with cancer and granulocytopenia. The International Antimicrobial Therapy Cooperative Group of the European Organization for Research and Treatment of Cancer. Ann Intern Med 1993;119(7 Pt 1):584–93.
47. Kliebe C, Nies BA, Meyer JF, et al. Evolution of plasmid-coded resistance to broad-spectrum cephalosporins. Antimicrob Agents Chemother 1985;28(2): 302–7.
48. Bush K. Extended-spectrum beta-lactamases in North America, 1987-2006. Clin Microbiol Infect 2008;14(Suppl 1):134–43.
49. Falagas ME, Karageorgopoulos DE. Extended-spectrum beta-lactamase-producing organisms. J Hosp Infect 2009;73(4):345–54.
50. Brun-Buisson C, Legrand P, Philippon A, et al. Transferable enzymatic resistance to third-generation cephalosporins during nosocomial outbreak of multiresistant Klebsiella pneumoniae. Lancet 1987;2(8554):302–6.
51. Babini GS, Livermore DM. Antimicrobial resistance amongst Klebsiella spp. collected from intensive care units in southern and western Europe in 1997-1998. J Antimicrob Chemother 2000;45(2):183–9.
52. Livermore DM, Yuan M. Antibiotic resistance and production of extended-spectrum beta-lactamases amongst Klebsiella spp. from intensive care units in Europe. J Antimicrob Chemother 1996;38(3):409–24.
53. Decre D, Gachot B, Lucet JC, et al. Clinical and bacteriologic epidemiology of extended-spectrum beta-lactamase-producing strains of Klebsiella pneumoniae in a medical intensive care unit. Clin Infect Dis 1998;27(4):834–44.
54. Pitout JD, Nordmann P, Laupland KB, et al. Emergence of enterobacteriaceae producing extended-spectrum beta-lactamases (ESBLs) in the community. J Antimicrob Chemother 2005;56(1):52–9.
55. Canton R, Coque TM. The CTX-M beta-lactamase pandemic. Curr Opin Microbiol 2006;9(5):466–75.

56. Hobson RP, MacKenzie FM, Gould IM. An outbreak of multiply-resistant Klebsiella pneumoniae in the Grampian region of Scotland. J Hosp Infect 1996;33(4): 249–62.
57. Borer A, Gilad J, Menashe G, et al. Extended-spectrum beta-lactamase-producing enterobacteriaceae strains in community-acquired bacteremia in southern Israel. Med Sci Monit 2002;8(1):CR44–7.
58. Goldstein FW, Pean Y, Gertner J. Resistance to ceftriaxone and other beta-lactams in bacteria isolated in the community. The Vigil'Roc Study Group. Antimicrob Agents Chemother 1995;39(11):2516–9.
59. Blomberg B, Jureen R, Manji KP, et al. High rate of fatal cases of pediatric septicemia caused by gram-negative bacteria with extended-spectrum beta-lactamases in Dar Es Salaam, Tanzania. J Clin Microbiol 2005;43(2):745–9.
60. Mirelis B, Navarro F, Miro E, et al. Community transmission of extended-spectrum beta-lactamase. Emerg Infect Dis 2003;9(8):1024–5.
61. Pitout JD, Hanson ND, Church DL, et al. Population-based laboratory surveillance for Escherichia coli-producing extended-spectrum beta-lactamases: importance of community isolates with blaCTX-M genes. Clin Infect Dis 2004; 38(12):1736–41.
62. Woodford N, Kaufmann ME, Karisik E, et al. Molecular epidemiology of multiresistant Escherichia coli isolates from community-onset urinary tract infections in Cornwall, England. J Antimicrob Chemother 2007;59(1):106–9.
63. Cormican M, Morris D, Corbett-Feeeney G, et al. Extended spectrum beta-lactamase production and fluorquinolone resistance in pathogens associated with community acquired urinary tract infection. Diagn Microbiol Infect Dis 1998;32(4):317–9.
64. Goldstein FW. Antibiotic susceptibility of bacterial strains isolated from patients with community-acquired urinary tract infections in france. Multicentre study group. Eur J Clin Microbiol Infect Dis 2000;19(2):112–7.
65. Centers for Disease Control and Prevention (CDC). Laboratory capacity to detect antimicrobial resistance, 1998. MMWR Morb Mortal Wkly Rep 2000; 48(51–52):1167–71.
66. Munoz-Price LS. Long-term acute care hospitals. Clin Infect Dis 2009;49(3): 438–43.
67. Denman SJ, Burton JR. Fluid intake and urinary tract infection in the elderly. JAMA 1992;267(16):2245–9.
68. de Medina T, Carmeli Y. The pivotal role of long-term care facilities in the epidemiology of Acinetobacter baumannii: another brick in the wall. Clin Infect Dis 2010;50(12):1617–8.
69. Marchaim D, Chopra T, Bogan C, et al. The burden of multidrug-resistant organisms on tertiary hospitals posed by patients with recent stays in long-term acute care facilities. Am J Infect Control 2012;40(8):760–5.
70. Adler A, Gniadkowski M, Baraniak A, et al. Transmission dynamics of ESBL-producing Escherichia coli clones in rehabilitation wards at a tertiary care centre. Clin Microbiol Infect 2012;18(12):E497–505.
71. Sengstock DM, Thyagarajan R, Apalara J, et al. Multidrug-resistant Acinetobacter baumannii: an emerging pathogen among older adults in community hospitals and nursing homes. Clin Infect Dis 2010;50(12):1611–6.
72. Ben-Ami R, Rodriguez-Bano J, Arslan H, et al. A multinational survey of risk factors for infection with extended-spectrum beta-lactamase-producing enterobacteriaceae in nonhospitalized patients. Clin Infect Dis 2009;49(5):682–90.

73. Rodriguez-Bano J, Alcala JC, Cisneros JM, et al. Community infections caused by extended-spectrum beta-lactamase-producing Escherichia coli. Arch Intern Med 2008;168(17):1897–902.
74. Rodriguez-Bano J, Lopez-Cerero L, Navarro MD, et al. Faecal carriage of extended-spectrum beta-lactamase-producing Escherichia coli: prevalence, risk factors and molecular epidemiology. J Antimicrob Chemother 2008;62(5): 1142–9.
75. Rodriguez-Bano J, Paterson DL. A change in the epidemiology of infections due to extended-spectrum beta-lactamase-producing organisms. Clin Infect Dis 2006;42(7):935–7.
76. Doi Y, Park YS, Rivera JI, et al. Community-associated extended-spectrum beta-lactamase-producing Escherichia coli infection in the United States. Clin Infect Dis 2013;56(5):641–8.
77. Hayakawa K, Gattu S, Marchaim D, et al. Epidemiology and risk factors for isolation of Escherichia coli producing CTX-M-type extended-spectrum beta-lactamase in a large U.S. medical center. Antimicrob Agents Chemother 2013;57(8):4010–8.
78. Wright GD. The antibiotic resistome: the nexus of chemical and genetic diversity. Nat Rev Microbiol 2007;5(3):175–86.
79. Rodriguez-Bano J, Navarro MD, Romero L, et al. Risk-factors for emerging bloodstream infections caused by extended-spectrum beta-lactamase-producing Escherichia coli. Clin Microbiol Infect 2008;14(2):180–3.
80. Schwaber MJ, Navon-Venezia S, Kaye KS, et al. Clinical and economic impact of bacteremia with extended-spectrum-beta-lactamase-producing enterobacteriaceae. Antimicrob Agents Chemother 2006;50(4):1257–62.
81. Schwaber MJ, Navon-Venezia S, Schwartz D, et al. High levels of antimicrobial coresistance among extended-spectrum-beta-lactamase-producing enterobacteriaceae. Antimicrob Agents Chemother 2005;49(5):2137–9.
82. Schwaber MJ, Carmeli Y. Mortality and delay in effective therapy associated with extended-spectrum beta-lactamase production in enterobacteriaceae bacteraemia: a systematic review and meta-analysis. J Antimicrob Chemother 2007; 60(5):913–20.
83. Apisarnthanarak A, Kiratisin P, Mundy LM. Clinical and molecular epidemiology of healthcare-associated infections due to extended-spectrum beta-lactamase (ESBL)-producing strains of Escherichia coli and Klebsiella pneumoniae that harbor multiple ESBL genes. Infect Control Hosp Epidemiol 2008;29(11): 1026–34.
84. Doi Y, Adams-Haduch JM, Paterson DL. Escherichia coli isolate coproducing 16s RRNA methylase and CTX-M-type extended-spectrum beta-lactamase isolated from an outpatient in the United States. Antimicrob Agents Chemother 2008;52(3):1204–5.
85. Doi Y, Adams-Haduch JM, Shivannavar CT, et al. Faecal carriage of CTX-M-15-producing Klebsiella pneumoniae in patients with acute gastroenteritis. Indian J Med Res 2009;129(5):599–602.
86. Doi Y, Paterson DL, Egea P, et al. Extended-spectrum and CMY-type beta-lactamase-producing Escherichia coli in clinical samples and retail meat from Pittsburgh, USA and Seville, Spain. Clin Microbiol Infect 2010;16(1):33–8.
87. Livermore DM, Hawkey PM. CTX-M: changing the face of ESBLs in the UK. J Antimicrob Chemother 2005;56(3):451–4.

88. Livermore DM, Hope R, Reynolds R, et al. Declining cephalosporin and fluoroquinolone non-susceptibility among bloodstream enterobacteriaceae from the UK: links to prescribing change? J Antimicrob Chemother 2013;68(11):2667–74.
89. Paterson DL. Extended-spectrum beta-lactamases: the European experience. Curr Opin Infect Dis 2001;14(6):697–701.
90. Poirel L, Nordmann P, Ducroz S, et al. Extended-spectrum beta-lactamase CTX-M-15-producing Klebsiella pneumoniae of sequence type st274 in companion animals. Antimicrob Agents Chemother 2013;57(5):2372–5.
91. Arpin C, Quentin C, Grobost F, et al. Nationwide survey of extended-spectrum {beta}-lactamase-producing enterobacteriaceae in the French community setting. J Antimicrob Chemother 2009;63(6):1205–14.
92. Djamdjian L, Naas T, Tande D, et al. CTX-M-93, a CTX-M variant lacking penicillin hydrolytic activity. Antimicrob Agents Chemother 2011;55(5):1861–6.
93. Bauernfeind A, Grimm H, Schweighart S. A new plasmidic cefotaximase in a clinical isolate of Escherichia coli. Infection 1990;18(5):294–8.
94. Canton R, Gonzalez-Alba JM, Galan JC. CTX-M enzymes: origin and diffusion. Front Microbiol 2012;3:110.
95. Bonnet R. Growing group of extended-spectrum beta-lactamases: the CTX-M enzymes. Antimicrob Agents Chemother 2004;48(1):1–14.
96. Navon-Venezia S, Chmelnitsky I, Leavitt A, et al. Dissemination of the CTX-M-25 family beta-lactamases among Klebsiella pneumoniae, Escherichia coli and Enterobacter cloacae and identification of the novel enzyme CTX-M-41 in Proteus mirabilis in Israel. J Antimicrob Chemother 2008;62(2):289–95.
97. Lytsy B, Lindback J, Torell E, et al. A case-control study of risk factors for urinary acquisition of Klebsiella pneumoniae producing CTX-M-15 in an outbreak situation in Sweden. Scand J Infect Dis 2010;42(6–7):439–44.
98. Azap OK, Arslan H, Serefhanoglu K, et al. Risk factors for extended-spectrum beta-lactamase positivity in uropathogenic Escherichia coli isolated from community-acquired urinary tract infections. Clin Microbiol Infect 2010;16(2): 147–51.
99. Apisarnthanarak A, Kiratisin P, Saifon P, et al. Clinical and molecular epidemiology of community-onset, extended-spectrum beta-lactamase-producing Escherichia coli infections in Thailand: a case-case-control study. Am J Infect Control 2007;35(9):606–12.
100. Calbo E, Romani V, Xercavins M, et al. Risk factors for community-onset urinary tract infections due to Escherichia coli harbouring extended-spectrum beta-lactamases. J Antimicrob Chemother 2006;57(4):780–3.
101. Rodriguez-Bano J, Navarro MD, Romero L, et al. Clinical and molecular epidemiology of extended-spectrum beta-lactamase-producing Escherichia coli as a cause of nosocomial infection or colonization: implications for control. Clin Infect Dis 2006;42(1):37–45.
102. Association AU. Best practice policy statement on urologic surgery antimicrobial prophylaxis; 2011.
103. Urology EAo. Guidelines on urological infections; 2013.
104. Lo E, Nicolle L, Classen D, et al. Strategies to prevent catheter-associated urinary tract infections in acute care hospitals. Infect Control Hosp Epidemiol 2008;29(Suppl 1):S41–50.
105. Wolf JS Jr, Bennett CJ, Dmochowski RR, et al. Best practice policy statement on urologic surgery antimicrobial prophylaxis. J Urol 2008;179(4):1379–90.

106. Grabe M, Botto H, Cek M, et al. Preoperative assessment of the patient and risk factors for infectious complications and tentative classification of surgical field contamination of urological procedures. World J Urol 2012;30(1):39–50.
107. Botelho LA, Kraychete GB, Costa ESJL, et al. Widespread distribution of CTX-M and plasmid-mediated AMPC beta-lactamases in Escherichia coli from Brazilian chicken meat. Mem Inst Oswaldo Cruz 2015;110(2):249–54.
108. Nagy B, Szmolka A, Smole Mozina S, et al. Virulence and antimicrobial resistance determinants of verotoxigenic Escherichia coli (VTEC) and of multidrug-resistant E. coli from foods of animal origin illegally imported to the EU by flight passengers. Int J Food Microbiol 2015;209:52–9.
109. Wong MH, Liu L, Yan M, et al. Dissemination of inci2 plasmids that harbor the blaCTX-M element among clinical salmonella isolates. Antimicrob Agents Chemother 2015;59(8):5026–8.
110. Xi M, Wu Q, Wang X, et al. Characterization of extended-spectrum beta-lactamase-producing Escherichia coli strains isolated from retail foods in Shaanxi Province, China. J Food Prot 2015;78(5):1018–23.
111. Capita R, Alonso-Calleja C. Antibiotic-resistant bacteria: a challenge for the food industry. Crit Rev Food Sci Nutr 2013;53(1):11–48.
112. Koluman A, Dikici A. Antimicrobial resistance of emerging foodborne pathogens: status quo and global trends. Crit Rev Microbiol 2013;39(1):57–69.
113. US supermarkets redefine antibiotic misuse. Lancet Infect Dis 2009;9(5):265.
114. Endimiani A, Bertschy I, Perreten V. Escherichia coli producing CMY-2 beta-lactamase in bovine mastitis milk. J Food Prot 2012;75(1):137–8.
115. Bortolaia V, Guardabassi L, Trevisani M, et al. High diversity of extended-spectrum beta-lactamases in Escherichia coli isolates from italian broiler flocks. Antimicrob Agents Chemother 2010;54(4):1623–6.
116. Kluytmans JA, Overdevest IT, Willemsen I, et al. Extended-spectrum beta-lactamase-producing Escherichia coli from retail chicken meat and humans: comparison of strains, plasmids, resistance genes, and virulence factors. Clin Infect Dis 2013;56(4):478–87.
117. Huijbers PM, de Kraker M, Graat EA, et al. Prevalence of extended-spectrum beta-lactamase-producing enterobacteriaceae in humans living in municipalities with high and low broiler density. Clin Microbiol Infect 2013;19(6):E256–9.
118. Leverstein-van Hall MA, Dierikx CM, Cohen Stuart J, et al. Dutch patients, retail chicken meat and poultry share the same ESBL genes, plasmids and strains. Clin Microbiol Infect 2011;17(6):873–80.
119. Jensen LB, Hasman H, Agerso Y, et al. First description of an oxyimino-cephalosporin-resistant, ESBL-carrying Escherichia coli isolated from meat sold in Denmark. J Antimicrob Chemother 2006;57(4):793–4.
120. Politi L, Tassios PT, Lambiri M, et al. Repeated occurrence of diverse extended-spectrum beta-lactamases in minor serotypes of food-borne Salmonella enterica subsp. enterica. J Clin Microbiol 2005;43(7):3453–6.
121. Leistner R, Meyer E, Gastmeier P, et al. Risk factors associated with the community-acquired colonization of extended-spectrum beta-lactamase (ESBL) positive Escherichia coli. An exploratory case-control study. PLoS One 2013;8(9):e74323.
122. Jourdan-da Silva N, Watrin M, Weill FX, et al. Outbreak of haemolytic uraemic syndrome due to shiga toxin-producing Escherichia coli o104:H4 among French tourists returning from Turkey, September 2011. Euro Surveill 2012;17(4).

123. Ullrich S, Bremer P, Neumann-Grutzeck C, et al. Symptoms and clinical course of EHEC o104 infection in hospitalized patients: a prospective single center study. PLoS One 2013;8(2):e55278.
124. Aurass P, Prager R, Flieger A. EHEC/EAEC o104:H4 strain linked with the 2011 German outbreak of haemolytic uremic syndrome enters into the viable but non-culturable state in response to various stresses and resuscitates upon stress relief. Environ Microbiol 2011;13(12):3139–48.
125. Costa D, Vinue L, Poeta P, et al. Prevalence of extended-spectrum beta-lactamase-producing Escherichia coli isolates in faecal samples of broilers. Vet Microbiol 2009;138(3–4):339–44.
126. Guenther S, Aschenbrenner K, Stamm I, et al. Comparable high rates of extended-spectrum-beta-lactamase-producing Escherichia coli in birds of prey from Germany and Mongolia. PLoS One 2012;7(12):e53039.
127. Guenther S, Bethe A, Fruth A, et al. Frequent combination of antimicrobial multiresistance and extraintestinal pathogenicity in Escherichia coli isolates from urban rats (Rattus norvegicus) in Berlin, Germany. PLoS One 2012;7(11):e50331.
128. Guenther S, Grobbel M, Beutlich J, et al. CTX-M-15-type extended-spectrum beta-lactamases-producing Escherichia coli from wild birds in Germany. Environ Microbiol Rep 2010;2(5):641–5.
129. Hiroi M, Yamazaki F, Harada T, et al. Prevalence of extended-spectrum beta-lactamase-producing Escherichia coli and Klebsiella pneumoniae in food-producing animals. J Vet Med Sci 2012;74(2):189–95.
130. Liu BT, Yang QE, Li L, et al. Dissemination and characterization of plasmids carrying oqxAB-bla CTX-M genes in Escherichia coli isolates from food-producing animals. PLoS One 2013;8(9):e73947.
131. Hordijk J, Schoormans A, Kwakernaak M, et al. High prevalence of fecal carriage of extended spectrum beta-lactamase/AMPC-producing enterobacteriaceae in cats and dogs. Front Microbiol 2013;4:242.
132. Dierikx C, van Essen-Zandbergen A, Veldman K, et al. Increased detection of extended spectrum beta-lactamase producing Salmonella enterica and Escherichia coli isolates from poultry. Vet Microbiol 2010;145(3–4):273–8.
133. Overdevest I, Willemsen I, Rijnsburger M, et al. Extended-spectrum beta-lactamase genes of Escherichia coli in chicken meat and humans, the Netherlands. Emerg Infect Dis 2011;17(7):1216–22.
134. Wassenberg MW, Bootsma MC, Troelstra A, et al. Transmissibility of livestock-associated methicillin-resistant Staphylococcus aureus (st398) in Dutch hospitals. Clin Microbiol Infect 2011;17(2):316–9.
135. Laupland KB, Church DL, Vidakovich J, et al. Community-onset extended-spectrum beta-lactamase (ESBL) producing Escherichia coli: importance of international travel. J Infect 2008;57(6):441–8.
136. Lewis JS 2nd, Herrera M, Wickes B, et al. First report of the emergence of CTX-M-type extended-spectrum beta-lactamases (ESBLs) as the predominant ESBL isolated in a U.S. health care system. Antimicrob Agents Chemother 2007;51(11):4015–21.
137. Moland ES, Black JA, Hossain A, et al. Discovery of CTX-M-like extended-spectrum beta-lactamases in Escherichia coli isolates from five US states. Antimicrob Agents Chemother 2003;47(7):2382–3.
138. Nicolas-Chanoine MH, Blanco J, Leflon-Guibout V, et al. Intercontinental emergence of Escherichia coli clone o25:H4-st131 producing CTX-M-15. J Antimicrob Chemother 2008;61(2):273–81.

139. Coque TM, Novais A, Carattoli A, et al. Dissemination of clonally related Escherichia coli strains expressing extended-spectrum beta-lactamase CTX-M-15. Emerg Infect Dis 2008;14(2):195–200.
140. Rodriguez-Bano J, Picon E, Gijon P, et al. Community-onset bacteremia due to extended-spectrum beta-lactamase-producing Escherichia coli: risk factors and prognosis. Clin Infect Dis 2010;50(1):40–8.
141. Cagnacci S, Gualco L, Debbia E, et al. European emergence of ciprofloxacin-resistant Escherichia coli clonal groups o25:H4-st 131 and o15:K52:H1 causing community-acquired uncomplicated cystitis. J Clin Microbiol 2008;46(8):2605–12.
142. Lau SH, Reddy S, Cheesbrough J, et al. Major uropathogenic Escherichia coli strain isolated in the northwest of England identified by multilocus sequence typing. J Clin Microbiol 2008;46(3):1076–80.
143. Dahbi G, Mora A, Lopez C, et al. Emergence of new variants of st131 clonal group among extraintestinal pathogenic Escherichia coli producing extended-spectrum beta-lactamases. Int J Antimicrob Agents 2013;42(4):347–51.
144. Peirano G, Pitout JD. Molecular epidemiology of Escherichia coli producing CTX-M beta-lactamases: the worldwide emergence of clone st131 o25:H4. Int J Antimicrob Agents 2010;35(4):316–21.
145. Clermont O, Bonacorsi S, Bingen E. Rapid and simple determination of the Escherichia coli phylogenetic group. Appl Environ Microbiol 2000;66(10):4555–8.
146. Clermont O, Johnson JR, Menard M, et al. Determination of Escherichia coli O types by allele-specific polymerase chain reaction: application to the O types involved in human septicemia. Diagn Microbiol Infect Dis 2007;57(2):129–36.
147. Pitout JD, Gregson DB, Campbell L, et al. Molecular characteristics of extended-spectrum-beta-lactamase-producing Escherichia coli isolates causing bacteremia in the Calgary health region from 2000 to 2007: emergence of clone st131 as a cause of community-acquired infections. Antimicrob Agents Chemother 2009;53(7):2846–51.
148. Rogers BA, Sidjabat HE, Paterson DL. Escherichia coli o25b-st131: a pandemic, multiresistant, community-associated strain. J Antimicrob Chemother 2011;66(1):1–14.
149. Petty NK, Ben Zakour NL, Stanton-Cook M, et al. Global dissemination of a multidrug resistant Escherichia coli clone. Proc Natl Acad Sci U S A 2014;111(15):5694–9.
150. Lopez-Cerero L, Navarro MD, Bellido M, et al. Escherichia coli belonging to the worldwide emerging epidemic clonal group o25b/st131: risk factors and clinical implications. J Antimicrob Chemother 2013;69(3):809–14.
151. Sherchan JB, Hayakawa K, Miyoshi-Akiyama T, et al. Clinical epidemiology and molecular analysis of extended-spectrum-beta-lactamase-producing Escherichia coli in Nepal: characteristics of sequence types 131 and 648. Antimicrob Agents Chemother 2015;59(6):3424–32.
152. Rattinger GB, Mullins CD, Zuckerman IH, et al. A sustainable strategy to prevent misuse of antibiotics for acute respiratory infections. PLoS One 2012;7(12):e51147.
153. Harris AD, Kotetishvili M, Shurland S, et al. How important is patient-to-patient transmission in extended-spectrum beta-lactamase Escherichia coli acquisition. Am J Infect Control 2007;35(2):97–101.
154. Arpin C, Dubois V, Coulange L, et al. Extended-spectrum beta-lactamase-producing enterobacteriaceae in community and private health care centers. Antimicrob Agents Chemother 2003;47(11):3506–14.

155. Arpin C, Dubois V, Maugein J, et al. Clinical and molecular analysis of extended-spectrum {beta}-lactamase-producing enterobacteria in the community setting. J Clin Microbiol 2005;43(10):5048–54.

156. Rodriguez-Bano J, Navarro MD, Romero L, et al. Epidemiology and clinical features of infections caused by extended-spectrum beta-lactamase-producing Escherichia coli in nonhospitalized patients. J Clin Microbiol 2004;42(3): 1089–94.

157. Banerjee R, Strahilevitz J, Johnson JR, et al. Predictors and molecular epidemiology of community-onset extended-spectrum beta-lactamase-producing Escherichia coli infection in a midwestern community. Infect Control Hosp Epidemiol 2013;34(9):947–53.

158. Soraas A, Sundsfjord A, Sandven I, et al. Risk factors for community-acquired urinary tract infections caused by ESBL-producing enterobacteriaceae–a case-control study in a low prevalence country. PLoS One 2013;8(7):e69581.

159. Freeman JT, Williamson DA, Heffernan H, et al. Comparative epidemiology of CTX-M-14 and CTX-M-15 producing Escherichia coli: association with distinct demographic groups in the community in New Zealand. Eur J Clin Microbiol Infect Dis 2012;31(8):2057–60.

160. Valverde A, Grill F, Coque TM, et al. High rate of intestinal colonization with extended-spectrum-beta-lactamase-producing organisms in household contacts of infected community patients. J Clin Microbiol 2008;46(8):2796–9.

161. Skippen I, Shemko M, Turton J, et al. Epidemiology of infections caused by extended-spectrum beta-lactamase-producing Escherichia coli and Klebsiella spp.: a nested case-control study from a tertiary hospital in London. J Hosp Infect 2006;64(2):115–23.

162. Pena C, Gudiol C, Tubau F, et al. Risk-factors for acquisition of extended-spectrum beta-lactamase-producing Escherichia coli among hospitalised patients. Clin Microbiol Infect 2006;12(3):279–84.

163. Graffunder EM, Preston KE, Evans AM, et al. Risk factors associated with extended-spectrum beta-lactamase-producing organisms at a tertiary care hospital. J Antimicrob Chemother 2005;56(1):139–45.

164. Friedman ND, Kaye KS, Stout JE, et al. Health care–associated bloodstream infections in adults: a reason to change the accepted definition of community-acquired infections. Ann Intern Med 2002;137(10):791–7.

165. Bratzler DW, Dellinger EP, Olsen KM, et al. Clinical practice guidelines for antimicrobial prophylaxis in surgery. Surg Infect (Larchmt) 2013;14(1):73–156.

166. Martin ET, Tansek R, Collins V, et al. The carbapenem-resistant enterobacteriaceae score: a bedside score to rule out infection with carbapenem-resistant enterobacteriaceae among hospitalized patients. Am J Infect Control 2013; 41(2):180–2.

167. Marchaim D, Chopra T, Bhargava A, et al. Recent exposure to antimicrobials and carbapenem-resistant enterobacteriaceae: the role of antimicrobial stewardship. Infect Control Hosp Epidemiol 2012;33(8):817–30.

168. Abbo A, Carmeli Y, Navon-Venezia S, et al. Impact of multi-drug-resistant Acinetobacter baumannii on clinical outcomes. Eur J Clin Microbiol Infect Dis 2007; 26(11):793–800.

169. Cosgrove SE, Sakoulas G, Perencevich EN, et al. Comparison of mortality associated with methicillin-resistant and methicillin-susceptible Staphylococcus aureus bacteremia: a meta-analysis. Clin Infect Dis 2003;36(1):53–9.

170. Aloush V, Navon-Venezia S, Seigman-Igra Y, et al. Multidrug-resistant Pseudomonas aeruginosa: risk factors and clinical impact. Antimicrob Agents Chemother 2006;50(1):43–8.
171. Carmeli Y, Samore MH, Huskins C. The association between antecedent vancomycin treatment and hospital-acquired vancomycin-resistant enterococci: a meta-analysis. Arch Intern Med 1999;159(20):2461–8.
172. Bogan C, Kaye KS, Chopra T, et al. Outcomes of carbapenem-resistant enterobacteriaceae isolation: matched analysis. Am J Infect Control 2014;42(6): 612–20.
173. Melzer M, Eykyn SJ, Gransden WR, et al. Is methicillin-resistant Staphylococcus aureus more virulent than methicillin-susceptible S. aureus? A comparative cohort study of British patients with nosocomial infection and bacteremia. Clin Infect Dis 2003;37(11):1453–60.
174. Sahly H, Navon-Venezia S, Roesler L, et al. Extended-spectrum beta-lactamase production is associated with an increase in cell invasion and expression of fimbrial adhesins in Klebsiella pneumoniae. Antimicrob Agents Chemother 2008;52(9):3029–34.
175. Rodriguez-Bano J, Mingorance J, Fernandez-Romero N, et al. Outcome of bacteraemia due to extended-spectrum beta-lactamase-producing Escherichia coli: impact of microbiological determinants. J Infect 2013;67(1):27–34.
176. Park YS, Adams-Haduch JM, Shutt KA, et al. Clinical and microbiologic characteristics of cephalosporin-resistant Escherichia coli at three centers in the United States. Antimicrob Agents Chemother 2012;56(4):1870–6.
177. Sidjabat HE, Paterson DL, Adams-Haduch JM, et al. Molecular epidemiology of CTX-M-producing Escherichia coli isolates at a tertiary medical center in western Pennsylvania. Antimicrob Agents Chemother 2009;53(11):4733–9.
178. Doi Y, Adams J, O'Keefe A, et al. Community-acquired extended-spectrum beta-lactamase producers, United States. Emerg Infect Dis 2007;13(7):1121–3.
179. Harris AD. Control group selection is an important but neglected issue in studies of antibiotic resistance. Ann Intern Med 2000;132(11):925.
180. Kaye KS, Harris AD, Samore M, et al. The case-case-control study design: addressing the limitations of risk factor studies for antimicrobial resistance. Infect Control Hosp Epidemiol 2005;26(4):346–51.
181. Rodriguez-Bano J, Pascual A. Clinical significance of extended-spectrum beta-lactamases. Expert Rev Anti Infect Ther 2008;6(5):671–83.
182. Tumbarello M, Sanguinetti M, Montuori E, et al. Predictors of mortality in patients with bloodstream infections caused by extended-spectrum-beta-lactamase-producing enterobacteriaceae: importance of inadequate initial antimicrobial treatment. Antimicrob Agents Chemother 2007;51(6):1987–94.
183. Tumbarello M, Spanu T, Sanguinetti M, et al. Bloodstream infections caused by extended-spectrum-beta-lactamase-producing Klebsiella pneumoniae: risk factors, molecular epidemiology, and clinical outcome. Antimicrob Agents Chemother 2006;50(2):498–504.
184. Paul M, Shani V, Muchtar E, et al. Systematic review and meta-analysis of the efficacy of appropriate empiric antibiotic therapy for sepsis. Antimicrob Agents Chemother 2010;54(11):4851–63.
185. Kumar A, Roberts D, Wood KE, et al. Duration of hypotension before initiation of effective antimicrobial therapy is the critical determinant of survival in human septic shock. Crit Care Med 2006;34(6):1589–96.
186. Tumbarello M, Trecarichi EM, Bassetti M, et al. Identifying patients harboring extended-spectrum-beta-lactamase-producing enterobacteriaceae on hospital

admission: derivation and validation of a scoring system. Antimicrob Agents Chemother 2011;55(7):3485–90.

187. Naas T, Cuzon G, Truong H, et al. Evaluation of a DNA microarray, the check-points ESBL/KPC array, for rapid detection of TEM, SHV, and CTX-M extended-spectrum beta-lactamases and KPC carbapenemases. Antimicrob Agents Chemother 2010;54(8):3086–92.
188. Oviano M, Fernandez B, Fernandez A, et al. Rapid detection of enterobacteriaceae producing extended spectrum beta-lactamases directly from positive blood cultures by matrix-assisted laser desorption ionization-time of flight mass spectrometry. Clin Microbiol Infect 2014;20(11):1146–57.
189. Johnson SW, Anderson DJ, May DB, et al. Utility of a clinical risk factor scoring model in predicting infection with extended-spectrum beta-lactamase-producing enterobacteriaceae on hospital admission. Infect Control Hosp Epidemiol 2013;34(4):385–92.
190. Vitkon-Barkay I, Yekutiel M, Martin ET, et al. Developing a score to shorten the time to initiation of appropriate therapy for extensively drug resistant gram-negative bacilli and avoid unnecessary use of polymixins. In: (ESCMID) ESoC-MaID, editor. European Congress of Clinical Microbiology and Infectious Diseases (ECCMID) Barcellona, Spain; 2014.
191. Harris PNA, Tambyah PA, Lye DC, et al. Effect of piperacillin-tazobactam vs meropenem on 30-day mortality for patients with E coli or Klebsiella pneumoniae bloodstream infection and ceftriaxone resistance: a randomized clinical trial. JAMA 2018;320(10):984–94.
192. Paterson DL, Ko WC, Von Gottberg A, et al. Antibiotic therapy for Klebsiella pneumoniae bacteremia: implications of production of extended-spectrum beta-lactamases. Clin Infect Dis 2004;39(1):31–7.
193. Vardakas KZ, Tansarli GS, Rafailidis PI, et al. Carbapenems versus alternative antibiotics for the treatment of bacteraemia due to enterobacteriaceae producing extended-spectrum beta-lactamases: a systematic review and meta-analysis. J Antimicrob Chemother 2012;67(12):2793–803.
194. Carmeli Y, Lidji SK, Shabtai E, et al. The effects of group 1 versus group 2 carbapenems on imipenem-resistant Pseudomonas aeruginosa: an ecological study. Diagn Microbiol Infect Dis 2011;70(3):367–72.
195. Dellinger RP, Levy MM, Carlet JM, et al. Surviving sepsis campaign: international guidelines for management of severe sepsis and septic shock: 2008. Crit Care Med 2008;36(1):296–327.
196. Schwaber MJ, Carmeli Y. Carbapenem-resistant enterobacteriaceae: a potential threat. JAMA 2008;300(24):2911–3.
197. Schwaber MJ, Lev B, Israeli A, et al. Containment of a country-wide outbreak of carbapenem-resistant Klebsiella pneumoniae in Israeli hospitals via a nationally implemented intervention. Clin Infect Dis 2011;52(7):848–55.
198. Lopez-Cerero L, Picon E, Morillo C, et al. Comparative assessment of inoculum effects on the antimicrobial activity of amoxycillin-clavulanate and piperacillin-tazobactam with extended-spectrum beta-lactamase-producing and extended-spectrum beta-lactamase-non-producing Escherichia coli isolates. Clin Microbiol Infect 2010;16(2):132–6.
199. Thomson KS, Moland ES. Cefepime, piperacillin-tazobactam, and the inoculum effect in tests with extended-spectrum beta-lactamase-producing enterobacteriaceae. Antimicrob Agents Chemother 2001;45(12):3548–54.
200. Zimhony O, Chmelnitsky I, Bardenstein R, et al. Endocarditis caused by extended-spectrum-beta-lactamase-producing Klebsiella pneumoniae:

emergence of resistance to ciprofloxacin and piperacillin-tazobactam during treatment despite initial susceptibility. Antimicrob Agents Chemother 2006; 50(9):3179–82.

201. Rodriguez-Bano J, Navarro MD, Retamar P, et al. Beta-lactam/beta-lactam inhibitor combinations for the treatment of bacteremia due to extended-spectrum beta-lactamase-producing Escherichia coli: a post hoc analysis of prospective cohorts. Clin Infect Dis 2012;54(2):167–74.
202. Perez F, Bonomo RA. Can we really use SS-lactam/SS-lactam inhibitor combinations for the treatment of infections caused by extended-spectrum SS-lactamase-producing bacteria? Clin Infect Dis 2012;54(2):175–7.
203. Dedeic-Ljubovic A, Hukic M, Pfeifer Y, et al. Emergence of CTX-M-15 extended-spectrum beta-lactamase-producing Klebsiella pneumoniae isolates in Bosnia and Herzegovina. Clin Microbiol Infect 2010;16(2):152–6.
204. Pfundstein J, Roghmann MC, Schwalbe RS, et al. A randomized trial of surgical antimicrobial prophylaxis with and without vancomycin in organ transplant patients. Clin Transplant 1999;13(3):245–52.
205. Hall JC, Christiansen K, Carter MJ, et al. Antibiotic prophylaxis in cardiac operations. Ann Thorac Surg 1993;56(4):916–22.
206. Tissera S, Lee SM. Isolation of extended spectrum beta-lactamase (ESBL) producing bacteria from urban surface waters in Malaysia. Malays J Med Sci 2013; 20(3):14–22.
207. Aslan AT, Akova M. Extended spectrum beta-lactamase producing enterobacteriaceae: carbapenem sparing options. Expert Rev Anti Infect Ther 2019; 17(12):969–81.
208. Ofer-Friedman H, Shefler C, Sharma S, et al. Carbapenems versus piperacillin-tazobactam for bloodstream infections of nonurinary source caused by extended-spectrum beta-lactamase-producing enterobacteriaceae. Infect Control Hosp Epidemiol 2015;36(8):981–5.
209. Tamma PD, Han JH, Rock C, et al. Carbapenem therapy is associated with improved survival compared with piperacillin-tazobactam for patients with extended-spectrum beta-lactamase bacteremia. Clin Infect Dis 2015;60(9): 1319–25.
210. Drawz SM, Papp-Wallace KM, Bonomo RA. New beta-lactamase inhibitors: a therapeutic renaissance in an MDR world. Antimicrob Agents Chemother 2014;58(4):1835–46.
211. Tehrani K, Martin NI. Beta-lactam/beta-lactamase inhibitor combinations: an update. Medchemcomm 2018;9(9):1439–56.
212. Castanheira M, Farrell SE, Krause KM, et al. Contemporary diversity of beta-lactamases among enterobacteriaceae in the nine U.S. census regions and ceftazidime-avibactam activity tested against isolates producing the most prevalent beta-lactamase groups. Antimicrob Agents Chemother 2014;58(2):833–8.
213. Castanheira M, Mills JC, Costello SE, et al. Ceftazidime-avibactam activity tested against enterobacteriaceae isolates from U.S. hospitals (2011 to 2013) and characterization of beta-lactamase-producing strains. Antimicrob Agents Chemother 2015;59(6):3509–17.
214. Hackel M, Kazmierczak KM, Hoban DJ, et al. Assessment of the in vitro activity of ceftazidime-avibactam against multidrug-resistant Klebsiella spp. collected in the inform global surveillance study, 2012 to 2014. Antimicrob Agents Chemother 2016;60(8):4677–83.

215. Ortiz de la Rosa JM, Nordmann P, Poirel L. ESBLs and resistance to ceftazidime/avibactam and ceftolozane/tazobactam combinations in Escherichia coli and Pseudomonas aeruginosa. J Antimicrob Chemother 2019;74(7):1934–9.
216. Livermore DM, Mushtaq S, Doumith M, et al. Selection of mutants with resistance or diminished susceptibility to ceftazidime/avibactam from ESBL- and AMPC-producing enterobacteriaceae. J Antimicrob Chemother 2018;73(12):3336–45.
217. Farrell DJ, Sader HS, Flamm RK, et al. Ceftolozane/tazobactam activity tested against gram-negative bacterial isolates from hospitalised patients with pneumonia in US and European medical centres (2012). Int J Antimicrob Agents 2014;43(6):533–9.
218. Popejoy MW, Paterson DL, Cloutier D, et al. Efficacy of ceftolozane/tazobactam against urinary tract and intra-abdominal infections caused by ESBL-producing Escherichia coli and Klebsiella pneumoniae: a pooled analysis of phase 3 clinical trials. J Antimicrob Chemother 2017;72(1):268–72.
219. Pfaller MA, Bassetti M, Duncan LR, et al. Ceftolozane/tazobactam activity against drug-resistant enterobacteriaceae and Pseudomonas aeruginosa causing urinary tract and intraabdominal infections in Europe: report from an antimicrobial surveillance programme (2012-15). J Antimicrob Chemother 2017;72(5):1386–95.
220. Pfaller MA, Shortridge D, Sader HS, et al. Ceftolozane/tazobactam activity against drug-resistant enterobacteriaceae and Pseudomonas aeruginosa causing healthcare-associated infections in the Asia-Pacific region (minus China, Australia and New Zealand): report from an antimicrobial surveillance programme (2013-2015). Int J Antimicrob Agents 2018;51(2):181–9.
221. Bin C, Hui W, Renyuan Z, et al. Outcome of cephalosporin treatment of bacteremia due to CTX-M-type extended-spectrum beta-lactamase-producing Escherichia coli. Diagn Microbiol Infect Dis 2006;56(4):351–7.
222. Paterson DL, Ko WC, Von Gottberg A, et al. Outcome of cephalosporin treatment for serious infections due to apparently susceptible organisms producing extended-spectrum beta-lactamases: implications for the clinical microbiology laboratory. J Clin Microbiol 2001;39(6):2206–12.
223. Wong-Beringer A, Hindler J, Loeloff M, et al. Molecular correlation for the treatment outcomes in bloodstream infections caused by Escherichia coli and Klebsiella pneumoniae with reduced susceptibility to ceftazidime. Clin Infect Dis 2002;34(2):135–46.
224. Kang CI, Kim SH, Park WB, et al. Bloodstream infections due to extended-spectrum beta-lactamase-producing Escherichia coli and Klebsiella pneumoniae: risk factors for mortality and treatment outcome, with special emphasis on antimicrobial therapy. Antimicrob Agents Chemother 2004;48(12):4574–81.
225. Institute CaLS, editor. CLSI. Performance standards for antimicrobial susceptibility testing. Nineteenth informational supplement. Approved standard m100-s20. Wayne (PA): CLSI; 2010.
226. Livermore DM, Andrews JM, Hawkey PM, et al. Are susceptibility tests enough, or should laboratories still seek ESBLs and carbapenemases directly? J Antimicrob Chemother 2012;67(7):1569–77.
227. Lee CH, Su LH, Tang YF, et al. Treatment of ESBL-producing Klebsiella pneumoniae bacteraemia with carbapenems or flomoxef: a retrospective study and laboratory analysis of the isolates. J Antimicrob Chemother 2006;58(5):1074–7.
228. Endimiani A, Luzzaro F, Perilli M, et al. Bacteremia due to Klebsiella pneumoniae isolates producing the TEM-52 extended-spectrum beta-lactamase: treatment

outcome of patients receiving imipenem or ciprofloxacin. Clin Infect Dis 2004; 38(2):243–51.

229. Rodriguez-Martinez JM, Diaz de Alba P, Briales A, et al. Contribution of OqxAB efflux pumps to quinolone resistance in extended-spectrum-beta-lactamase-producing Klebsiella pneumoniae. J Antimicrob Chemother 2013;68(1):68–73.
230. Kritsotakis EI, Tsioutis C, Roumbelaki M, et al. Antibiotic use and the risk of carbapenem-resistant extended-spectrum-{beta}-lactamase-producing Klebsiella pneumoniae infection in hospitalized patients: results of a double case-control study. J Antimicrob Chemother 2011;66(6):1383–91.
231. Lu PL, Liu YC, Toh HS, et al. Epidemiology and antimicrobial susceptibility profiles of gram-negative bacteria causing urinary tract infections in the Asia-Pacific region: 2009-2010 results from the Study for Monitoring Antimicrobial Resistance Trends (SMART). Int J Antimicrob Agents 2012;40(Suppl):S37–43.
232. Hawser SP, Bouchillon SK, Lascols C, et al. Susceptibility of European Escherichia coli clinical isolates from intra-abdominal infections, extended-spectrum beta-lactamase occurrence, resistance distribution, and molecular characterization of ertapenem-resistant isolates (SMART 2008-2009). Clin Microbiol Infect 2012;18(3):253–9.
233. Hoban DJ, Bouchillon SK, Hawser SP, et al. Susceptibility of gram-negative pathogens isolated from patients with complicated intra-abdominal infections in the United States, 2007-2008: results of the Study for Monitoring Antimicrobial Resistance Trends (SMART). Antimicrob Agents Chemother 2010;54(7):3031–4.
234. Rotschafer JC, Zabinski RA, Walker KJ. Pharmacodynamic factors of antibiotic efficacy. Pharmacotherapy 1992;12(6 Pt 2):64S–70S.
235. Gupta K, Hooton TM, Naber KG, et al. International clinical practice guidelines for the treatment of acute uncomplicated cystitis and pyelonephritis in women: a 2010 update by the Infectious Diseases Society of America and the European Society for Microbiology and Infectious Diseases. Clin Infect Dis 2011;52(5): e103–20.
236. Pakyz AL, MacDougall C, Oinonen M, et al. Trends in antibacterial use in US academic health centers: 2002 to 2006. Arch Intern Med 2008;168(20):2254–60.
237. Klastersky J, Thys JP, Mombelli G. Comparative studies of intermittent and continuous administration of aminoglycosides in the treatment of bronchopulmonary infections due to gram-negative bacteria. Rev Infect Dis 1981;3(1): 74–83.
238. Falagas ME, Maraki S, Karageorgopoulos DE, et al. Antimicrobial susceptibility of multidrug-resistant (MDR) and extensively drug-resistant (XDR) enterobacteriaceae isolates to fosfomycin. Int J Antimicrob Agents 2010;35(3):240–3.
239. FDA. Drug safety communication - increased risk of death with tygacil (tigecycline) compared to other antibiotics used to treat similar infections. Washington DC: FDA; 2010.
240. Pogue JM, Lee J, Marchaim D, et al. Incidence of and risk factors for colistin-associated nephrotoxicity in a large academic health system. Clin Infect Dis 2011;53(9):879–84.
241. Pogue JM, Cohen DA, Marchaim D. Editorial commentary: polymyxin-resistant Acinetobacter baumannii: urgent action needed. Clin Infect Dis 2015;60(9): 1304–7.
242. Chen PC, Chang LY, Lu CY, et al. Drug susceptibility and treatment response of common urinary tract infection pathogens in children. J Microbiol Immunol Infect 2013;47(6):478–83.

243. Kurtaran B, Candevir A, Tasova Y, et al. Antibiotic resistance in community-acquired urinary tract infections: prevalence and risk factors. Med Sci Monit 2010;16(5):CR246–51.
244. Yamamoto S, Higuchi Y, Nojima M. Current therapy of acute uncomplicated cystitis. Int J Urol 2010;17(5):450–6.
245. Kim ME, Ha US, Cho YH. Prevalence of antimicrobial resistance among uropathogens causing acute uncomplicated cystitis in female outpatients in South Korea: a multicentre study in 2006. Int J Antimicrob Agents 2008;31(Suppl 1): S15–8.
246. Ilic T, Gracan S, Arapovic A, et al. Changes in bacterial resistance patterns in children with urinary tract infections on antimicrobial prophylaxis at university hospital in Split. Med Sci Monit 2011;17(7):CR355–61.
247. Lowe CF, McGeer A, Muller MP, et al. Decreased susceptibility to noncarbapenem antimicrobials in extended-spectrum-beta-lactamase-producing Escherichia coli and Klebsiella pneumoniae isolates in Toronto, Canada. Antimicrob Agents Chemother 2012;56(7):3977–80.
248. Puerto AS, Fernandez JG, del Castillo Jde D, et al. In vitro activity of beta-lactam and non-beta-lactam antibiotics in extended-spectrum beta-lactamase-producing clinical isolates of Escherichia coli. Diagn Microbiol Infect Dis 2006;54(2): 135–9.
249. de Cueto M, Lopez L, Hernandez JR, et al. In vitro activity of fosfomycin against extended-spectrum-beta-lactamase-producing Escherichia coli and Klebsiella pneumoniae: comparison of susceptibility testing procedures. Antimicrob Agents Chemother 2006;50(1):368–70.
250. Arslan H, Azap OK, Ergonul O, et al. Risk factors for ciprofloxacin resistance among Escherichia coli strains isolated from community-acquired urinary tract infections in Turkey. J Antimicrob Chemother 2005;56(5):914–8.

Multidrug-Resistant Bacteria in the Community

An Update

David van Duin, MD, PhD[a,*], David L. Paterson, MD, PhD[b]

KEYWORDS

• Carbapenem resistant Enterobacteriaceae • *K pneumoniae* • Gonococcus • MRSA

KEY POINTS

- Multidrug-resistant bacteria are among the most important current threats to public health.
- The community spread of multidrug-resistant bacteria, more typically associated with health care environments, is also a crucial development. Methicillin-resistant *S aureus* and extended-spectrum beta-lactamase–producing *E coli* are the most prevalent of such bacteria.
- The prevalence of these is driven by person to person transmission in the community and, in the case of extended-spectrum beta-lactamase–producing *E coli* by the use of antibiotics in agriculture.
- An important global threat on the horizon is represented by production of carbapenemases by community-acquired hypervirulent *K pneumoniae*.
- Such strains have already been found in Asia, Europe, and North America. Prevention is of the utmost importance and will require a multidisciplinary approach involving all stakeholders.

INTRODUCTION

Multidrug-resistant (MDR) bacteria are well-recognized to be one of the most important current public health problems. More than 2.8 million antibiotic-resistant infections occur in the United States each year, accounting for 35,000 deaths.[1] Rising rates of antibacterial resistance have an impact on all aspects of modern medicine, and compromise the results of cancer care, transplantation, and surgical procedures.[2] Although difficult to accurately calculate, there are also substantial economic costs to

Portions of this article were previously published in van Duin D, Paterson DL. Multidrug-Resistant Bacteria in the Community: Trends and Lessons Learned. Infect Dis Clin North Am 2016; 30(2): 377-390.

[a] Division of Infectious Diseases, University of North Carolina, CB 7030, 130 Mason Farm Road, Chapel Hill, NC 27599, USA; [b] University of Queensland Centre for Clinical Research, Royal Brisbane & Women's Hospital Campus, Building 71/918, Herston, Queensland 4029, Australia
* Corresponding author.
E-mail address: david_vanduin@med.unc.edu

Infect Dis Clin N Am 34 (2020) 709–722
https://doi.org/10.1016/j.idc.2020.08.002

antibiotic resistance. This may result from extended duration of hospital stay, the need for greater outpatient follow-up, and the higher costs of new drugs needed to treat MDR bacteria.[1] Unfortunately, the occurrence of specific MDR bacteria is closely linked to the use of broad-spectrum antibiotics, both for empiric as well as for definitive therapy.[3] This increased use in turn leads to even higher rates of MDR bacteria, thus creating a vicious cycle.

Typically, MDR bacteria were associated with nosocomial infections. However, some MDR bacteria have become quite prevalent causes of community-acquired infections. This development is important, because the community spread of MDR bacteria leads to a large increase of the population at risk, and subsequently an increase in the number of infections caused by MDR bacteria. In addition, when the incidence of a certain resistance pattern in bacteria causing community-acquired infections exceeds a specific threshold, broader spectrum antibacterials and/or combination antibacterial therapy are indicated for the empiric treatment of community-acquired infections. In this review, we outline the trends in and epidemiology of community prevalence of various MDR bacteria.

COMMUNITY-ASSOCIATED, HEALTH CARE–ASSOCIATED, AND NOSOCOMIAL INFECTIONS

Infections can be divided into community onset and nosocomial acquisition. The widely used cut-off to distinguish between these 2 categories is whether the onset of infection was within the first 48 hours of hospitalization (community onset) or later (nosocomial). Limitations of this division include the arbitrary nature of the 48-hour time point, as well as the dependence on the timing of diagnosis. If cultures are performed earlier during hospitalization, more infections are likely to be labeled as community onset.

The category of community onset can then be further subdivided into community acquired and health care associated, based on work pioneered by Morin and Hadler[4] and Friedman and colleagues.[5] Generally, an infection is deemed to be health care associated if a patient was hospitalized in an acute care hospital for 2 or more days within 90 days of the infection; resided in a nursing home or long-term care facility; received recent intravenous antibiotic therapy, chemotherapy, or wound care within the past 30 days of the current infection; or attended a hospital or hemodialysis clinic.[6]

The remaining category includes those patients who have a community-onset infection and who do not meet any of these criteria for a health care–associated infection. These infections are considered to be community acquired. However, for the purposes of evaluating MDR bacteria in the community, these definitions may not tell the whole story. Patients tend to get infected with organisms with which they were previously colonized. Therefore, it is the timing of colonization, rather than the timing of diagnosis of infection, that is crucially important to determine the origin of the MDR bacteria. Studies that have used screening of noninfected individuals have addressed these questions for some MDR bacteria in certain populations.

ANTIBIOTIC RESISTANCE IN BACTERIA TYPICALLY REGARDED AS COMMUNITY ACQUIRED

Antibiotic-Resistant Sexually Transmitted Infections

Multidrug-resistant bacteria that cause sexually transmitted infections have become increasingly prominent in recent years. Drug-resistant *N gonorrhoeae* is now regarded by the Centers for Disease Control and Prevention as an urgent threat (**Table 1**) and is estimated to infect 550,000 Americans annually.[1] Although antibiotic

Table 1
Multidrug resistant bacteria observed in the community, classified according to the Centers for Disease Control and Prevention threat level

MDR Phenotype	Epidemiologic Setting of Community-Onset Infections
Urgent threats	
Carbapenem-resistant *Acinetobacter baumannii*	Extremely rare
Candida auris	Extremely rare
Clostridioides difficile	Prior antibiotic exposure; nursing homes
CRE	Rare at present; emerging in India and China
Drug-resistant *Neisseria gonorrhoeae*	Exclusively community onset
Serious threats	
Drug-resistant *Campylobacter*	Exclusively community onset
Drug-resistant *Candida*	Rare at present; prior azole exposure typical
ESBL + Enterobacterales	Endemic in most parts of the world
VRE	Rare except in nursing home residents
Carbapenem-resistant *Pseudomonas aeruginosa*	Extremely rare, except in those with suppurative lung disease and extensive antibiotic use
Drug-resistant nontyphoidal *Salmonella*	Exclusively community onset
Drug-resistant *Salmonella* serotype Typhi	Exclusively community onset
Drug-resistant Shigella	Exclusively community onset
MRSA	Household colonization; farm animal exposure
Drug-resistant *Streptococcus pneumononiae*	Almost exclusively community onset
Drug-resistant tuberculosis	Predominantly community onset

resistance in *Chlamydia trachomatis* and *Treponema pallidum* does occasionally occur, these organisms are not renowned as being MDR. In contrast, an emerging pathogen, drug resistant *Mycoplasma genitalium*, is on the Centers for Disease Control and Prevention's watch list owing to its propensity for multidrug resistance. It should also be noted that bacteria that cause gastrointestinal illness may be sexually transmitted; MDR shigellosis is increasingly recognized as an issue for men who have sex with men.[7]

There are a number of reasons why MDR in bacteria that cause sexually transmitted infections has become so prominent. This includes the availability of antibiotics without a prescription in many parts of the world and reliance of treatment that is typically empiric, either based on symptoms or culture independent methods for laboratory diagnosis. In recent years, molecular methods for rapid diagnosis of antibiotic resistance genes in *N gonorrhoeae* and *M genitalium* have been developed.[8,9] This factor could improve surveillance and may allow more targeted treatment choices.

Antibiotic-Resistant Gastrointestinal Infections

Clostridioides difficile is regarded by the Centers for Disease Control and Prevention as an urgent antimicrobial resistance threat. Further discussion on this pathogen is beyond the scope of this article. Drug-resistant *Campylobacter*, nontyphoidal *Salmonella*, and *Shigella* are all serious antimicrobial resistance threats. They infect more than 700,000 people in the United States annually. The use of antibiotics in agriculture with subsequent entry of antimicrobial-resistant pathogens (or genes) into human food is the usual means by which these MDR pathogens infect humans. In contrast, in the United States and Western Europe, patients with drug-resistant *Salmonella* serotype Typhi have typically traveled internationally.

One of the key challenges associated with treatment of antibiotic-resistant gastrointestinal infections and sexually transmitted infections is provision of alternatives to orally administered fluoroquinolones and macrolides when resistance is present. Some new antibiotic options are now under development, and are hoped to address this need.

Antibiotic-Resistant Respiratory Infections

S pneumoniae is the most common cause of community-acquired pneumonia and drug-resistant *S pneumoniae* infects more than 900,000 Americans annually. In response to this threat, new antibiotics, including delafloxacin, omadacycline, lefamulin, solithromycin, nemonoxacin, and ceftaroline, have recently been approved or are in clinical development.[10] Drug-resistant tuberculosis, an enormous global health problem, is beyond the scope of this article.

ANTIBIOTIC-RESISTANT ORGANISMS CLASSICALLY DESCRIBED IN HOSPITALS BUT NOW FOUND IN THE COMMUNITY

Methicillin-Resistant Staphylococcus aureus

Methicillin-resistant *Staphylococcus aureus* (MRSA) is probably the best example of a prevalent and important MDR bacterium that has successfully transitioned from an almost exclusively nosocomial setting to being widespread in the community. The epidemiology of community-associated MRSA (CA-MRSA) has been extensively reviewed elsewhere.[11,12] Here, we will give a brief overview of MRSA in the community because it may be predictive of the behavior of other MDR bacteria.

As early as 1982, an outbreak of CA-MRSA was reported in Detroit.[13] In this outbreak, more than one-half of patients were intravenous drug users, and the remaining patients had several comorbidities that put them at risk. Importantly, various different strains were found in this outbreak.[13] It was not until the early 1990s that more genuine CA-MRSA outbreaks began to be reported. These outbreaks occurred in populations without specific risk factors. The MRSA strains involved were generally monoclonal or oligoclonal and rather than being extensively multidrug resistant, such as nosocomial MRSA strains at that time, these CA-MRSA strains were susceptible to many non–β-lactam antibiotics. In the early 2000s, a new strain of CA-MRSA—USA300—became the predominant CA-MRSA in the United States, effectively replacing the previous USA400 CA-MRSA strain.[11] This USA300 strain is characterized by the presence of the staphylococcal cassette chromosome mec type IV as well as genes encoding for Panton-Valentine leucocidin toxins.[14] Households are an important reservoir for the USA300 strain. In a recent study that used whole genome sequencing data, USA300 MRSA was shown to persist in households between 2 and 8 years before the admission of a symptomatic patient from that household, and to continue to persist for at least another year after that.[15] This and other evidence shows conclusively that this specific strain of MRSA has been able to become entrenched in a community setting in the absence of ongoing antibiotic pressure. In addition, specific strains of CA-MRSA have been shown to be associated with exposure to livestock; so-called livestock-associated MRSA. The ST398 livestock-associated MRSA is predominantly found in Europe and America, whereas ST9 livestock-associated MRSA is encountered in Asia.[16]

Vancomycin-Resistant Enterococci

Vancomycin-resistant enterococci (VRE) emerged in the late 1980s, and became a common cause of nosocomial infections in the 1990s.[17] Studies in the 1990s did not detect the presence of vancomycin resistance in enterococci isolated from subjects without health care exposure in the United States.[18,19] In contrast, in European studies from the same time period, VRE was detected in the stool of healthy volunteers.[20] In addition, VRE was commonly found in European food animals.[21,22] The underlying reason for this difference between Europe and the United States is the use of avoparcin—a glycopeptide antibiotic—for the purpose of promoting growth in food animals. Avoparcin was never approved for use in the United States or Canada, but its use was widespread in Europe up to 1997.[22] After a ban on avoparcin in animal husbandry, rates of VRE in both animal samples, as well as in samples from human volunteers, started to decrease.[20,22] These important data illustrate the critical link between antibiotic use in the food industry and antimicrobial resistance rates in humans. It also indicates that it is never too late to make a change, and that banning antimicrobials from our food chain may have an almost instantaneous positive—and cost-saving—effect.

Around 2000, community-associated VRE began to appear in the United States. In a screening study of patients attending an ambulatory care clinic in Nashville, Tennessee, 3 patients tested positive for VRE out of 100 patients screened. One of these patients came in for her annual check-up and had no prior health care exposures.[23] Also, VRE was found in wastewater from a semiclosed agri-food system.[24] Nonetheless, VRE remains an uncommon pathogen in community-associated infections. In 289 patients with community-onset VRE, 85% of patients had been hospitalized, and 71% had antimicrobial exposure in the last 3 months.[25] In another study that included 81 patients with community-onset VRE bacteremia, 79% of patients had prior hospitalizations.[26] These data indicate that, even in those patients where VRE is detected on admission or early during hospitalization, acquisition likely occurred in the health care setting. This acquisition was driven by traditional risk factors of antimicrobial exposure, health care exposure, chronic illness, indwelling devices, malignancies, and immunosuppression.[25,26]

The discrepancy between the community spread of MRSA and VRE is notable, because both *S aureus* and enterococci are common human colonizers. However, overall colonization with enterococci is much more universal than with *S aureus*, and *S aureus* is not truly a commensal. Apparently—in contrast with MRSA—the high prevalence of current strains of VRE in the community requires either an ongoing incoming supply of VRE into the shared community gut microbiome through the food chain or a high level of antibiotic pressure. The fitness cost of maintaining a vancomycin-resistant phenotype would be an intuitive explanation for the relative lack of true community-associated VRE infections. However, the fitness cost of vancomycin resistance seems to be minimal for enterococci, especially in the context of inducible resistance.[27,28] A recent study suggests that pheromone-mediated killing of VRE may account for why vancomycin-susceptible commensal enterococci outcompete VRE in the human gut.[29] In this study, the prototype MDR clinical isolate strain *Enterococcus faecalis* V583 was killed by human fecal flora, whereas commensal antibiotic-susceptible *E faecalis* was able to survive in the presence of flora. The killing effect was traced to pheromone production by commensal *E faecalis* strains.[29]

Carbapenem-Resistant Acinetobacter baumannii

Acinetobacter baumannii infections are commonly encountered in hospitalized patients, especially in the intensive care.[30] However, community-associated *A. baumannii* infections have been well-described especially in (sub-) tropical climates, including Asia and Australia.[31] These infections are generally associated with pharyngeal carriage and are linked to alcohol abuse and smoking.[31] These infections are serious and the attributable mortality in 80 patients with bacteremia and/or pneumonia from various case series was reported at 56%.[31] Community reservoirs for *A baumannii* include environmental sources such as soil and vegetables, as well as human and animal skin and throat carriage. Furthermore, *A baumannii* has also been recovered from human lice.[32]

A baumannii is intrinsically resistant to several antibiotic classes. In addition, carbapenem resistance may occur through acquisition of carbapenemases such as IMP-like carbapenemases and/or oxacillinases.[33] The rate of carbapenem resistance in clinical isolates of *A baumannii* increased sharply from 9% to 40% between 1995 and 2004 in the United States.[30] More recent studies suggest that this rate has remained at around 40%.[34,35] In contrast, the rate of carbapenem resistance in *Acinetobacter* infections isolated from community-dwelling patients has remained around 4%.[34] Similarly, resistance to carbapenems was detected in only 1 of 23 community-dwelling volunteers who had *A baumannii* isolated from their hands.[36] In an Australian study of 36 patients with community-onset bacteremic *Acinetobacter* pneumonia, all tested isolates were susceptible to carbapenems.[37] A more worrisome report from China described 32 patients with community-acquired pneumonia caused by *A baumannii*. Three and 6 isolates were nonsusceptible to meropenem and imipenem, respectively. In addition, $bla_{\text{OXA-23}}$ was found in 12 of 15 tested isolates, some of which tested susceptible to both meropenem and imipenem.[38] Of note, 87% of patients with MDR *A baumannii* had a hospitalization history, suggesting that these did not truly represent community-associated infections.[38]

In summary, community-associated carbapenem-resistant *A baumannii* seems to remain uncommon, likely reflecting the natural habitats of *Acinetobacter* species, and the differences between true community strains found to cause infections in Asia and Australia and hospital-associated strains. Of concern is the potential for acquisition of carbapenemases by such a community strain, especially in high antibiotic use areas in Asia.

Multidrug-Resistant Pseudomonas aeruginosa

P aeruginosa is a common cause of nosocomial infections, including bloodstream infections and pneumonia. It prefers moist environments and can be found in a large variety of places in the hospital, including sink traps and aerators, various equipment such as scopes and respiratory gear, and contaminated solutions.[39] In addition, *P aeruginosa* may be present on fresh fruit and vegetables as well as on the fingernails of health care providers.[39]

Similar to *A baumannii*, *P aeruginosa* is intrinsically resistant to many antibiotic classes. Furthermore, additional acquired antibiotic resistance arises relatively easily and quickly after antibiotic exposure. Some patients have chronic biofilm-mediated pseudomonal colonization; patients with cystic fibrosis are an important example.[40] In these patients, repeated antibiotic courses are the rule, as is the subsequent development of MDR strains. Although these patients are often community dwelling, these infections are clearly health care associated. Nonetheless, spread of MDR isolates between patients with cystic fibrosis has been well-described and is an important infection control risk.[41]

True community-associated infections with MDR *P aeruginosa* fortunately remain very uncommon.[42,43] In a cohort of 60 patients with community-acquired bloodstream infections with *P aeruginosa*, 100% of isolates were meropenem susceptible, and 95% were susceptible to piperacillin/tazobactam and ceftazidime.[44] A case report from Turkey describes a young man without health care exposure who presented with a pyogenic liver abscess caused by a *P aeruginosa* strain that was only susceptible to imipenem, amikacin, and colistin.[45]

Enterobacteriaceae that Produce Extended Spectrum β-lactamases

Enterobacteriaceae are very common causes of community-associated infections, including urinary tract infections and bacteremia. Unfortunately—in contrast with the situation described elsewhere in this article with *P aeruginosa* and *A baumannii*—there is widespread resistance in community-associated Enterobacteriaceae isolates mediated by extended spectrum β-lactamases (ESBL).[46] This is a global phenomenon and involves patients of all ages including pediatric populations. In a multicenter, prospective US study over a 1-year period in 2009 to 2010, 4% of *E coli* community-onset isolates were ESBL producers.[47] The majority reflected urinary tract infections such as cystitis or pyelonephritis. The most common ESBL encountered were of the CTX-M group (91%), the remaining ESBLs were either SHV (8%) or CMY-2 (1%). Most isolates (54%) belonged to the ST131 clonal group.[47] *Escherichia coli* ST131 is a globally disseminated MDR clone, and is characterized by resistance to fluoroquinolones in addition to production of CTX-M type ESBL.[48]

In Asia, the Middle East, South America, and some parts of Europe, community-onset infection with ESBL-producing *E coli* is extraordinarily frequent. Lower prevalence regions include North America, some parts of Northern Europe, Australia, and New Zealand. Specific risk factors for community-onset ESBL-producing *E coli* infections have been found in these low prevalence regions. Reported risk factors from a Chicago-based study for ESBL-producing *E coli* included travel to India (odds ratio [OR], 14.4), advancing age (OR, 1.04 per year), and prior use of ciprofloxacin (OR, 3.92).[49] In a German survey-based study, risk factors for ESBL-positive *E coli* colonization included an Asian language being the primary language spoken in the household (OR, 13.4) and frequent pork consumption (OR, 3.5).[50] A population-based study in London also suggested South Asian ethnicity and older age as risk factors for ESBL-positive *E coli* bacteriuria.[51] A study performed in Australia and New Zealand also found that birth on the Indian subcontinent or travel to Southeast Asia, China, India, Africa, or the Middle East were risk factors for community-onset third-generation cephalosporin-resistant *E coli* infections.[52]

A significant problem in Asia is disseminated infection with hypervirulent *K pneumoniae* strains. These hypermucoviscous strains have a propensity to cause community-onset pyogenic liver abscess and sometimes metastatic infections, including meningitis.[53] Although these strains were typically susceptible to multiple antibiotics, community-onset ESBL-producing strains are now well-described and seem to be increasing.[54]

Community-associated ESBL-producing Enterobacteriaceae are of specific concern, because treatment requires broad-spectrum antibiotics. A randomized controlled trial to address the question of comparative efficacy of piperacillin-tazobactam versus meropenem to treat bloodstream infections caused by ceftriaxone nonsusceptible *E coli* and *Klebsiella* spp showed that carbapenems were the more reliable choice.[55] Whether carbapenems are always indicated for infections caused by ESBL-producing organisms remains controversial. Tamma and Cosgrove[56] in a recent observational study showed that piperacillin plus tazobactam was as effective as carbapenems for complicated urinary tract infection in the absence of bloodstream infection. A number of trials of carbapenem-sparing options for ESBL-producing organisms are now planned or underway.[57]

Carbapenemase-Producing Enterobacteriaceae

Carbapenem-resistant Enterobacteriaceae (CRE) represent an immediate public health threat that requires urgent and aggressive action.[58,1] CRE are resistant to most antibiotics and clinical outcomes after CRE infections are generally poor.[59–64] Although less frequent than carbapenem-resistant *K pneumoniae*, carbapenem-resistant *E coli* constitute an important subset of CRE, and are increasing globally; outbreaks have been reported in the United States.[65,66] To date, most CRE infections in the United States and Europe are health care associated, with patients from long-term care facilities at especially high risk.[67] Although data from Asia are somewhat sparse, carbapenemases have been found in bacteria recovered from drinking water in India and in food-producing animals in China.[68,69] This finding raises the specter of huge numbers of people in these large countries being colonized with CRE. It is now clear that hypervirulent *Klebsiella* can be carbapenem resistant. This phenomenon has been found in both Asia and elsewhere in the world, and has been associated both with *K pneumoniae* carbapenem and other carbapenemase types.[70–75] A worrying development has been the finding of a transmissible plasmid that augments virulence in *K pneumoniae*.[76] Disturbingly, this plasmid could be conjugated to carbapenem resistant strains, enabling them to simultaneously express carbapenem resistance and hypervirulence.

Given the rapid global spread of ESBL-producing *E coli* ST131, another obvious concern is for this highly successful clone to acquire a carbapenemase. Indeed, several reports of carbapenemase-producing *E coli* ST131 have been published.[77–79] In a study from India, ST131 clinical isolates were compared with non-ST131 clinical isolates. Overall 20% of clinical isolates were positive for metallo-β-lactamases such as $bla_{NDM\text{-}1}$, which was evenly distributed between ST131 and non-ST131 *E coli*.[78] Because the epidemiology of ESBL is estimated to be about 10 years ahead of that of the carbapenemases, it is likely that community-associated carbapenem-resistant ST131 *E coli* will become a major threat in the near future.

PREVENTION

Prevention of the further spread of MDR bacteria in the community is one of the most urgent public health challenges. Unfortunately, national or even regional data on antibiotic susceptibilities are often limited. In addition, when these data are available in some form, the accompanying epidemiologic metadata are usually too restricted to determine which isolates are truly community associated. Furthermore, clinical infections are generally the tip of the proverbial iceberg and once a signal is generated that is sufficient in amplitude to get the attention of policymakers, subclinical spread has already occurred.

Any successful prevention strategy will have to consist of a multipronged approach and involve all stakeholders. In addition to human clinical antimicrobial stewardship, we need to remove antibiotics from the food chain. Furthermore, we need to limit the amount of xenobiotics such as quaternary ammonium compounds that reach the environment.[80] Another challenging step in limiting exposure of bacteria to antibiotics is the treatment of contaminated wastewater such as that generated by pharmaceutical factories and medical facilities. For instance, a study evaluated samples collected from a wastewater treatment plant in India that received water from 90 regional bulk drug manufacturers containing—among other compounds—higher concentrations of ciprofloxacin than are generally found in the blood of patients who are being treated with this agent. Bacteria recovered from this water were tested against 39 antibiotics. Approximately 30% of bacteria were resistant 29 to 32 antibiotics tested, and approximately another 20% were resistant to 33 to 36 antibiotics.[81] The magnitude of this effect, combined with the knowledge that soil-dwelling bacteria will pass on resistance genes to more clinically relevant bacteria, illustrates the importance of limiting this contamination.[82]

Antimicrobial stewardship is developing rapidly as a hospital specialty. Stewardship teams often will combine strengths from infectious disease medical specialist and doctors of pharmacy to evaluate the appropriateness of choice and duration of antibiotic strategies.[83] However, most antibiotics are prescribed in ambulatory care settings and more attention is needed in this realm to really impact overall community antibiotic exposure.[84] This effort will not only require a paradigm shift in the behavior of prescribers, but also a cultural shift in the public on the risks and benefits of antibiotics. Rapid diagnostic testing to identify MDR bacteria more quickly and thus limit the empiric use of unnecessarily broad antibiotics will be of great significance. Also, rapid testing to diagnose alternative, nonbacterial etiologies is important.

An important question is whether any interventions can address the issue of chronic colonization with MDR bacteria. Obviously, decolonizing these patients would decrease the risk of transmission. In addition, the burden on the individual patient of this condition should not be underestimated. In many health care systems, patients with MRSA or CRE are labeled as carriers for life, resulting in the institution of isolation precautions whenever they are admitted to the hospital. This practice has multiple adverse effects and leads to decreased patient satisfaction.[85] For these reasons, decolonization is a theoretically attractive option. However, most decolonizing strategies involve the use of antibiotics. For MRSA decolonization, most strategies involve some combination of intranasal mupirocin with topical chlorhexidine.[86] This approach has been shown to be effective in decreasing infections after surgery.[87] However, the effect is generally short lived and recurrence of colonization is the rule. For enteric bacteria, no good options are currently available. Various selective gut decontamination strategies have been described, but none have shown true promise. In addition, with growing knowledge of the role of the gut microbiome in the defense against MDR bacteria, it would seem counterintuitive to give even more antibiotics. Modulating the gut microbiome either through probiotics or through fecal microbiota transplantation is a promising, but as of yet an experimental method of decolonizing patients.

SUMMARY

Antibiotic resistance is clearly increasing in bacterial pathogens typically regarded as community acquired. Additionally, there is community spread of common nosocomial MDR pathogens. The success of these pathogens in the community is likely secondary to a number of factors that include the natural habitats of the bacteria and the competition present in those niches. In addition, certain strains of bacteria seem to be much more able to maintain their MDR phenotype and spread throughout the community. This finding is most likely secondary to additional genetic content that compensates for the relative fitness cost of the expression of genes associated with antibacterial resistance. Community spread of MDR bacteria is an important public health threat that should be approached urgently and proactively.

ACKNOWLEDGMENTS

D. van Duin was supported by the National Institute of Allergy and Infectious Diseases of the National Institutes of Health under Award Number R01AI143910.

REFERENCES

1. Centers for Disease Control and Prevention. Antibiotic resistance threats in the United States. U.S. Department of Health and Human Services 2019. Available at: www.cdc.gov/DrugResistance/Biggest-Threats.html. Accessed May 1, 2020.
2. Perez F, van Duin D. Carbapenem-resistant Enterobacteriaceae: a menace to our most vulnerable patients. Cleve Clin J Med 2013;80:225–33.
3. Ena J, Dick RW, Jones RN, et al. The epidemiology of intravenous vancomycin usage in a university hospital. A 10-year study. JAMA 1993;269:598–602.
4. Morin CA, Hadler JL. Population-based incidence and characteristics of community-onset Staphylococcus aureus infections with bacteremia in 4 metropolitan Connecticut areas, 1998. J Infect Dis 2001;184:1029–34.
5. Friedman ND, Kaye KS, Stout JE, et al. Health care–associated bloodstream infections in adults: a reason to change the accepted definition of community-acquired infections. Ann Intern Med 2002;137:791–7.
6. American Thoracic Society and Infectious Diseases Society of America. Guidelines for the management of adults with hospital-acquired, ventilator-associated, and healthcare-associated pneumonia. Am J Respir Crit Care Med 2005;171:388–416.
7. Williamson D, Ingle D, Howden B. Extensively Drug-Resistant Shigellosis in Australia among Men Who Have Sex with Men. N Engl J Med 2019;381:2477–9.
8. Namraj G, Monica ML, Marcus C, et al. Molecular approaches to enhance surveillance of gonococcal antimicrobial resistance. Nat Rev Microbiol 2014;12:223.
9. Su M, Satola S, Read T. Genome-Based Prediction of Bacterial Antibiotic Resistance. J Clin Microbiol 2019;57:e01405-18.
10. Kollef HM, Betthauser DK. New antibiotics for community-acquired pneumonia. Curr Opin Infect Dis 2019;32:169–75.
11. DeLeo FR, Otto M, Kreiswirth BN, et al. Community-associated methicillin-resistant Staphylococcus aureus. Lancet 2010;375:1557–68.
12. Witte W. Community-acquired methicillin-resistant Staphylococcus aureus: what do we need to know? Clin Microbiol Infect 2009;15(Suppl 7):17–25.
13. Saravolatz LD, Pohlod DJ, Arking LM. Community-acquired methicillin-resistant Staphylococcus aureus infections: a new source for nosocomial outbreaks. Ann Intern Med 1982;97:325–9.
14. Thurlow LR, Joshi GS, Richardson AR. Virulence strategies of the dominant USA300 lineage of community-associated methicillin-resistant Staphylococcus aureus (CA-MRSA). FEMS Immunol Med Microbiol 2012;65:5–22.
15. Alam MT, Read TD, Petit RA 3rd, et al. Transmission and microevolution of USA300 MRSA in U.S. households: evidence from whole-genome sequencing. mBio 2015;6:e00054.
16. Graveland H, Duim B, van Duijkeren E, et al. Livestock-associated methicillin-resistant Staphylococcus aureus in animals and humans. Int J Med Microbiol 2011;301:630–4.
17. Murray BE. Vancomycin-resistant enterococcal infections. N Engl J Med 2000;342:710–21.
18. Coque TM, Tomayko JF, Ricke SC, et al. Vancomycin-resistant enterococci from nosocomial, community, and animal sources in the United States. Antimicrob Agents Chemother 1996;40:2605–9.
19. Silverman J, Thal LA, Perri MB, et al. Epidemiologic evaluation of antimicrobial resistance in community-acquired enterococci. J Clin Microbiol 1998;36:830–2.

20. Bruinsma N, Stobberingh E, de Smet P, et al. Antibiotic use and the prevalence of antibiotic resistance in bacteria from healthy volunteers in the Dutch community. Infection 2003;31:9–14.
21. Bates J. Epidemiology of vancomycin-resistant enterococci in the community and the relevance of farm animals to human infection. J Hosp Infect 1997;37:89–101.
22. Klare I, Badstubner D, Konstabel C, et al. Decreased incidence of VanA-type vancomycin-resistant enterococci isolated from poultry meat and from fecal samples of humans in the community after discontinuation of avoparcin usage in animal husbandry. Microb Drug Resist 1999;5:45–52.
23. D'Agata EM, Jirjis J, Gouldin C, et al. Community dissemination of vancomycin-resistant Enterococcus faecium. Am J Infect Control 2001;29:316–20.
24. Poole TL, Hume ME, Campbell LD, et al. Vancomycin-resistant Enterococcus faecium strains isolated from community wastewater from a semiclosed agri-food system in Texas. Antimicrob Agents Chemother 2005;49:4382–5.
25. Omotola AM, Li Y, Martin ET, et al. Risk factors for and epidemiology of community-onset vancomycin-resistant Enterococcus faecalis in southeast Michigan. Am J Infect Control 2013;41:1244–8.
26. Wolfe CM, Cohen B, Larson E. Prevalence and risk factors for antibiotic-resistant community-associated bloodstream infections. J Infect Public Health 2014;7:224–32.
27. Foucault ML, Depardieu F, Courvalin P, et al. Inducible expression eliminates the fitness cost of vancomycin resistance in enterococci. Proc Natl Acad Sci U S A 2010;107:16964–9.
28. Johnsen PJ, Townsend JP, Bohn T, et al. Retrospective evidence for a biological cost of vancomycin resistance determinants in the absence of glycopeptide selective pressures. J Antimicrob Chemother 2011;66:608–10.
29. Gilmore MS, Rauch M, Ramsey MM, et al. Pheromone killing of multidrug-resistant Enterococcus faecalis V583 by native commensal strains. Proc Natl Acad Sci U S A 2015;112:7273–8.
30. Munoz-Price LS, Weinstein RA. Acinetobacter infection. N Engl J Med 2008;358:1271–81.
31. Falagas ME, Karveli EA, Kelesidis I, et al. Community-acquired Acinetobacter infections. Eur J Clin Microbiol Infect Dis 2007;26:857–68.
32. Eveillard M, Kempf M, Belmonte O, et al. Reservoirs of Acinetobacter baumannii outside the hospital and potential involvement in emerging human community-acquired infections. Int J Infect Dis 2013;17:e802–5.
33. Poirel L, Nordmann P. Carbapenem resistance in Acinetobacter baumannii: mechanisms and epidemiology. Clin Microbiol Infect 2006;12:826–36.
34. Sengstock DM, Thyagarajan R, Apalara J, et al. Multidrug-resistant Acinetobacter baumannii: an emerging pathogen among older adults in community hospitals and nursing homes. Clin Infect Dis 2010;50:1611–6.
35. Queenan AM, Pillar CM, Deane J, et al. Multidrug resistance among Acinetobacter spp. in the USA and activity profile of key agents: results from CAPITAL Surveillance 2010. Diagn Microbiol Infect Dis 2012;73:267–70.
36. Zeana C, Larson E, Sahni J, et al. The epidemiology of multidrug-resistant Acinetobacter baumannii: does the community represent a reservoir? Infect Control Hosp Epidemiol 2003;24:275–9.
37. Davis JS, McMillan M, Swaminathan A, et al. A 16-year prospective study of community-onset bacteremic Acinetobacter pneumonia: low mortality with appropriate initial empirical antibiotic protocols. Chest 2014;146:1038–45.

38. Peng C, Zong Z, Fan H. Acinetobacter baumannii isolates associated with community-acquired pneumonia in West China. Clin Microbiol Infect 2012;18: E491–3.
39. Paterson DL. The epidemiological profile of infections with multidrug-resistant Pseudomonas aeruginosa and Acinetobacter species. Clin Infect Dis 2006; 43(Suppl 2):S43–8.
40. Hassett DJ, Sutton MD, Schurr MJ, et al. Pseudomonas aeruginosa hypoxic or anaerobic biofilm infections within cystic fibrosis airways. Trends Microbiol 2009;17:130–8.
41. O'Malley CA. Infection control in cystic fibrosis: cohorting, cross-contamination, and the respiratory therapist. Respir Care 2009;54:641–57.
42. Rodriguez-Bano J, Lopez-Prieto MD, Portillo MM, et al. Epidemiology and clinical features of community-acquired, healthcare-associated and nosocomial bloodstream infections in tertiary-care and community hospitals. Clin Microbiol Infect 2010;16:1408–13.
43. Anderson DJ, Moehring RW, Sloane R, et al. Bloodstream infections in community hospitals in the 21st century: a multicenter cohort study. PLoS One 2014;9: e91713.
44. Hattemer A, Hauser A, Diaz M, et al. Bacterial and clinical characteristics of health care- and community-acquired bloodstream infections due to Pseudomonas aeruginosa. Antimicrob Agents Chemother 2013;57:3969–75.
45. Ulug M, Gedik E, Girgin S, et al. Pyogenic liver abscess caused by community-acquired multidrug resistance Pseudomonas aeruginosa. Braz J Infect Dis 2010; 14:218.
46. Pitout JD. Enterobacteriaceae that produce extended-spectrum beta-lactamases and AmpC beta-lactamases in the community: the tip of the iceberg? Curr Pharm Des 2013;19:257–63.
47. Doi Y, Park YS, Rivera JI, et al. Community-associated extended-spectrum beta-lactamase-producing Escherichia coli infection in the United States. Clin Infect Dis 2013;56:641–8.
48. Petty NK, Ben Zakour NL, Stanton-Cook M, et al. Global dissemination of a multidrug resistant Escherichia coli clone. Proc Natl Acad Sci U S A 2014;111:5694–9.
49. Banerjee R, Strahilevitz J, Johnson JR, et al. Predictors and molecular epidemiology of community-onset extended-spectrum beta-lactamase-producing Escherichia coli infection in a Midwestern community. Infect Control Hosp Epidemiol 2013;34:947–53.
50. Leistner R, Meyer E, Gastmeier P, et al. Risk factors associated with the community-acquired colonization of extended-spectrum beta-lactamase (ESBL) positive Escherichia Coli. an exploratory case-control study. PLoS One 2013;8: e74323.
51. Gopal Rao G, Batura D, Batura N, et al. Key demographic characteristics of patients with bacteriuria due to extended spectrum beta-lactamase (ESBL)-producing Enterobacteriaceae in a multiethnic community, in North West London. Infect Dis (Lond) 2015;47(10):719–24.
52. Rogers BA, Ingram PR, Runnegar N, et al. Community-onset Escherichia coli infection resistant to expanded-spectrum cephalosporins in low-prevalence countries. Antimicrob Agents Chemother 2014;58:2126–34.
53. Ko WC, Paterson DL, Sagnimeni AJ, et al. Community-acquired Klebsiella pneumoniae bacteremia: global differences in clinical patterns. Emerg Infect Dis 2002; 8:160–6.

54. Li W, Sun G, Yu Y, et al. Increasing occurrence of antimicrobial-resistant hypervirulent (hypermucoviscous) Klebsiella pneumoniae isolates in China. Clin Infect Dis 2014;58:225–32.
55. Harris PNA, Tambyah PA, Lye DC, et al. Effect of piperacillin-tazobactam vs meropenem on 30-day mortality for patients with E coli or Klebsiella pneumoniae bloodstream infection and ceftriaxone resistance: a randomized clinical trial. JAMA 2018;320:984.
56. Tamma PD, Cosgrove SE. Unlikely bedfellows: the partnering of antibiotic stewardship programs and the pharmaceutical industry. Clin Infect Dis 2020;71(3): 682–4.
57. Paterson DL, Henderson A, Harris PNA. Current evidence for therapy of ceftriaxone-resistant Gram-negative bacteremia. Curr Opin Infect Dis 2020;33:78–85.
58. Spellberg B, Blaser M, Guidos RJ, et al. Combating antimicrobial resistance: policy recommendations to save lives. Clin Infect Dis 2011;52(Suppl 5):S397–428.
59. Yigit H, Queenan AM, Anderson GJ, et al. Novel carbapenem-hydrolyzing beta-lactamase, KPC-1, from a carbapenem-resistant strain of Klebsiella pneumoniae. Antimicrob Agents Chemother 2001;45:1151–61.
60. Nordmann P, Cuzon G, Naas T. The real threat of Klebsiella pneumoniae carbapenemase-producing bacteria. Lancet Infect Dis 2009;9:228–36.
61. Schwaber MJ, Carmeli Y. Carbapenem-resistant Enterobacteriaceae: a potential threat. JAMA 2008;300:2911–3.
62. Hirsch EB, Tam VH. Detection and treatment options for *Klebsiella pneumoniae* carbapenemases (KPCs): an emerging cause of multidrug-resistant infection. J Antimicrob Chemother 2010;65(6):1119–25.
63. Neuner EA, Yeh JY, Hall GS, et al. Treatment and outcomes in carbapenem-resistant Klebsiella pneumoniae bloodstream infections. Diagn Microbiol Infect Dis 2011;69:357–62.
64. van Duin D, Kaye KS, Neuner EA, et al. Carbapenem-resistant Enterobacteriaceae: a review of treatment and outcomes. Diagn Microbiol Infect Dis 2013; 75:115–20.
65. Epstein L, Hunter JC, Arwady MA, et al. New Delhi metallo-beta-lactamase-producing carbapenem-resistant Escherichia coli associated with exposure to duodenoscopes. JAMA 2014;312:1447–55.
66. Khajuria A, Praharaj AK, Kumar M, et al. Emergence of Escherichia coli, Co-Producing NDM-1 and OXA-48 Carbapenemases, in Urinary Isolates, at a Tertiary Care Centre at Central India. J Clin Diagn Res 2014;8:DC01–4.
67. Bhargava A, Hayakawa K, Silverman E, et al. Risk factors for colonization due to carbapenem-resistant Enterobacteriaceae among patients exposed to long-term acute care and acute care facilities. Infect Control Hosp Epidemiol 2014;35: 398–405.
68. Walsh TR, Weeks J, Livermore DM, et al. Dissemination of NDM-1 positive bacteria in the New Delhi environment and its implications for human health: an environmental point prevalence study. Lancet Infect Dis 2011;11:355–62.
69. Wang Y, Wu C, Zhang Q, et al. Identification of New Delhi metallo-beta-lactamase 1 in Acinetobacter lwoffii of food animal origin. PloS one 2012;7:e37152.
70. Gu D, Dong N, Zheng Z, et al. A fatal outbreak of ST11 carbapenem-resistant hypervirulent Klebsiella pneumoniae in a Chinese hospital: a molecular epidemiological study. Lancet Infect Dis 2018;18:37–46.
71. Huang Y-H, Chou S-H, Liang S-W, et al. Emergence of an XDR and carbapenemase-producing hypervirulent Klebsiella pneumoniae strain in Taiwan. J Antimicrob Chemother 2018;73:2039–46.

72. Karlsson M, Stanton RA, Ansari U, et al. Identification of a Carbapenemase-Producing Hypervirulent Klebsiella pneumoniae Isolate in the United States. Antimicrob Agents Chemother 2019;63.
73. Liu Y, Long D, Xiang T-X, et al. Whole genome assembly and functional portrait of hypervirulent extensively drug-resistant NDM-1 and KPC-2 co-producing Klebsiella pneumoniae of capsular serotype K2 and ST86. J Antimicrob Chemother 2019;74:1233–40.
74. Roulston KJ, Bharucha T, Turton JF, et al. A case of NDM-carbapenemase-producing hypervirulent Klebsiella pneumoniae sequence type 23 from the UK. JMM Case Rep 2018;5.
75. Zhang Y, Jin L, Ouyang P, et al. Evolution of hypervirulence in carbapenem-resistant Klebsiella pneumoniae in China: a multicentre, molecular epidemiological analysis. J Antimicrob Chemother 2019;75:327–36.
76. Zheng R, Zhang Q, Guo Y, et al. Outbreak of plasmid-mediated NDM-1-producing Klebsiella pneumoniae ST105 among neonatal patients in Yunnan, China.(Report). Ann Clin Microbiol Antimicrob 2016;15.
77. Pannaraj PS, Bard JD, Cerini C, et al. Pediatric carbapenem-resistant Enterobacteriaceae in Los Angeles, California, a high-prevalence region in the United States. Pediatr Infect Dis J 2015;34:11–6.
78. Hussain A, Ranjan A, Nandanwar N, et al. Genotypic and phenotypic profiles of Escherichia coli isolates belonging to clinical sequence type 131 (ST131), clinical non-ST131, and fecal non-ST131 lineages from India. Antimicrob Agents Chemother 2014;58:7240–9.
79. Peirano G, Schreckenberger PC, Pitout JD. Characteristics of NDM-1-producing Escherichia coli isolates that belong to the successful and virulent clone ST131. Antimicrob Agents Chemother 2011;55:2986–8.
80. Hawkey PM, Jones AM. The changing epidemiology of resistance. J Antimicrob Chemother 2009;64(Suppl 1):i3–10.
81. Marathe NP, Regina VR, Walujkar SA, et al. A treatment plant receiving waste water from multiple bulk drug manufacturers is a reservoir for highly multi-drug resistant integron-bearing bacteria. PLoS One 2013;8:e77310.
82. Forsberg KJ, Reyes A, Wang B, et al. The shared antibiotic resistome of soil bacteria and human pathogens. Science 2012;337:1107–11.
83. Wagner B, Filice GA, Drekonja D, et al. Antimicrobial stewardship programs in inpatient hospital settings: a systematic review. Infect Control Hosp Epidemiol 2014;35:1209–28.
84. Gangat MA, Hsu JL. Antibiotic stewardship: a focus on ambulatory care. South Dakota Med 2015;(Spec No):44–8.
85. Vinski J, Bertin M, Sun Z, et al. Impact of isolation on hospital consumer assessment of healthcare providers and systems scores: is isolation isolating? Infect Control Hosp Epidemiol 2012;33:513–6.
86. Coates T, Bax R, Coates A. Nasal decolonization of Staphylococcus aureus with mupirocin: strengths, weaknesses and future prospects. J Antimicrob Chemother 2009;64:9–15.
87. Chen AF, Wessel CB, Rao N. Staphylococcus aureus screening and decolonization in orthopaedic surgery and reduction of surgical site infections. Clin Orthop Relat Res 2013;471:2383–99.

Agents of Last Resort

An Update on Polymyxin Resistance

Qiwen Yang, MD[a,*], Jason M. Pogue, PharmD[b], Zekun Li, BS[a], Roger L. Nation, PhD[c], Keith S. Kaye, MD, MPH[d], Jian Li, PhD[e]

KEYWORDS

- Polymyxin resistance • Gram-negative pathogens • Risk factors
- Infection prevention • Bacterial stewardship

KEY POINTS

- Polymyxins are considered as last-line antibiotic for Pandrug-resistant organisms.
- Effective prevention of deterioration of polymyxin resistance requires both further comprehension of its mechanisms and systematic measures in surveillance, infection control and administration.
- Novel methodologies improved efficiency of polymyxin resistance control while optimization of polymyxin susceptibility testing and therapeutic options is still demanded.

INTRODUCTION

The polymyxins, colistin (also known as polymyxin E) and polymyxin B, have a unique and interesting history. Originally introduced in the 1950s for the treatment of infections owing to gram-negative organisms, the polymyxins fell out of favor by the mid-1970s because of high rates of nephrotoxicity (approaching 50%) and neurotoxicity and the advent of less toxic alternatives, notably the antipseudomonal aminoglycosides. By the mid-1990s, the polymyxins were reintroduced into clinical practice, not because of an enhanced safety profile, but rather owing to the development of

---

Portions of this article were previously published in Kaye KS, Pogue JM, Tran TB, et al. Agents of Last Resort: Polymyxin Resistance. Infect Dis Clin North Am 2016; 30(2): 391-414. This work was supported by the National Key Research and Development Program of China (2018YFC1200100 , 2018YFC1200105).

[a] Department of Clinical Laboratory, Peking Union Medical College Hospital, Peking Union Medical College, Chinese Academy of Medical Sciences, No.9 Dongdan Santiao, Dongcheng District, Beijing, China; [b] Department of Clinical Pharmacy, University of Michigan College of Pharmacy, 428 Church Street, Ann Arbor, MI 48109, USA; [c] Drug Delivery, Disposition and Dynamics, Monash Institute of Pharmaceutical Sciences, Faculty of Pharmacy and Pharmaceutical Sciences, Monash University, Victoria 3052, Australia; [d] Department of Internal Medicine, University of Michigan Medical School, 1301 Catherine Street, Ann Arbor, MI 48109, USA; [e] Laboratory of Antimicrobial Systems Pharmacology, Department of Microbiology, Monash University, Victoria 3800, Australia

* Corresponding author.

E-mail address: yangqiwen81@vip.163.com

Infect Dis Clin N Am 34 (2020) 723–750
https://doi.org/10.1016/j.idc.2020.08.003

extensively drug-resistant (XDR) gram-negative bacilli resistant to all other treatment options.[1,2] The polymyxins now serve a critical role in the antimicrobial armamentarium, because they are one of few, and sometimes the only, antimicrobial agent retaining activity against carbapenem-resistant *Pseudomonas aeruginosa*, carbapenem-resistant *Acinetobacter baumannii*, and carbapenem-resistant Enterobacteriaceae (CRE), organisms that frequently cause life-threatening infections in the most vulnerable of patient populations. These pathogens have been recognized by the Centers for Disease Control and Prevention as serious or urgent threats to human health and mortality rates in invasive infections owing to these pathogens can exceed 50%.[2,3] The relatively dry antimicrobial pipeline for the treatment of infections caused by these organisms magnifies the importance of the polymyxins. Given the critical role of the polymyxins in the care of hospitalized patients, an understanding of both the epidemiology of polymyxin resistance as well as strategies to prevent resistance are paramount. Therefore, this article introduces similarities and differences between the 2 clinically available polymyxins, discusses the mechanism of action and resistance to these agents, describes the clinical epidemiology of polymyxin-resistant organisms, and finally suggests strategies to minimize the development and spread of polymyxin resistance.

Colistin and polymyxin B are nearly structurally identical, differing by only 1 amino acid at position 6 (**Fig. 1**). They are considered to be very similar microbiologically and cross-resistance exists. Both polymyxins are products of fermentation and therefore are multicomponent mixtures. Colistin and polymyxin B have 2 major components (colistin A and B; polymyxin B1 and B2) that slightly differ at the site of the *N*-terminal fatty acyl tail.[4] The polymyxins are amphipathic molecules, consisting of both hydrophilic and hydrophobic regions (see **Fig. 1**) and these properties are essential to their antimicrobial activity (described elsewhere in this article). Although polymyxin B is administered directly as its sulfate salt, colistin is administered in the form of its inactive prodrug colistimethate sodium (CMS, also known as colistin methanesulfonate).[5] CMS is synthesized by sulfomethylation of active colistin, and although CMS is considered to exist in its fully penta-methanesulfonated form, recent analyses have shown that the material reconstituted for use in patients likely exists as a combination of a large number of fully or partially methanesulfonated derivatives.[6,7] As is described in detail elsewhere in this article, the administration of colistin as an inactive prodrug has a significant impact on the pharmacokinetics (PK) of colistin in patients and is an important differentiator between the 2 polymyxins. Both polymyxins are associated with nephrotoxicity rates in the 30% to 50% range,[1] and all strategies for optimal use need to be taken in the context of the dose, and subsequent concentration-dependent toxicity that may be seen.

MECHANISM OF ACTION

The precise mechanism of antibacterial activity of polymyxins is not completely understood; however, it is well-known that polymyxins kill bacteria by disrupting the bacterial outer membrane through the self-promoted uptake pathway.[8] Polymyxins initially bind to the lipopolysaccharides (LPS) in the outer membrane of gram-negative bacteria, and both electrostatic and hydrophobic interactions are essential in the disorganization of the outer membrane.[4] Electrostatic interaction via the positively charged diaminobutyric acid residues of the polymyxin (see **Fig. 1**) and the negatively charged phosphate groups on the lipid A moiety of LPS leads to displacement of divalent cations (Mg^{2+} and Ca^{2+}) that bridge the lipid A phosphoesters, thereby destabilizing the outer membrane.[9] This event allows the polymyxin to insert its hydrophobic regions

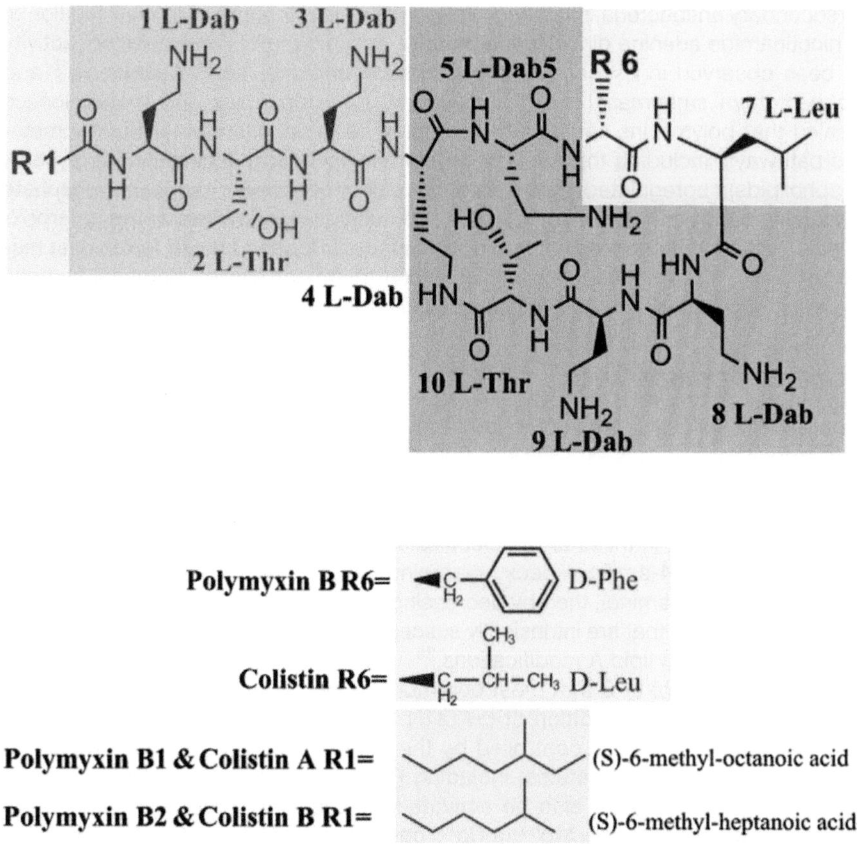

Fig. 1. Chemical structures of polymyxin B and colistin. The functional segments of polymyxins are colored as follows: yellow, fatty acyl chain; green, linear tripeptide segment; red, the polar residues of the heptapeptide; blue, the hydrophobic motif within the hepta-peptide ring. (Reprinted with permission from Velkov T, Thompson PE, Nation RL, et al. Structure–activity relationships of polymyxin antibiotics. J Med Chem 2010;53(5):1898. Copyright © 2010 American Chemical Society.)

(fatty acyl tail and amino acids at positions 6 and 7) into the bacterial outer membrane to interact with the fatty acyl chains of lipid A; this hydrophobic interaction causes further outer membrane disruption that promotes the uptake of other polymyxin molecules.[8,10] It has been proposed that after transiting the outer membrane, polymyxins mediate the fusion of the inner leaflet of the outer membrane with the outer leaflet of the cytoplasmic membrane, which induces phospholipid exchange and causes osmotic imbalance that leads to cell death[11]; however, strong experimental data to prove this hypothesis are lacking. The amphipathic property of polymyxins (ie, presence of both cationic and hydrophobic regions) is necessary for the killing of gram-negative bacteria. Polymyxin B nonapeptide (ie, polymyxin B lacking the fatty acyl tail and the diaminobutyric acid residue at position 1) and colistimethate (in which the diaminobutyric acid residues are masked by negatively charged methanesulfonate moieties) do not possess antibacterial activity.[5,12] In addition to their membrane-disrupting effect in gram-negative bacteria, binding of polymyxins to lipid A also neutralizes the toxicity of endotoxins.[13,14]

A secondary antibacterial mechanism of polymyxins is thought to be via inhibition of the nicotinamide adenine dinucleotide oxidase enzyme family. This inhibitory activity has been observed in *Escherichia coli*, *Klebsiella pneumoniae*, *A baumannii*,[15] and *Mycobacterium smegmatis*.[16] In *A baumannii*, transcriptomics and metabolomics revealed that polymyxins cause rapid, complex perturbations of multiple key metabolic pathways, including the levels of membrane lipids (predominantly the glycerophospholipids); upregulated fluxes through gluconeogenesis, pentose phosphate pathway, and biosynthesis of amino acids and nucleotides; downregulated tricarboxylic acid cycle and biogenesis of peptidoglycan and LPS; and altered fluxes over respiratory chain.[17–20] In *P aeruginosa*, polymyxin treatment causes potential osmotic imbalance and decreases the synthesis of LPS and peptidoglycan.[21]

MECHANISMS OF RESISTANCE

As reviewed previously, the interaction of polymyxins with LPS is essential for their antimicrobial activity. This explains why polymyxin B and colistin are not active against gram-positive bacteria. In gram-negative bacteria, which are intrinsically resistant to polymyxins, this interaction is diminished owing to LPS, which has a lower binding affinity for polymyxins. In these LPS molecules, lipid A usually contains modified phosphate groups (eg, 4-amino-4-deoxy-L-arabinose [L-Ara4N], phosphoethanolamine [pEtN], and galactosamine), thereby decreasing their overall net negative charge.[22–24] Likewise, in bacteria that are intrinsically susceptible to polymyxins, resistance is usually acquired through lipid A modifications.[25]

The modification of LPS that most commonly leads to polymyxin resistance in *P aeruginosa* involves the addition of L-Ara4N to the phosphate groups in lipid A.[25] This modification is usually controlled by the *arn* (*pmr*) operon, which is regulated by several 2-component systems, including PmrA/PmrB and PhoP/PhoQ.[26] These 2-component systems can also be activated by changes in the environment (eg, high Fe^{3+} concentration, low Mg^{2+} or Ca^{2+} concentrations, and low pH) and the lipid A modification can lead to decreased bridging of adjacent lipid A molecules via divalent cations.[27–29] PmrB and PhoQ are cytoplasmic membrane-bound sensor kinases that phosphorylate their respective regulator proteins PmrA and PhoP on activation. Once phosphorylated, PmrA and PhoP promote the upregulation of the *arn* operon leading to the addition of L-Ara4N to the phosphate groups of lipid A.[30] Resistance to polymyxins can develop when mutations occur in the PmrA/PmrB and PhoP/PhoQ systems.[31] In addition, lipid A modification with pEtN has been reported in polymyxin-resistant *P aeruginosa*, which is controlled by the ColR/ColS 2-component system and upregulated in the presence of excess extracellular Zn^{2+}.[32] Interestingly, polymyxins can also induce lipid A deacylation in polymyxin-resistant *P aeruginosa*, which perturbs polymyxin penetration and confers high-level resistance.[33]

In *A baumannii*, L-Ara4N biosynthesis is generally lacking and polymyxin resistance is often achieved by the modification of lipid A with pEtN.[34] This modification can be caused by mutations in *pmrA* and/or *pmrB* that induce the autoregulation of the promoter region of the *pmrCAB* operon.[31] It was also reported that polymyxin resistance in *A baumannii* clinical isolates can occur via the modification of lipid A with galactosamine, although the precise regulatory pathway is not yet understood.[35] Apart from LPS modifications, *A baumannii* also possesses a unique polymyxin resistance mechanism that involves the loss of LPS.[36] This phenotype can be caused by mutations in lipid A biosynthesis genes. In these highly polymyxin-resistant *A baumannii* isolates, genes responsible for the transport of phospholipids/lipoproteins and production of poly-ß-1,6-*N*-acetylglucosamine are upregulated to compensate for the missing LPS in the outer leaflet of the outer membrane.[37]

In *K pneumoniae*, resistance to polymyxins may involve several different strategies, and the major resistance mechanism involves the modification of lipid A by the addition of either L-Ara4N or pEtN.[31] These modifications can be caused by mutations in *pmrAB* or *phoPQ*.[38–40] It has also been reported that the upregulation of the PhoP/PhoQ and PmrA/PmrB systems can be caused by mutations in *mgrB*, a negative regulator of PhoPQ.[41,42] Another polymyxin resistance mechanism in *K pneumoniae* is overproduction of surface capsular polysaccharides. It is believed that the capsular polysaccharides may act as a barrier to limit the interaction of polymyxins with lipid A,[43] by trapping polymyxins.[44] It is also reported that the AcrAB-TolC efflux pump may play a role in polymyxin resistance in *K pneumoniae*.[45]

A plasmid-mediated polymyxin resistance gene, *mcr-1*, was first discovered in *E coli* and *K pneumoniae* from animals and humans in China in November 2015.[46] Subsequently, isolates carrying *mcr* genes, mainly *mcr-1* and less commonly *mcr-2* to *-9*, have been reported worldwide.[47–50] The *mcr* genes confer resistance to polymyxins by the modification of lipid A via pEtN[48–50]; fortunately, the majority of *mcr*-carrying isolates reported to date are not multidrug- resistant (MDR). Nevertheless, the global dissemination of *mcr* genes has highlighted a potential threat to the last-line polymyxins.

Phenotypically, resistance to polymyxins also can be developed in polymyxin-heteroresistant bacteria. The minimum inhibitory concentrations (MICs) of polymyxins in these bacteria are 2 mg/L or less (ie, the current susceptibility breakpoint); however, there is a subpopulation of bacterial cells that can survive in the presence of more than 2 mg/L of a polymyxin. This nature leads to the amplification of the resistant subpopulation in the presence of polymyxins alone and the eventual development of polymyxin resistance.[51] Recent studies indicate that polymyxin heteroresistance in *P aeruginosa* is infrequent[52]; however, it is very common in both MDR *K pneumoniae*[53] and *A baumannii*.[54]

Laboratory studies have indicated that resistance to polymyxins in *A baumannii* may compromise the resistance to other classes of antibiotics.[55,56] In a study with *A baumannii* that compared the antibiograms of MDR colistin-susceptible clinical isolates with those of the respective laboratory-generated colistin-resistant paired strains,[55] the polymyxin-resistant strains were more susceptible to other antibiotics compared with their parent polymyxin-susceptible strains. These findings suggested that polymyxin combinations may be useful to prevent polymyxin resistance in MDR bacteria. However, the clinical relevance of this finding remains to be determined, as in clinical practice most polymyxin-resistant gram-negative bacteria are usually resistant to a broad range of other antibiotics.

Resistance to polymyxins may also come at a fitness cost. *A baumannii* isolates with polymyxin resistance usually grow at a much slower rate and are less capable of causing infection.[57,58] Studies that compared the fitness cost of lipid A modification and LPS loss in *A baumannii* isolates showed that a decrease in biological fitness associated with LPS loss was greater than with pEtN addition.[57,59] Impaired virulence in *A baumannii* is also linked to decreased expression of metabolic proteins and of the OmpA porin.[60] Significant biological fitness cost owing to polymyxin resistance has yet to be observed in *P aeruginosa* and *K pneumoniae*.

CLINICAL EPIDEMIOLOGY OF POLYMYXIN-RESISTANT GRAM-NEGATIVE BACILLI

As discussed elsewhere in this article, the primary clinical role for the polymyxins is for the treatment of infections owing to carbapenem-resistant *A baumannii, P aeruginosa*, or CRE (most notably carbapenem-resistant *K pneumoniae*), when no other reliable treatment options are available. Fortunately, colistin has excellent in vitro activity in this setting, and most isolates are susceptible at the susceptibility breakpoint of 2 mg/L. However, there are regional variations in susceptibility rates and clinicians should be aware of local susceptibility data. Although it is not the focus of this article, it is important for the reader to be aware of a few important points. First, not all published analyses have used the same susceptibility breakpoint for colistin to define resistance. Second, the current susceptibility breakpoints might not be ideal from a pharmacokinetic or pharmacodynamic standpoint. Third, there are unique complexities that exist with regard to the determination of the colistin MIC via conventional methods. Because disk diffusion and E-test cannot reliably detect resistance (ie, false susceptibility can occur), publications that determine susceptibility by of these methods might overstate susceptibility rates.[61] For the purposes of this section, a susceptibility breakpoint of 2 mg/L is used. Polymyxin B susceptibility is not routinely performed and colistin is used as a categorical surrogate for susceptibility.

Published data regarding rates of colistin-resistant *P aeruginosa* are relatively scarce; however, most published rates are between 0% and 10% with some geographic variance.[62,63] In the United States, surveillance data from the SENTRY database from 2011 to 2017 place colistin resistance at less than 1%.[64] Recent epidemiologic data from ERAS-Net, demonstrated that 4% of overall *P aeruginosa* isolates were resistant to colistin in Europe in 2016.[65] In South Korea, Wi and colleagues[66] reported 7.4% (16/215) of *P aeruginosa* isolates in patients hospitalized with sepsis or a urinary tract infection were colistin resistant during 2012 to 2013. Data from India assessing *P aeruginosa* isolates found that 8 of 95 (8%) were resistant to colistin,[67] whereas data from 385 *P aeruginosa* in patients with cystic fibrosis patients in Germany[68] found colistin resistance in 35 of 229 nonmucoid strains (15%) and 5 of 156 mucoid strains (3%), for an overall resistance rate of 10.4%.

Despite the widespread nature of carbapenem resistance in *A baumannii* and the increasingly common use of polymyxins as one of the only therapeutic options, wide-spread polymyxin resistance in this organism has not been reported. Data from the Sentry Antimicrobial Surveillance database, which include isolates from the United States, Europe, Latin America, and the Asia-Pacific region, have shown resistance between 0.9% and 3.3% from 2001 to 2011.[69–71] Although some individual reports have shown higher numbers, rarely do rates exceed 5%[72] and, when they do, there are notable methodologic limitations. Many studies reporting high rates of colistin resistance include isolates that are carbapenem susceptible and/or do not include all *Acinetobacter* isolates in a given institution. For example, a frequently cited report that showed colistin resistance to be 16.7% is limited because it included only 18 isolates, 3 of which were colistin resistant.[73] Additionally, the vast majority (17/18) were actually susceptible to carbapenems. Similarly, although Ko and colleagues[74] reported an extremely high rate of colistin resistance of 31% in 214 *A baumannii* isolates in Korea, of the 83 polymyxin-resistant strains, only 5 were resistant to imipenem. Although Arroyo and colleagues[75] reported a rate of colistin resistance of 19.1% in Spain (21/115 isolates), it is unclear how these isolates were selected and whether or not they represented all isolates in their institution. Similarly, in another report published by the same group in Spain that described a 41% rate of colistin resistance, the analysis did not consist of all *Acinetobacter* isolates from their institution and was specifically chosen to assess the in vitro activities of various other antimicrobials against both multidrug and pan-drug–resistant isolates.[76] Although these studies might overstate the incidence of colistin resistance in carbapenem-resistant *A baumannii*, they clearly demonstrate that colistin-resistant *A baumannii* exists in various geographic locales and some reports have shown the incidence to be increasing, albeit still at low overall numbers.[77]

The most alarming epidemiologic trend with regard to carbapenem-resistant gram-negative bacilli has been the increase and worldwide spread of CRE, primarily, but not exclusively, driven by the *K pneumoniae* carbapenemase (KPC) enzyme.[78] Although KPC is most commonly produced in *K pneumoniae*, it can be produced by other *Enterobacteriaceae*, as well as by nonfermenting organisms. Rates of KPC production among clinical isolates of *K pneumoniae* vary worldwide, but staggering numbers have been reported in some regions. For example, in Italy, surveillance data pertaining to *K pneumoniae* bloodstream isolates demonstrated an increase in carbapenem resistance from 1% to 2% in 2006 to 2009, to 30% in 2011.[78] Furthermore, a recent publication from Italy showed a continual increase in the rates of carbapenem resistance in *K pneumoniae* bloodstream infections from a rate of 3% in 2009 to 42% in 2011 and to 66% in 2013.[79] Similar rates have been reported in neighboring Greece.[78] Although rates have been lower in general in the United States, endemic areas have occurred. In the New York area hospitals, the incidence of KPC *K pneumoniae* isolates reached 36% in 2006, and significantly decreased to 13% in 2013 to 2014.[80]

Unfortunately, but perhaps unsurprisingly, immediately after the increase in KPCs worldwide, case reports and series describing clusters and outbreaks of colistin-resistant KPC producers began to appear in the literature. Additionally, rates of colistin resistance in *Klebsiella* spp. from surveillance studies have varied greatly and interpretation of these studies is complicated because many of them do not focus solely on KPC- producing isolates.[81] However, the rates of colistin resistance in carbapenem-resistant *K pneumoniae*, unlike what has been described with other carbapenem-resistant organisms, seem to be increasing at a much higher rate. Surveillance data examining worldwide rates of colistin resistance among carbapenem-resistant as well as carbapenem-susceptible *Klebsiella* isolates generally place the rate at approximately 7%.[81] However, data from Greece from the mid to late 2000s place the rate at 10.5% to 20.0%.[82,83] Additionally, 2 reports, one from Austria and one from the Netherlands, showed rates of approximately 50% in extended-spectrum β-lactamase (ESBL)-producing *Klebsiella* spp. It is notable that these studies were done in the setting of oral colistin administration for selective gut decontamination.[84,85] Most concerning, however, have been reports of extremely high rates of colistin resistance from regions in which KPC producers have become endemic. Rates of colistin resistance in carbapenemase-producing *Klebsiella* have ranged from 14% to 25% in Greece.[86–90] Colistin resistance in KPC-producing *K pneumoniae* in São Paulo has increased from 0% to 27.1% during 2011 to 2015.[91] In Italy, reported rates have been even higher. Multiple publications have reported colistin resistance exceeding 30% in carbapenem-resistant *K pneumoniae*.[81] One study of *Klebsiella* resistance in bloodstream infections in an Italian hospital reported 66% of strains to be carbapenem resistant, and 57% to 65% of those carbapenem-resistant *K pneumoniae* strains were also resistant to colistin.[79] To put these resistant rates in clinical perspective, if a patient was to develop a *Klebsiella* spp. bloodstream infection, there would be approximately a 43% chance that it would be both colistin resistant and carbapenem resistant. Similarly, data examining 191 carbapenemase-producing Enterobacteriaceae in 21 hospitals in Italy from November 2013 to April 2014 reported 76 (43%) to also be colistin resistant.[92] Moubareck and colleagues[93] reported a high colistin resistant rate of 31.4% in carbapenem-resistant *K pneumoniae* isolates in Dubai during 2015 to 2016. As the authors mentioned, although these data indicated a concerning situation pertaining to colistin resistance, their data only represented the CRE in certain hospitals which might affect the generalizability of the results throughout the region.[93]

Importantly however, since the first New Delhi metallo-β-lactamases (bla_{NDM}) related carbapenem-resistant *K pneumoniae* was reported in India in 2009,[94] β-lactamases other than KPC have also been recognized as important carbapenem-resistant mechanisms recently. NDM has been reported mainly in Asia and has been the second most frequently found carbapenemase gene in China.[95] Malchione and colleagues[96] analyzed 114 data reports of carbapenem resistant *Enterobacteriaceae* in nine Southeast countries and found that the most common carbapenemases were NDM and OXA β-lactamase, whereas NDM was most prevalent in *E coli*. Although NDM has flourished, other metallo β-lactamases, VIM and IMP, have remained relatively uncommon in Enterobacteriaceae. VIM has been reported sporadically in Greece, Mexico, Russia, South Africa, Iran and some Southeast Asian countries in Enterobacteriaceae and *P aeruginosa*. IMP was mainly reported in Japan and Taiwan, China.[95–98] In America, metallo β-lactamase–induced carbapenem resistance is still uncommon. As of 2016, 25 states reported 157 Enterobacteriaceae isolates harboring NDM to the Centers for Disease Control and Prevention, whereas for VIM- and IMP-producing *Enterobacteriaceae* were discovered 17 and 10 isolates from 7 and 5 states, respectively.[99] In 2017, of 4442 CRE and *P aeruginosa* isolates collected from National Healthcare Safety Network, the positive rate of NDM, VIM, and IMP was 2.4%, 0.6% and 0.4%, respectively.[100] In addition to metallo β-lactamases, oxacillinase-48 (OXA-48)–like enzymes have emerged as a mechanism of carbapenem resistance in Enterobacteriaceae with the first case was reported in Turkey in 2001.[101] According to SMART global surveillance data from 2008 to 2014, OXA-48–like has been the second most common carbapenemase gene present in carbapenemase-producing Enterobacteriaceae. As for geographic distribution of OXA-48–like, it has been spread worldwide expect for the Antarctic continent and importantly it has become the most common carbapenemase detected in Africa and the second most common in Europe.[102,103] In the United States, OXA is still a relatively uncommon etiology for Enterobacteriaceae carbapenem resistance. According the Centers for Disease Control and Prevention data, as of 2015, only 43 cases of OXA-48–like CPEs were reported.[99,100]

Unfortunately, data reporting on colistin resistance rates in metallo β-lactamases or OXA-48–like producers remains scarce. Bradford and colleagues[104] demonstrated a 16% rate of colistin resistance in OXA-48–producing isolates worldwide. In China, a nationwide epidemiologic surveillance program collected 1868 CRE isolates and identified 14 *E coli* coexpressing bla_{NDM} and mcr1, among which the combination of $bla_{NDM\text{-}5}$ and mcr-1 was predominant (n = 11).[105]

Although most available data assessing rates of colistin resistance in gram-negative bacilli represent nonclinical surveillance data, there are a few reports assessing risk factors for isolation of colistin-resistant gram-negative bacilli. Although polymyxin exposure is frequently identified as a risk factor, this finding is not universal. Qureshi and colleagues[106] described the characteristics of 20 patients with colistin-resistant *A baumannii* isolated from their institution over a 7-year period. Nineteen of 20 patients (95%) had prior isolation of genetically related colistin-susceptible isolates and significant prior intravenous and inhaled colistin exposure was present in all but 1 of the 20 patients. Similarly, Papadimitriou-Olivgeris and colleagues[90] described their experience in 254 patients who were not colonized with colistin-resistant KPC-producing isolates on admission to the intensive care unit (ICU). Of the 254 patients, 62 (24.4%) became colonized with colistin-resistant KPC-producing organisms, whereas in the ICU, with the primary risk factor for isolation being colistin exposure (odds ratio, 13.5; 95% confidence interval, 6.1–30.2). Other risk factors for isolation of colistin-resistant KPC producers were corticosteroid use and number of patients with colistin-resistant KPC-producing–positive organisms treated in nearby beds per day, suggesting the importance of horizontal transmission and colonization pressure as well. Other risk factors that have been identified for colistin resistant organisms have been age, ICU residence, and mechanical ventilation.[107]

Meletis and colleagues[108] evaluated colistin use over time and its association with colistin-resistant gram-negative bacilli. Colistin use increased significantly over the period of the study from 7 defined daily doses per 1000 patient-days in 2007 to 27 defined daily doses per 1000 patient-days in 2013 and a likewise significant increase in colistin-resistant KPC was seen from 0% in 2007 to 2010, to 16% in 2010 to 2013. This increase was most notable among ICU isolates, where a colistin-resistant KPC-producing organism was reported in 20 of 92 (22%) isolates. What is most interesting is that although there was a dramatic increase in colistin-resistant KPC over the study period, there was no parallel increase in colistin resistance in carbapenem-resistant *A baumannii* or *P aeruginosa*. Rates of colistin-resistant carbapenem-resistant *A baumannii* were 0% over the entire study period, and rates of colistin resistance in *P aeruginosa* actually decreased from 5% in 2007 to 2010, to 2% in 2010 to 2013. This finding is consistent with the overall data presented in this section that colistin resistance in KPC producers seems to be developing at an alarming rate, whereas colistin resistance rates in the nonfermenters remain relatively low and stable.

These findings are interesting in light of a recent publication by Giani and colleagues,[79] in which the investigators described their experience with an outbreak of 93 bloodstream infections with colistin-resistant KPC over a 4-year period, in an area in Italy where KPC is endemic (the investigators reported that two-thirds of all *Klebsiella* were carbapenem resistant, and carbapenem resistance was largely mediated by KPC production). Data on previous colistin exposure were available for 38 patients, 35 (92%) of whom did not receive colistin before isolation of their colistin-resistant pathogen. Of the 59 patients in whom genotyping was performed, the *mgrB* gene deletion was present in 50 of 59 (85%) isolates; and in a subset of 19 patients for whom colistin data were available, 18 (95%) had not had prior colistin exposure. Although the outbreak was initially tied to increased colistin use at the institution, the continued spread in the absence of colistin exposure suggested clonal expansion of a single strain (ie, patient-to-patient spread) and also suggested that this particular mechanism may not have been associated with decreased strain fitness of survival. This finding is in line with another report that associates *mgrB* inactivation with a lack of fitness cost in *A baumannii*.[59]

In summary, although overall rates of colistin resistance among carbapenem-resistant *A baumannii*, *P aeruginosa*, and *K pneumoniae* remain relatively low, certain institutions and regions have higher rates. In addition, polymyxin exposure remains high in some institutions because of the need for active treatment of these carbapenem-resistant pathogens. This continued use of polymyxins is likely to promote the continued emergence of resistance. Additionally, particularly in *K pneumoniae*, there is mounting evidence that a stable form of resistance is emerging that might be seen in the absence of polymyxin exposure. Thus, clonal expansion throughout a given unit or institution can occur in some cases leading to rapid widespread colistin resistance. These findings, when taken together, stress the critical need for optimal stewardship strategies for the use of polymyxins, as well as for effective infection control processes to preserve these critical, last-line agents.

STRATEGIES TO MINIMIZE POLYMYXIN RESISTANCE

As discussed elsewhere in this article, there are 2 polymyxins currently being used in the clinic: colistin and polymyxin B.[109,110] Colistin is administered parenterally in the form of an inactive prodrug, the sodium salt of colistin methanesulfonate (CMS, also known as colistimethate).[5,111] A parenteral formulation of polymyxin B (as its sulfate salt) is available in a number of countries, including the United States, but is not available in Europe, Australia, and several other countries.[10,110] Polymyxin B is administered directly in its active antibacterial form, whereas CMS requires conversion in vivo to generate the active entity, colistin. This difference in the form administered to patients has a major effect on the clinical pharmacologic profile of the 2 polymyxins, an understanding of which is critical to their optimal clinical use.[110,112–116]

Because of the limited therapeutic options for these pathogens and potential for development of resistance with polymyxin monotherapy, it is important that both polymyxins are used optimally to maximize their efficacy and minimize resistance and nephrotoxicity. Unfortunately, because polymyxins were approved for clinical use before the introduction of the contemporary drug development and regulatory approval processes, the prescribing information of both polymyxin products has been limited and not supported by solid pharmacologic data.[110] Fortunately, this situation has been changing over the past decade. Indeed, the polymyxins have been the first of the old antibiotics to be subjected to a redevelopment process, largely led by academic and clinical researchers.[110,116] To optimize their dosage regimens, it is essential to understand their PK, pharmacodynamics (PD), and toxicodynamics (TD), and the relationships between exposure and desired and undesired responses (ie, PK/PD and PK/TD).[116–123] There are a number of approaches that may minimize resistance development to polymyxins, in particular optimizing their dosage regimens in patients using PK, PD, and TD; use of rational combinations; and limiting clinical use to patients with MDR/XDR gram-negative infections. As discussed elsewhere in this article, there is a paucity of clinical evidence supporting these strategies as a means to minimize development of polymyxin resistance.

Optimizing Dosing Regimens

Currently, there are 2 different labeling systems in use for parenteral CMS.[109,110,116] In Europe and some other regions, the international unit is used for CMS, whereas colistin base activity is used in North America, South America, and Southeast Asia. One million international units is equivalent to approximately 33 mg of colistin base activity.[116,124] It is crucial that clinicians are aware of the labeling differences and proper conversions are achieved before implementing at the local level dosage regimens reported in journal articles.[110,116]

Over the past decade, significant preclinical and clinical pharmacologic data have been generated to inform clinicians on optimizing the use of colistin and polymyxin B in patients.[125] The PK/PD index that best predicts the activity of colistin has been identified as the ratio of the area under the unbound (free) plasma colistin concentration versus time curve across 24 hours to the MIC. This was shown with colistin against *P aeruginosa* and *K pneumoniae* using dose-fractionation studies in an in vitro PK/PD model and in other in vitro investigations.[118,126,127] In vivo studies using murine thigh and lung infection models have confirmed this finding for parenteral colistin against *P aeruginosa* and *A baumannii*,[117] and for direct pulmonary administration of colistin against *P aeruginosa*, *A baumannii* and *K pneumoniae* lung infections in mice.[128,129] The data from the mouse thigh infection studies involving parenteral administration of colistin,[117] when translated to the clinic after accounting for interspecies differences in plasma protein binding, suggest that the average steady-state plasma colistin concentration ($C_{ss,avg}$) required for antibacterial effect in a patient receiving intravenous CMS corresponds to the MIC of the organism causing the infection.[130,131] It is important, however, to keep in mind that the risk of nephrotoxicity in patients increases as the plasma colistin concentration increases, especially at concentrations or more than approximately 2.5 mg/L.[121–123] The colistin MIC may not be known at initiation of therapy and even if it is the reported MIC may be inaccurate owing to well recognized problems with susceptibility testing.[132,133] For these reasons a target plasma colistin $C_{ss,avg}$ of 2 mg/L is considered appropriate for intravenous CMS regimens, especially in view of the known link between inadequate initial antibiotic therapy and clinical outcome.[134–136] Thus, there is substantial overlap in the plasma concentrations associated with the desired and undesired effects of the drug; it is very clear that colistin is an antibiotic with a very narrow therapeutic window. It is important to note that, in murine models, infections in the lung were substantially less responsive to systemic administration of colistin than those in the thigh.[117] Although a plasma colistin $C_{ss,avg}$ target of 2 mg/L for intravenous CMS regimens might be suboptimal for lower respiratory tract infections, it should be considered as a maximum tolerable exposure owing to concerns around risk of nephrotoxicity.[116,131]

Designing an intravenous dosage regimen to achieve a desired target plasma colistin concentration requires knowledge of the PK of the administered inactive prodrug (CMS) and the active entity, colistin, that is, subsequently formed within the patient. After initiating CMS therapy in critically ill patients, plasma colistin concentrations have been reported to increase slowly over many hours or even days,[137–140] although more rapid increases have also been reported.[141] This variability in the rate of formation of colistin may be caused by brand-to-brand or even batch-to-batch variability in the composition of parenteral CMS.[7,110] It is expected that the case for a loading dose would be greatest for a brand or batch that undergoes slow conversion. Unfortunately, there is no a priori way of knowing the rate of in vivo conversion for a particular batch. Thus, there is a general recommendation in recently promulgated international consensus polymyxin guidelines that intravenous CMS regimens commence with a loading dose.[116]

Clinical studies conducted over the first one and one-half decades of this century revealed that the daily maintenance dose of intravenous CMS required to sustain a desired plasma colistin $C_{ss,avg}$ is determined by the renal function of the patient.[131,139,140] Even though colistin is excreted in urine to only a small extent, the prodrug CMS has a high renal clearance.[109,142] Two major PK outcomes arise from these characteristics. Firstly, in a patient with good kidney function, only approximately 20% of each dose of CMS is converted to colistin. This conversion occurs because the rate of renal clearance of the prodrug is substantially greater than the conversion clearance of CMS to colistin. Second, in patients with diminished renal function, the excretion of CMS by the kidney is decreased and a greater fraction of each administered dose of CMS is available within the body for conversion to colistin.[109,112,131] This factor means that the apparent clearance of formed colistin depends on renal function. The corresponding clinical outcomes of this PK behavior are as follows. First, in patients with a creatinine clearance of greater than 80 mL/min, only a small proportion of patients achieve a plasma colistin $C_{ss,avg}$ of 2 mg/L, even with a daily dose of intravenous CMS at the upper level of those approved by the US Food and Drug Administration and the European Medicines Agency.[131,139] This occurs because avid renal clearance of CMS decreases the proportion of each dose of the prodrug that is available for conversion to colistin. Substantial escalation of the CMS daily dose in an attempt to compensate for the diminished fraction converted is not an option because this strategy may increase the risk of colistin-associated nephrotoxicity. The international consensus guidelines indicate that a high creatinine clearance is a reason to consider active colistin combination therapy[116]; this is discussed elsewhere in this article. Second, the impact of renal function on the PK of CMS and formed colistin explains the need to decrease the daily dose of CMS in renally impaired patients who are not receiving renal replacement therapy,[131] as recommended in the international consensus guidelines.[116] CMS and formed colistin are efficiently cleared from the body by various forms of intermittent and continuous renal replacement therapy.[131,143–151] The consensus guidelines provide recommendations for dosage regimens of intravenous CMS in patients receiving different types of renal replacement, including supplemental doses in patients on intermittent dialysis.[116]

Clinicians should be aware that a very large degree of interpatient variability exists in the apparent clearance of formed colistin and, consequently, the plasma colistin $C_{ss,avg}$ achieved from the same daily dose of intravenous CMS.[131] This large variability is observed even among patients with similar renal function, possibly related to brand-to-brand or batch-to-batch variability across CMS parenteral products in the extent of conversion of CMS to colistin.[7,110] This factor complicates and renders difficult the clinical use of intravenous colistin, especially in view of its narrow therapeutic window. Therefore, although the use of dosage recommendations[116,131] is encouraged, whenever possible ongoing adjustment of the daily dose of CMS should be guided by measurement of plasma colistin concentration to enable therapeutic drug management (TDM).[110,116]

In regard to polymyxin B, fewer PK/PD and PK/TD studies have been undertaken to inform a target plasma concentration. Preclinical PK/PD investigations of polymyxin B against *P aeruginosa* in an in vitro dynamic model, and of parenteral polymyxin B against *K pneumoniae* in a murine thigh infection model, and intratracheal administration against *P aeruginosa* lung infection in mice showed that area under the unbound (free) plasma colistin concentration versus time curve across 24 hours/MIC was the most predictive PK/PD index of the antibacterial activity.[119,120,152] Parenteral administration of polymyxin B was ineffective against infection in the lung in contrast with the thigh.[119] A recent PK/TD meta-analysis of previously reported nephrotoxicity rates in patients treated with polymyxin B revealed a statistically significant linear relationship between the percentage of patients with a 25% or greater decrease in creatinine clearance during treatment and the predicted plasma polymyxin B $C_{ss,avg}$.[153] The $C_{ss,avg}$ associated with rates of mild nephrotoxicity ($\leq$25% decrease in creatinine clearance) in 40% or more of patients was estimated to be approximately 4 mg/L. On the basis of the PK/PD data for parenteral colistin against *P aeruginosa* and *A baumannii* in murine infection models,[117] assuming similar in vivo antibacterial effects of colistin and polymyxin B, and more recent PK/PD data for parenteral polymyxin B against *K pneumoniae* thigh infection in mice,[119] some experts have recommended a target therapeutic range for plasma polymyxin B $C_{ss,avg}$ of approximately 2 to 4 mg/L.[116,153]

The first reports on the clinical PK of intravenous polymyxin B since its resurgence in use this century were in 2008.[154,155] Subsequently, additional studies have been conducted to characterize the PK and explore potential patient factors that modulate the PK.[156–160] These studies have revealed the following key aspects. First, although the administration of a loading dose of polymyxin B may be less important than for CMS (because the former is not administered as an inactive prodrug), Monte Carlo simulations conducted as part of a population PK analysis indicated that a polymyxin B loading dose can decrease the time to achieve steady-state plasma concentrations.[156] Second, the clearance of polymyxin B is not influenced to a clinically important extent by the renal function of the patient,[156–158,160,161] in keeping with the very small proportion of each dose that is excreted in urine as unchanged polymyxin B.[155,156] This factor indicates that renal dose adjustments are not indicated for intravenous polymyxin B, which is contrary to the decades-old suggestion in the US Food and Drug Administration product label that the daily dose should be decreased in patients with impaired kidney function. Third, a very limited amount of PK data on the impact of continuous renal replacement therapy on removal of polymyxin B from the body suggest that extracorporeal clearance is very low relative to the residual natural clearance by the patient.[156,162,163] These findings informed the intravenous dosage recommendations in the international consensus guidelines.[116] Population PK studies indicate that the extent of interpatient variability in the clearance of polymyxin B is substantially less than that for colistin after the administration of CMS.[156,158] Nevertheless, because of the narrow therapeutic window, TDM and adaptive feedback control are recommended to guide intravenous dosing of polymyxin B.[116,153]

As noted elsewhere in this article, a major difference between polymyxin B and colistin is that the former is administered in its active form. Owing to the different formulations of the parenteral products of colistin and polymyxin B, the 2 products are considered pharmacokinetically as "chalk and cheese" rather than "peas in a pod."[112–114] In most clinical applications where intravenous administration is used, polymyxin B would be regarded as having superior clinical pharmacologic properties. For example, it is possible to more quickly and reliably achieve and maintain plasma concentrations that may be effective, even in patients with high creatinine clearance.[112,116] Both polymyxins have narrow therapeutic windows and, as discussed elsewhere in this article, TDM and adaptive feedback control are recommended. Because of the stringent sample handling procedures required to minimize the ongoing conversion of CMS to colistin in collected plasma samples, TDM and adaptive feedback control are regarded as more feasible for polymyxin B.[110,112,153] In addition, clinical data that have emerged over the past decade suggest that the risk of nephrotoxicity may be lower with polymyxin B than CMS,[164–170] although as reviewed elsewhere some of these studies may have been subject to bias.[115] For these reasons, a recommendation of the international consensus guidelines is that polymyxin B is the preferred agent for routine systemic use in invasive infections.[116] It is further recommended that clinicians have access to parenteral products of both CMS and polymyxin B, as there are some circumstances where CMS may be the preferred agent (eg, for treatment of lower urinary tract infection as CMS is extensively eliminated by the renal pathway and degrades to colistin within the urinary tract; intraventricular or intrathecal administration for the treatment of meningitis or ventriculitis because there is limited clinical experience with polymyxin B).[116]

Essentially, all studies that have examined the impact of polymyxin dosing modality on development of resistance have been conducted in laboratory-based experiments. A very common finding in studies conducted in in vitro PK and PD models is that with colistin or polymyxin B monotherapy dosage regimens at the upper end of clinically relevant exposures with intravenous administration, early bacterial killing of susceptible strains is followed by regrowth associated with amplification of resistant subpopulations.[171] In regard to possible impact of colistin or polymyxin B dosage interval, results from a study conducted using a 1-compartment PK/PD model that examined the effect of once-daily, twice-daily, and thrice-daily dosing of colistin on the emergence of colistin resistance in *P aeruginosa* suggested the 8-hourly regimen to be the most effective at minimizing emergence of resistance.[172] Similar observations were obtained for a study that investigated polymyxin B against *P aeruginosa* in a hollow fiber infection model.[120] These findings run parallel with current preclinical and clinical data that suggest it is prudent to divide the daily dose to minimize the risk of polymyxin-associated nephrotoxicity.[173]

Combination Therapy

Across the spectrum of infectious diseases, combination antimicrobial therapy has been used clinically for many years for 1 or more reasons that include achieving a synergistic or enhanced antimicrobial effect, preventing emergence or amplification of resistant populations, and decreasing the risk of toxicity by using lower doses.[174] These reasons underpin the substantial interest in using polymyxin combinations against gram-negative pathogens. There is abundant evidence from preclinical studies in in vitro PK/PD models and animal infection models that some polymyxin combinations can achieve enhanced antibacterial effect and suppression of resistance against strains of *P aeruginosa*, *A baumannii*, and *K pneumoniae.* Space does not permit presentation of the details of the many preclinical studies that have been conducted, and readers are referred to very extensive reviews.[171,175–177] Notwithstanding the evidence that has accrued from preclinical models for enhanced antibacterial activity and resistance suppression for some combinations against certain gram-negative organisms, the role of polymyxin combinations in patient care has been hotly debated. Indeed, the question of whether or not to combine a polymyxin with other antibiotics was the most contentious topic encountered by members of the committee that formulated the international consensus guidelines for the optimal use of the polymyxins. The reader is directed to the polymyxin guidelines for a comprehensive review on the strengths and limitations of the clinical observational studies and randomized controlled trials that have examined the efficacy of polymyxin combination therapy versus monotherapy.[116] This article focuses primarily on the evidence relating to resistance development.

Very few of the observational studies and randomized controlled trials that have examined polymyxin monotherapy versus polymyxin combination therapy have assessed the emergence of polymyxin resistance. Two randomized controlled trials, the first involving colistin combined with rifampicin and the second with meropenem, reported no difference in emergence of colistin resistance between monotherapy and combination therapy groups.[178,179] Such a finding may have been influenced by the use in those studies of MIC measurement methods other than the broth microdilution method approved by the Clinical and Laboratory Standards Institute and the European Committee on Antimicrobial Susceptibility Testing. More recently, broth microdilution was used to monitor emergence of colistin resistance in rectal swabs collected from patients in the above-mentioned colistin and meropenem randomized controlled trial.[180] In that study, only patients with colistin-susceptible infection site index cultures by broth microdilution were included. Rectal swabs taken on day 7 or later were evaluated for the presence of new colistin-resistant organisms and the emergence of colistin-resistant Enterobacteriaceae. Emergent colistin-resistant organisms were detected overall in 10.3% of the 214 patients included in the analysis. No difference was observed between patients randomized to treatment with colistin monotherapy (10/106% [9.4%]) versus patients randomized to colistin-meropenem combination therapy (12/108% [11.1%]; $P = .669$).[180] Colistin-resistant Enterobacteriaceae were detected overall in 7.2% of the patients available for analysis with no difference between the monotherapy (6/128% [4.7%]) and combination (12/121 [9.9%]; $P = .111$) treatment arms. Having acknowledged limitations of the study, the investigators concluded that meropenem-colistin combination therapy did not reduce the incidence of colistin resistance emergence in patients with infections owing to colistin-susceptible and carbapenem-resistant organisms.[180] More evidence from well-designed clinical studies is needed to assess the impact of polymyxin monotherapy versus combination therapy for resistance development.

In formulating recommendations on the use of polymyxin combination therapy, the international consensus guidelines committee considered the available clinical studies, most of which had focused on clinical effectiveness.[116] In addition, the committee recognized the abundant preclinical data demonstrating that polymyxin combinations can both enhance bacterial killing and decrease the emergence of polymyxin resistance.[171,175–177] Based on these considerations, the international guidelines committee reached the following consensus recommendation for invasive infections owing to CRE, *A baumannii* or *P aeruginosa*: intravenous polymyxin B or colistin should be used in combination with 1 or more additional agents to which the pathogen displays a susceptible MIC.[116] The committee had secondary recommendations for each of these organisms in the event that a second active agent to which the infecting organism displays a susceptible MIC is unavailable. Readers should consult the international consensus guidelines for further information on the recommendations concerning use of polymyxin combination therapy.[116]

Infection Control

Polymyxin MIC testing is typically performed only for XDR pathogens, and thus, most identified polymyxin-resistant pathogens are XDR and, as a result, patients often have already been placed in enhanced infection control precautions. As the polymyxins are last-line therapeutic options, polymyxin-resistant XDR pathogens represent an urgent threat, and an outbreak could lead to temporary closure of a hospital ward or floor. Patients colonized with polymyxin-resistant MDR or XDR pathogens should be managed as an infection control emergency and serious efforts should be made to prevent hospital spread of these pathogens.

In addition to standard precautions (eg, hand hygiene), enhanced infection control precautions for patients colonized with polymyxin-resistant MDR pathogens often involve contact precautions (ie, use of gowns and gloves and dedicated medical equipment, such as stethoscopes) and placement of a patient in a private room.[181,182] Extrapolating from experience in controlling CRE,[183] cohorting patients colonized with polymyxin-resistant MDR pathogens and when hospital resources permit, cohorting health care workers caring for those patients (so that certain health care workers care for colonized and/or infected patients only) are warranted in outbreaks or in hyperendemic settings. Active surveillance screening (eg, of rectal swabs for CRE), coupled with contact precautions, has been useful in containing MDR gram-negative pathogens, including CRE,[184] and could be used in a similar way to identify patients asymptomatically colonized with polymyxin-resistant MDR pathogens. Chlorhexidine bathing of patients has also been reported to be effective in decreasing the risk for spread of MDR pathogens.[184,185] Prevention bundles used to effectively control CRE have included active surveillance, contact precautions, chlorhexidine bathing, and cohorting of patients. A similar bundle of strategies would likely be effective in preventing the spread of polymyxin-resistant gram-negative pathogens.[184–186] A recent report by Ben-Chetrit and colleagues[187] showed that several interventions significantly decreased an ICU-related carbapenem-resistant *A baumannii* infection from 54.6 cases per 1000 admissions to 1.9 cases per 1000 admissions after the intervention. Their control program included sodium hypochlorite cleaning of contaminated ICU structures, use of a virtual boundary on each unit with conspicuous markings, and relatively positioned equipment in each patient's area.[187] Although decontamination was considered helpful in ICU management, a recent study indicated that selective digestive tract decontamination or selective oropharyngeal decontamination was not efficacious in the prevention of blood stream infections with antibiotic-resistant microbes, including colistin-resistant gram-negative bacteria.[188]

Antimicrobial Stewardship

Antimicrobial stewardship strategies are an important component of prevention strategies to limit the emergence of antimicrobial resistance among gram-negative bacteria.[189] Although avoidance of polymyxin use whenever possible will likely help to prevent the emergence and spread of polymyxin resistance, timely and appropriate use can have a positive impact on clinical outcomes. In some instances, when patients are at increased risk for infection owing to XDR gram-negative bacteria pathogens, empiric polymyxin use is warranted. Certain patient characteristics, such as a prior history of XDR gram-negative bacteria infection or admission from a long-term acute care center where XDR gram-negative bacteria pathogens are common, in addition to assessment of level of acute severity of illness, can help to identify patients who have an increased risk for life-threatening XDR gram-negative bacteria infection, and who might be appropriate candidates for empiric polymyxin therapy. Using formal clinical scores to identify patients at high risk for infection owing to an XDR pathogen and who is an appropriate candidate for empiric polymyxin therapy have, unfortunately, not been shown to be accurate or effective.[189] As an alternative and/or complement to empiric polymyxin therapy, rapid diagnostics can be used to more quickly identify XDR gram-negative bacteria pathogens and more rapidly implement polymyxin therapy.

Additionally, negative results from rapid diagnostic tests can be used to quickly discontinue polymyxins. If polymyxins are empirically prescribed, then rapid de-escalation should be practiced whenever possible to limit unnecessary polymyxin use. De-escalation is modification of empiric therapy (when appropriate) based on a patient's clinical status and available culture results.[190] Typically, de-escalation occurs at approximately day 3 of antimicrobial therapy. If patients have microbiologic data indicating that an XDR pathogen is not present, then more often than not, polymyxin therapy can be stopped. De-escalation can help to limit unnecessary polymyxin use and prevent both toxicity and emergence of polymyxin resistance. If a full course of polymyxins is needed to treat an infection, then the duration of therapy should be monitored and the shortest effective duration should be prescribed. Careful attention to the "day of polymyxin therapy," and to the patient's clinical response to therapy, can help to minimize the duration of therapy whenever possible, to avoid unnecessarily long polymyxin courses and to prevent the emergence of polymyxin resistance. In addition, with multiple newer agents now available for the treatment of XDR gram-negative bacteria, in many instances, when appropriate, use of these newer agents instead of polymyxins can often reduce nephrotoxicity, improve clinical outcomes and decrease selective antibiotic pressure leading to polymyxin resistance.

Finally, because the polymyxins represent a last-line therapeutic option, and resistance to these agents will in many cases leave clinicians with no viable treatment alternatives, the use of polymyxins for selective gut decontamination strategies for ESBL-producing organisms or other gram-negative pathogens, should be avoided. Multiple analyses looking at ESBL gut decontamination strategies with colistin showed both a failure to eradicate the ESBL-producing pathogens and even more concerning, an astounding increase in the rate of colistin resistance from essentially zero to greater than 50%.[84,85]

SUMMARY

Polymyxin resistance is a major public health threat, because the polymyxins represent last-line therapeutics for gram-negative pathogens resistant to essentially all other antibiotics. Minimizing any potential emergence and dissemination of polymyxin resistance relies on an improved understanding of mechanisms of and risk factors for polymyxin resistance, infection prevention and stewardship strategies, together with optimization of dosing of polymyxins (eg, combination regimens).

REFERENCES

1. Ortwine JK, Kaye KS, Li J, et al. Colistin: understanding and applying recent pharmacokinetic advances. Pharmacotherapy 2015;35(1):11–6.
2. Prevention CfDCa. Antibiotic resistant threats in the United States, 2013. 2013. Available at: http://www.cdc.gov/drugresistance/pdf/ar-threats-2013-508.pdf. Accessed March, 16, 2016.
3. Morrill HJ, Pogue JM, Kaye KS, et al. Treatment options for carbapenem-resistant enterobacteriaceae infections. Open Forum Infect Dis 2015;2(2): ofv050.
4. Velkov T, Thompson PE, Nation RL, et al. Structure–activity relationships of polymyxin antibiotics. J Med Chem 2010;53(5):1898–916.
5. Bergen PJ, Li J, Rayner CR, et al. Colistin methanesulfonate is an inactive prodrug of colistin against Pseudomonas aeruginosa. Antimicrob Agents Chemother 2006;50(6):1953–8.
6. Metcalf AP, Hardaker LEA, Hatley RHM. A simple method for assaying colistimethate sodium in pharmaceutical aerosol samples using high performance liquid chromatography. J Pharm Biomed Anal 2017;142:15–8.
7. He H, Li JC, Nation RL, et al. Pharmacokinetics of four different brands of colistimethate and formed colistin in rats. J Antimicrob Chemother 2013;68(10): 2311–7.
8. Hancock RE. Peptide antibiotics. Lancet 1997;349(9049):418–22.
9. Hancock RE, Chapple DS. Peptide antibiotics. Antimicrob Agents Chemother 1999;43(6):1317–23.
10. Velkov T, Roberts KD, Nation RL, et al. Pharmacology of polymyxins: new insights into an 'old' class of antibiotics. Future Microbiol 2013;8(6):711–24.
11. Cajal Y, Rogers J, Berg OG, et al. Intermembrane molecular contacts by polymyxin B mediate exchange of phospholipids. Biochemistry 1996;35(1):299–308.
12. Dixon RA, Chopra I. Polymyxin B and polymyxin B nonapeptide alter cytoplasmic membrane permeability in Escherichia coli. J Antimicrob Chemother 1986;18(5):557–63.
13. Vincent JL, Laterre PF, Cohen J, et al. A pilot-controlled study of a polymyxin B-immobilized hemoperfusion cartridge in patients with severe sepsis secondary to intra-abdominal infection. Shock 2005;23(5):400–5.
14. Nishibori M, Takahashi HK, Katayama H, et al. Specific removal of monocytes from peripheral blood of septic patients by polymyxin B-immobilized filter column. Acta Med Okayama 2009;63(1):65–9.
15. Deris ZZ, Akter J, Sivanesan S, et al. A secondary mode of action of polymyxins against Gram-negative bacteria involves the inhibition of NADH-quinone oxidoreductase activity. J Antibiot (Tokyo) 2014;67(2):147–51.
16. Mogi T, Murase Y, Mori M, et al. Polymyxin B identified as an inhibitor of alternative NADH dehydrogenase and malate: quinone oxidoreductase from the Gram-positive bacterium Mycobacterium smegmatis. J Biochem 2009;146(4):491–9.
17. Cheah SE, Johnson MD, Zhu Y, et al. Polymyxin resistance in Acinetobacter baumannii: genetic mutations and transcriptomic changes in response to clinically relevant dosage regimens. Sci Rep 2016;6:26233.

18. Henry R, Crane B, Powell D, et al. The transcriptomic response of Acinetobacter baumannii to colistin and doripenem alone and in combination in an in vitro pharmacokinetics/pharmacodynamics model. J Antimicrob Chemother 2015; 70(5):1303–13.
19. Maifiah MH, Creek DJ, Nation RL, et al. Untargeted metabolomics analysis reveals key pathways responsible for the synergistic killing of colistin and doripenem combination against Acinetobacter baumannii. Sci Rep 2017;7:45527.
20. Zhu Y, Zhao J, Maifiah MHM, et al. Metabolic Responses to Polymyxin Treatment in Acinetobacter baumannii ATCC 19606: integrating transcriptomics and metabolomics with genome-scale metabolic modeling. mSystems 2019;4(1). e00157-18.
21. Han ML, Zhu Y, Creek DJ, et al. Comparative metabolomics and transcriptomics reveal multiple pathways associated with polymyxin killing in pseudomonas aeruginosa. mSystems 2019;4(1). e00149-18.
22. Basu S, Radziejewska-Lebrecht J, Mayer H. Lipopolysaccharide of Providencia rettgeri. Chemical studies and taxonomical implications. Arch Microbiol 1986; 144(3):213–8.
23. Boll M, Radziejewska-Lebrecht J, Warth C, et al. 4-Amino-4-deoxy-L-arabinose in LPS of enterobacterial R-mutants and its possible role for their polymyxin reactivity. FEMS Immunol Med Microbiol 1994;8(4):329–41.
24. Vinogradov E, Lindner B, Seltmann G, et al. Lipopolysaccharides from Serratia marcescens possess one or two 4-amino-4-deoxy-L-arabinopyranose 1-phosphate residues in the lipid A and D-glycero-D-talo-oct-2-ulopyranosonic acid in the inner core region. Chemistry 2006;12(25):6692–700.
25. Kline T, Trent MS, Stead CM, et al. Synthesis of and evaluation of lipid A modification by 4-substituted 4-deoxy arabinose analogs as potential inhibitors of bacterial polymyxin resistance. Bioorg Med Chem Lett 2008;18(4):1507–10.
26. Miller AK, Brannon MK, Stevens L, et al. PhoQ mutations promote lipid A modification and polymyxin resistance of Pseudomonas aeruginosa found in colistin-treated cystic fibrosis patients. Antimicrob Agents Chemother 2011;55(12): 5761–9.
27. Breazeale SD, Ribeiro AA, McClerren AL, et al. A formyltransferase required for polymyxin resistance in Escherichia coli and the modification of lipid A with 4-Amino-4-deoxy-L-arabinose. Identification and function oF UDP-4-deoxy-4-formamido-L-arabinose. J Biol Chem 2005;280(14):14154–67.
28. Gunn JS, Lim KB, Krueger J, et al. PmrA-PmrB-regulated genes necessary for 4-aminoarabinose lipid A modification and polymyxin resistance. Mol Microbiol 1998;27(6):1171–82.
29. McPhee JB, Lewenza S, Hancock RE. Cationic antimicrobial peptides activate a two-component regulatory system, PmrA-PmrB, that regulates resistance to polymyxin B and cationic antimicrobial peptides in Pseudomonas aeruginosa. Mol Microbiol 2003;50(1):205–17.
30. McPhee JB, Bains M, Winsor G, et al. Contribution of the PhoP-PhoQ and PmrA-PmrB two-component regulatory systems to Mg2+-induced gene regulation in Pseudomonas aeruginosa. J Bacteriol 2006;188(11):3995–4006.
31. Olaitan AO, Morand S, Rolain JM. Mechanisms of polymyxin resistance: acquired and intrinsic resistance in bacteria. Front Microbiol 2014;5:643.
32. Nowicki EM, O'Brien JP, Brodbelt JS, et al. Extracellular zinc induces phosphoethanolamine addition to Pseudomonas aeruginosa lipid A via the ColRS two-component system. Mol Microbiol 2015;97(1):166–78.

33. Han ML, Velkov T, Zhu Y, et al. Polymyxin-induced lipid A deacylation in pseudomonas aeruginosa perturbs polymyxin penetration and confers high-level resistance. ACS Chem Biol 2018;13(1):121–30.
34. Adams MD, Nickel GC, Bajaksouzian S, et al. Resistance to colistin in Acinetobacter baumannii associated with mutations in the PmrAB two-component system. Antimicrob Agents Chemother 2009;53(9):3628–34.
35. Pelletier MR, Casella LG, Jones JW, et al. Unique structural modifications are present in the lipopolysaccharide from colistin-resistant strains of Acinetobacter baumannii. Antimicrob Agents Chemother 2013;57(10):4831–40.
36. Moffatt JH, Harper M, Harrison P, et al. Colistin resistance in Acinetobacter baumannii is mediated by complete loss of lipopolysaccharide production. Antimicrob Agents Chemother 2010;54(12):4971–7.
37. Henry R, Vithanage N, Harrison P, et al. Colistin-resistant, lipopolysaccharide-deficient Acinetobacter baumannii responds to lipopolysaccharide loss through increased expression of genes involved in the synthesis and transport of lipoproteins, phospholipids, and poly-beta-1,6-N-acetylglucosamine. Antimicrob Agents Chemother 2012;56(1):59–69.
38. Cannatelli A, Di Pilato V, Giani T, et al. In vivo evolution to colistin resistance by PmrB sensor kinase mutation in KPC-producing Klebsiella pneumoniae is associated with low-dosage colistin treatment. Antimicrob Agents Chemother 2014; 58(8):4399–403.
39. Jayol A, Poirel L, Brink A, et al. Resistance to colistin associated with a single amino acid change in protein PmrB among Klebsiella pneumoniae isolates of worldwide origin. Antimicrob Agents Chemother 2014;58(8):4762–6.
40. Olaitan AO, Diene SM, Kempf M, et al. Worldwide emergence of colistin resistance in Klebsiella pneumoniae from healthy humans and patients in Lao PDR, Thailand, Israel, Nigeria and France owing to inactivation of the PhoP/PhoQ regulator mgrB: an epidemiological and molecular study. Int J Antimicrob Agents 2014;44(6):500–7.
41. Cannatelli A, Giani T, D'Andrea MM, et al. MgrB inactivation is a common mechanism of colistin resistance in KPC-producing Klebsiella pneumoniae of clinical origin. Antimicrob Agents Chemother 2014;58(10):5696–703.
42. Pitt ME, Elliott AG, Cao MD, et al. Multifactorial chromosomal variants regulate polymyxin resistance in extensively drug-resistant Klebsiella pneumoniae. Microb Genom 2018;4(3):e000158.
43. Campos MA, Vargas MA, Regueiro V, et al. Capsule polysaccharide mediates bacterial resistance to antimicrobial peptides. Infect Immun 2004;72(12): 7107–14.
44. Llobet E, Tomas JM, Bengoechea JA. Capsule polysaccharide is a bacterial decoy for antimicrobial peptides. Microbiology 2008;154(Pt 12):3877–86.
45. Padilla E, Llobet E, Domenech-Sanchez A, et al. Klebsiella pneumoniae AcrAB efflux pump contributes to antimicrobial resistance and virulence. Antimicrob Agents Chemother 2010;54(1):177–83.
46. Liu YY, Wang Y, Walsh TR, et al. Emergence of plasmid-mediated colistin resistance mechanism MCR-1 in animals and human beings in China: a microbiological and molecular biological study. Lancet Infect Dis 2016;16(2):161–8.
47. Carroll LM, Gaballa A, Guldimann C, et al. Identification of novel mobilized colistin resistance gene mcr-9 in a multidrug-resistant, colistin-susceptible salmonella enterica serotype typhimurium isolate. mBio 2019;10(3):e00853-19.
48. Nang SC, Li J, Velkov T. The rise and spread of mcr plasmid-mediated polymyxin resistance. Crit Rev Microbiol 2019;45(2):131–61.

49. Poirel L, Madec JY, Lupo A, et al. Antimicrobial Resistance in Escherichia coli. Microbiol Spectr 2018;6(4).
50. Zhang H, Srinivas S, Xu Y, et al. Genetic and biochemical mechanisms for bacterial lipid A modifiers associated with polymyxin resistance. Trends Biochem Sci 2019;44(11):973–88.
51. Li J, Rayner CR, Nation RL, et al. Heteroresistance to colistin in multidrug-resistant Acinetobacter baumannii. Antimicrob Agents Chemother 2006;50(9): 2946–50.
52. Hermes DM, Pormann Pitt C, Lutz L, et al. Evaluation of heteroresistance to polymyxin B among carbapenem-susceptible and -resistant Pseudomonas aeruginosa. J Med Microbiol 2013;62(Pt 8):1184–9.
53. Poudyal A, Howden BP, Bell JM, et al. In vitro pharmacodynamics of colistin against multidrug-resistant Klebsiella pneumoniae. J Antimicrob Chemother 2008;62(6):1311–8.
54. Barin J, Martins AF, Heineck BL, et al. Hetero- and adaptive resistance to polymyxin B in OXA-23-producing carbapenem-resistant Acinetobacter baumannii isolates. Ann Clin Microbiol Antimicrob 2013;12:15.
55. Li J, Nation RL, Owen RJ, et al. Antibiograms of multidrug-resistant clinical Acinetobacter baumannii: promising therapeutic options for treatment of infection with colistin-resistant strains. Clin Infect Dis 2007;45(5):594–8.
56. Vidaillac C, Benichou L, Duval RE. In vitro synergy of colistin combinations against colistin-resistant Acinetobacter baumannii, Pseudomonas aeruginosa, and Klebsiella pneumoniae isolates. Antimicrob Agents Chemother 2012; 56(9):4856–61.
57. Beceiro A, Moreno A, Fernandez N, et al. Biological cost of different mechanisms of colistin resistance and their impact on virulence in Acinetobacter baumannii. Antimicrob Agents Chemother 2014;58(1):518–26.
58. Hraiech S, Roch A, Lepidi H, et al. Impaired virulence and fitness of a colistin-resistant clinical isolate of Acinetobacter baumannii in a rat model of pneumonia. Antimicrob Agents Chemother 2013;57(10):5120–1.
59. Wand ME, Bock LJ, Bonney LC, et al. Retention of virulence following adaptation to colistin in Acinetobacter baumannii reflects the mechanism of resistance. J Antimicrob Chemother 2015;70(8):2209–16.
60. Lopez-Rojas R, Dominguez-Herrera J, McConnell MJ, et al. Impaired virulence and in vivo fitness of colistin-resistant Acinetobacter baumannii. J Infect Dis 2011;203(4):545–8.
61. Humphries RM. Susceptibility testing of the polymyxins: where are we now? Pharmacotherapy 2015;35(1):22–7.
62. Morrow BJ, Pillar CM, Deane J, et al. Activities of carbapenem and comparator agents against contemporary US Pseudomonas aeruginosa isolates from the CAPITAL surveillance program. Diagn Microbiol Infect Dis 2013;75(4):412–6.
63. Tunyapanit W, Pruekprasert P, Laoprasopwattana K, et al. In vitro activity of colistin against multidrug-resistant Pseudomonas aeruginosa isolates from patients in Songklanagarind Hospital, Thailand. Southeast Asian J Trop Med Public Health 2013;44(2):273–80.
64. Pogue JM, Jones RN, Bradley JS, et al. Polymyxin susceptibility testing and interpretive breakpoints: recommendations from the united states committee on antimicrobial susceptibility testing (USCAST). Antimicrob Agents Chemother 2020;64(2):e01495-19.

65. Control ECfDPa. Surveillance of Antimicrobial Resistance in Europe 2017. 2018. Available at: https://ecdc.europa.eu/en/publicationsdata/surveillance-antimicrobial-resistance-europe-2017. Accessed August 25, 2019.
66. Wi YM, Choi JY, Lee JY, et al. Emergence of colistin resistance in Pseudomonas aeruginosa ST235 clone in South Korea. Int J Antimicrob Agents 2017;49(6):767–9.
67. Mohanty S, Maurya V, Gaind R, et al. Phenotypic characterization and colistin susceptibilities of carbapenem-resistant of Pseudomonas aeruginosa and Acinetobacter spp. J Infect Dev Ctries 2013;7(11):880–7.
68. Schulin T. In vitro activity of the aerosolized agents colistin and tobramycin and five intravenous agents against Pseudomonas aeruginosa isolated from cystic fibrosis patients in southwestern Germany. J Antimicrob Chemother 2002;49(2):403–6.
69. Yau W, Owen RJ, Poudyal A, et al. Colistin hetero-resistance in multidrug-resistant Acinetobacter baumannii clinical isolates from the Western Pacific region in the SENTRY antimicrobial surveillance programme. J Infect 2009;58(2):138–44.
70. Gales AC, Jones RN, Sader HS. Global assessment of the antimicrobial activity of polymyxin B against 54 731 clinical isolates of Gram-negative bacilli: report from the SENTRY antimicrobial surveillance programme (2001-2004). Clin Microbiol Infect 2006;12(4):315–21.
71. Gales AC, Reis AO, Jones RN. Contemporary assessment of antimicrobial susceptibility testing methods for polymyxin B and colistin: review of available interpretative criteria and quality control guidelines. J Clin Microbiol 2001;39(1):183–90.
72. Cai Y, Chai D, Wang R, et al. Colistin resistance of Acinetobacter baumannii: clinical reports, mechanisms and antimicrobial strategies. J Antimicrob Chemother 2012;67(7):1607–15.
73. Dobrewski R, Savov E, Bernards AT, et al. Genotypic diversity and antibiotic susceptibility of Acinetobacter baumannii isolates in a Bulgarian hospital. Clin Microbiol Infect 2006;12(11):1135–7.
74. Ko KS, Suh JY, Kwon KT, et al. High rates of resistance to colistin and polymyxin B in subgroups of Acinetobacter baumannii isolates from Korea. J Antimicrob Chemother 2007;60(5):1163–7.
75. Arroyo LA, Garcia-Curiel A, Pachon-Ibanez ME, et al. Reliability of the E-test method for detection of colistin resistance in clinical isolates of Acinetobacter baumannii. J Clin Microbiol 2005;43(2):903–5.
76. Arroyo LA, Mateos I, Gonzalez V, et al. In vitro activities of tigecycline, minocycline, and colistin-tigecycline combination against multi- and pandrug-resistant clinical isolates of Acinetobacter baumannii group. Antimicrob Agents Chemother 2009;53(3):1295–6.
77. Baadani AM, Thawadi SI, El-Khizzi NA, et al. Prevalence of colistin and tigecycline resistance in Acinetobacter baumannii clinical isolates from 2 hospitals in Riyadh Region over a 2-year period. Saudi Med J 2013;34(3):248–53.
78. Munoz-Price LS, Poirel L, Bonomo RA, et al. Clinical epidemiology of the global expansion of Klebsiella pneumoniae carbapenemases. Lancet Infect Dis 2013;13(9):785–96.
79. Giani T, Arena F, Vaggelli G, et al. Large nosocomial outbreak of colistin-resistant, carbapenemase-producing klebsiella pneumoniae traced to clonal expansion of an mgrB deletion mutant. J Clin Microbiol 2015;53(10):3341–4.

80. Abdallah M, Olafisoye O, Cortes C, et al. Rise and fall of KPC-producing Klebsiella pneumoniae in New York City. J Antimicrob Chemother 2016;71(10):2945–8.
81. Ah YM, Kim AJ, Lee JY. Colistin resistance in Klebsiella pneumoniae. Int J Antimicrob Agents 2014;44(1):8–15.
82. Neonakis IK, Samonis G, Messaritakis H, et al. Resistance status and evolution trends of Klebsiella pneumoniae isolates in a university hospital in Greece: ineffectiveness of carbapenems and increasing resistance to colistin. Chemotherapy 2010;56(6):448–52.
83. Kontopidou F, Plachouras D, Papadomichelakis E, et al. Colonization and infection by colistin-resistant Gram-negative bacteria in a cohort of critically ill patients. Clin Microbiol Infect 2011;17(11):E9–11.
84. Strenger V, Gschliesser T, Grisold A, et al. Orally administered colistin leads to colistin-resistant intestinal flora and fails to prevent faecal colonisation with extended-spectrum beta-lactamase-producing enterobacteria in hospitalised newborns. Int J Antimicrob Agents 2011;37(1):67–9.
85. Halaby T, Al Naiemi N, Kluytmans J, et al. Emergence of colistin resistance in Enterobacteriaceae after the introduction of selective digestive tract decontamination in an intensive care unit. Antimicrob Agents Chemother 2013;57(7):3224–9.
86. Meletis G, Tzampaz E, Sianou E, et al. Colistin heteroresistance in carbapenemase-producing Klebsiella pneumoniae. J Antimicrob Chemother 2011;66(4):946–7.
87. Samonis G, Maraki S, Karageorgopoulos DE, et al. Synergy of fosfomycin with carbapenems, colistin, netilmicin, and tigecycline against multidrug-resistant Klebsiella pneumoniae, Escherichia coli, and Pseudomonas aeruginosa clinical isolates. Eur J Clin Microbiol Infect Dis 2012;31(5):695–701.
88. Souli M, Galani I, Antoniadou A, et al. An outbreak of infection due to beta-Lactamase Klebsiella pneumoniae Carbapenemase 2-producing K. pneumoniae in a Greek University Hospital: molecular characterization, epidemiology, and outcomes. Clin Infect Dis 2010;50(3):364–73.
89. Souli M, Kontopidou FV, Papadomichelakis E, et al. Clinical experience of serious infections caused by Enterobacteriaceae producing VIM-1 metallo-beta-lactamase in a Greek University Hospital. Clin Infect Dis 2008;46(6):847–54.
90. Papadimitriou-Olivgeris M, Christofidou M, Fligou F, et al. The role of colonization pressure in the dissemination of colistin or tigecycline resistant KPC-producing Klebsiella pneumoniae in critically ill patients. Infection 2014;42(5):883–90.
91. Sampaio JL, Gales AC. Antimicrobial resistance in Enterobacteriaceae in Brazil: focus on beta-lactams and polymyxins. Braz J Microbiol 2016;47(Suppl 1):31–7.
92. Monaco M, Giani T, Raffone M, et al. Colistin resistance superimposed to endemic carbapenem-resistant Klebsiella pneumoniae: a rapidly evolving problem in Italy, November 2013 to April 2014. Euro Surveill 2014;19(42):20939.
93. Moubareck CA, Mouftah SF, Pal T, et al. Clonal emergence of Klebsiella pneumoniae ST14 co-producing OXA-48-type and NDM carbapenemases with high rate of colistin resistance in Dubai, United Arab Emirates. Int J Antimicrob Agents 2018;52(1):90–5.
94. Yong D, Toleman MA, Giske CG, et al. Characterization of a new metallo-beta-lactamase gene, bla(NDM-1), and a novel erythromycin esterase gene carried on a unique genetic structure in Klebsiella pneumoniae sequence type 14 from India. Antimicrob Agents Chemother 2009;53(12):5046–54.

95. Cui X, Zhang H, Du H. Carbapenemases in enterobacteriaceae: detection and antimicrobial therapy. Front Microbiol 2019;10:1823.
96. Malchione MD, Torres LM, Hartley DM, et al. Carbapenem and colistin resistance in Enterobacteriaceae in Southeast Asia: review and mapping of emerging and overlapping challenges. Int J Antimicrob Agents 2019;54(4): 381–99.
97. Edelstein MV, Skleenova EN, Shevchenko OV, et al. Spread of extensively resistant VIM-2-positive ST235 Pseudomonas aeruginosa in Belarus, Kazakhstan, and Russia: a longitudinal epidemiological and clinical study. Lancet Infect Dis 2013;13(10):867–76.
98. Emami A, Pirbonyeh N, Keshavarzi A, et al. Evaluation of the Saliva of Burn ICU patients for resistant bacteria harbor metallo-beta-lactamase genes. J Burn Care Res 2020;41(3):647–51.
99. van Duin D, Doi Y. The global epidemiology of carbapenemase-producing Enterobacteriaceae. Virulence 2017;8(4):460–9.
100. Woodworth KR, Walters MS, Weiner LM, et al. Vital signs: containment of novel multidrug-resistant organisms and resistance mechanisms - United States, 2006-2017. MMWR Morb Mortal Wkly Rep 2018;67(13):396–401.
101. Poirel L, Heritier C, Tolun V, et al. Emergence of oxacillinase-mediated resistance to imipenem in Klebsiella pneumoniae. Antimicrob Agents Chemother 2004;48(1):15–22.
102. Karlowsky JA, Lob SH, Kazmierczak KM, et al. In vitro activity of imipenem against carbapenemase-positive enterobacteriaceae isolates collected by the SMART Global Surveillance Program from 2008 to 2014. J Clin Microbiol 2017;55(6):1638–49.
103. Pitout JDD, Peirano G, Kock MM, et al. The Global Ascendency of OXA-48-type carbapenemases. Clin Microbiol Rev 2019;33(1). e00102-19.
104. Bradford PA, Kazmierczak KM, Biedenbach DJ, et al. Correlation of beta-Lactamase Production and Colistin Resistance among Enterobacteriaceae Isolates from a Global Surveillance Program. Antimicrob Agents Chemother 2015; 60(3):1385–92.
105. Oikonomou O, Sarrou S, Papagiannitsis CC, et al. Rapid dissemination of colistin and carbapenem resistant Acinetobacter baumannii in Central Greece: mechanisms of resistance, molecular identification and epidemiological data. BMC Infect Dis 2015;15:559.
106. Qureshi ZA, Hittle LE, O'Hara JA, et al. Colistin-resistant Acinetobacter baumannii: beyond carbapenem resistance. Clin Infect Dis 2015;60(9):1295–303.
107. Li Z, Cao Y, Yi L, et al. Emergent polymyxin resistance: end of an era? Open Forum Infect Dis 2019;6(10):ofz368.
108. Meletis G, Oustas E, Botziori C, et al. Containment of carbapenem resistance rates of Klebsiella pneumoniae and Acinetobacter baumannii in a Greek hospital with a concomitant increase in colistin, gentamicin and tigecycline resistance. New Microbiol 2015;38(3):417–21.
109. Li J, Nation RL, Turnidge JD, et al. Colistin: the re-emerging antibiotic for multidrug-resistant Gram-negative bacterial infections. Lancet Infect Dis 2006; 6(9):589–601.
110. Nation RL, Li J, Cars O, et al. Framework for optimisation of the clinical use of colistin and polymyxin B: the Prato polymyxin consensus. Lancet Infect Dis 2015;15(2):225–34.
111. Barnett M, Bushby SR, Wilkinson S. Sodium sulphomethyl derivatives of polymyxins. Br J Pharmacol Chemother 1964;23:552–74.

112. Nation RL, Velkov T, Li J. Colistin and Polymyxin B: peas in a pod, or chalk and cheese? Clin Infect Dis 2014;59:88–94.
113. Kwa A, Kasiakou SK, Tam VH, et al. Polymyxin B: similarities to and differences from colistin (polymyxin E). Expert Rev Anti Infect Ther 2007;5(5):811–21.
114. Cai Y, Lee W, Kwa AL. Polymyxin B versus colistin: an update. Expert Rev Anti Infect Ther 2015;13(12):1481–97.
115. Zavascki AP, Nation RL. Nephrotoxicity of polymyxins: is there any difference between colistimethate and polymyxin B? Antimicrob Agents Chemother 2017;61(3):61, e02319-02316.
116. Tsuji BT, Pogue JM, Zavascki AP, et al. International Consensus Guidelines for the Optimal Use of the Polymyxins: endorsed by the American College of Clinical Pharmacy (ACCP), European Society of Clinical Microbiology and Infectious Diseases (ESCMID), Infectious Diseases Society of America (IDSA), International Society for Anti-infective Pharmacology (ISAP), Society of Critical Care Medicine (SCCM), and Society of Infectious Diseases Pharmacists (SIDP). Pharmacotherapy 2019;39(1):10–39.
117. Cheah SE, Wang J, Nguyen VT, et al. New pharmacokinetic/pharmacodynamic studies of systemically administered colistin against Pseudomonas aeruginosa and Acinetobacter baumannii in mouse thigh and lung infection models: smaller response in lung infection. J Antimicrob Chemother 2015;70(12):3291–7.
118. Bergen PJ, Bulitta JB, Forrest A, et al. Pharmacokinetic/pharmacodynamic investigation of colistin against Pseudomonas aeruginosa using an in vitro model. Antimicrob Agents Chemother 2010;54(9):3783–9.
119. Landersdorfer CB, Wang J, Wirth V, et al. Pharmacokinetics/pharmacodynamics of systemically administered polymyxin B against Klebsiella pneumoniae in mouse thigh and lung infection models. J Antimicrob Chemother 2018;73(2):462–8.
120. Tam VH, Schilling AN, Vo G, et al. Pharmacodynamics of polymyxin B against Pseudomonas aeruginosa. Antimicrob Agents Chemother 2005;49(9):3624–30.
121. Sorli L, Luque S, Grau S, et al. Trough colistin plasma level is an independent risk factor for nephrotoxicity: a prospective observational cohort study. BMC Infect Dis 2013;13:380.
122. Horcajada JP, Sorli L, Luque S, et al. Validation of a colistin plasma concentration breakpoint as a predictor of nephrotoxicity in patients treated with colistin methanesulfonate. Int J Antimicrob Agents 2016;48(6):725–7.
123. Forrest A, Garonzik SM, Thamlikitkul V, et al. Pharmacokinetic/toxicodynamic analysis of colistin-associated acute kidney injury in critically ill patients. Antimicrob Agents Chemother 2017;61(11):61, e01367-01317.
124. European Medicines Agency. Assessment report on polymyxin-based products. Referral under Article 31 of Directive 2001/83/EC. 2014. Available at: http://www.ema.europa.eu/docs/en_GB/document_library/Referrals_document/Polymyxin_31/WC500179664.pdf Last. Accessed October 14, 2019.
125. Nation RL, Forrest A. Clinical pharmacokinetics, pharmacodynamics and toxicodynamics of polymyxins: implications for therapeutic use. Adv Exp Med Biol 2019;1145:219–49.
126. Khan DD, Friberg LE, Nielsen EI. A pharmacokinetic-pharmacodynamic (PKPD) model based on in vitro time-kill data predicts the in vivo PK/PD index of colistin. J Antimicrob Chemother 2016;71(7):1881–4.
127. Tsala M, Vourli S, Georgiou PC, et al. Exploring colistin pharmacodynamics against Klebsiella pneumoniae: a need to revise current susceptibility breakpoints. J Antimicrob Chemother 2018;73(4):953–61.

128. Lin YW, Zhou QT, Cheah SE, et al. Pharmacokinetics/pharmacodynamics of pulmonary delivery of colistin against pseudomonas aeruginosa in a mouse lung infection model. Antimicrob Agents Chemother 2017;61(3). e02025-16.
129. Lin YW, Zhou QT, Han ML, et al. Elucidating the pharmacokinetics/pharmacodynamics of aerosolized colistin against multidrug-resistant Acinetobacter baumannii and klebsiella pneumoniae in a mouse lung infection model. Antimicrob Agents Chemother 2018;62(2). e01790-17.
130. Nation RL, Garonzik SM, Li J, et al. Updated US and European dose recommendations for intravenous colistin: how do they perform? Clin Infect Dis 2016;62(5): 552–8.
131. Nation RL, Garonzik SM, Thamlikitkul V, et al. Dosing guidance for intravenous colistin in critically ill patients. Clin Infect Dis 2017;64(5):565–71.
132. Mouton JW, Meletiadis J, Voss A, et al. Variation of MIC measurements: the contribution of strain and laboratory variability to measurement precision-authors' response. J Antimicrob Chemother 2019;74(6):1761–2.
133. Mouton JW, Muller AE, Canton R, et al. MIC-based dose adjustment: facts and fables. J Antimicrob Chemother 2018;73(3):564–8.
134. Kumar A, Roberts D, Wood KE, et al. Duration of hypotension before initiation of effective antimicrobial therapy is the critical determinant of survival in human septic shock. Crit Care Med 2006;34(6):1589–96.
135. Luna CM, Aruj P, Niederman MS, et al. Appropriateness and delay to initiate therapy in ventilator-associated pneumonia. Eur Respir J 2006;27(1):158–64.
136. Kumar A, Ellis P, Arabi Y, et al. Initiation of inappropriate antimicrobial therapy results in a fivefold reduction of survival in human septic shock. Chest 2009; 136(5):1237–48.
137. Plachouras D, Karvanen M, Friberg LE, et al. Population pharmacokinetic analysis of colistin methanesulfonate and colistin after intravenous administration in critically ill patients with infections caused by gram-negative bacteria. Antimicrob Agents Chemother 2009;53(8):3430–6.
138. Mohamed AF, Karaiskos I, Plachouras D, et al. Application of a loading dose of colistin methanesulfonate in critically ill patients: population pharmacokinetics, protein binding, and prediction of bacterial kill. Antimicrob Agents Chemother 2012;56(8):4241–9.
139. Karaiskos I, Friberg LE, Pontikis K, et al. Colistin population pharmacokinetics after application of a loading dose of 9 MU colistin methanesulfonate in critically ill patients. Antimicrob Agents Chemother 2015;59(12):7240–8.
140. Garonzik SM, Li J, Thamlikitkul V, et al. Population pharmacokinetics of colistin methanesulfonate and formed colistin in critically ill patients from a multicenter study provide dosing suggestions for various categories of patients. Antimicrob Agents Chemother 2011;55(7):3284–94.
141. Gregoire N, Mimoz O, Megarbane B, et al. New colistin population pharmacokinetic data in critically ill patients suggesting an alternative loading dose rational. Antimicrob Agents Chemother 2014;58(12):7324–30.
142. Couet W, Gregoire N, Gobin P, et al. Pharmacokinetics of colistin and colistimethate sodium after a single 80-mg intravenous dose of CMS in young healthy volunteers. Clin Pharmacol Ther 2011;89(6):875–9.
143. Marchand S, Frat JP, Petitpas F, et al. Removal of colistin during intermittent haemodialysis in two critically ill patients. J Antimicrob Chemother 2010;65(8): 1836–7.

144. Markou N, Fousteri M, Markantonis SL, et al. Colistin pharmacokinetics in intensive care unit patients on continuous venovenous haemodiafiltration: an observational study. J Antimicrob Chemother 2012;67(10):2459–62.
145. Karvanen M, Plachouras D, Friberg LE, et al. Colistin methanesulfonate and colistin pharmacokinetics in critically ill patients receiving continuous venovenous hemodiafiltration. Antimicrob Agents Chemother 2013;57(1):668–71.
146. Luque S, Sorli L, Li J, et al. Effective removal of colistin methanesulphonate and formed colistin during intermittent haemodialysis in a patient infected by polymyxin-only-susceptible Pseudomonas aeruginosa. J Chemother 2014; 26(2):122–4.
147. Mariano F, Leporati M, Carignano P, et al. Efficient removal of colistin A and B in critically ill patients undergoing CVVHDF and sorbent technologies. J Nephrol 2015;28(5):623–31.
148. Jacobs M, Gregoire N, Megarbane B, et al. Population pharmacokinetics of colistin methanesulphonate (CMS) and colistin in critically ill patients with acute renal failure requiring intermittent haemodialysis. Antimicrob Agents Chemother 2016;60(3):1788–93.
149. Karaiskos I, Friberg LE, Galani L, et al. Challenge for higher colistin dosage in critically ill patients receiving continuous venovenous haemodiafiltration. Int J Antimicrob Agents 2016;48(3):337–41.
150. Strunk AK, Schmidt JJ, Baroke E, et al. Single- and multiple-dose pharmacokinetics and total removal of colistin in a patient with acute kidney injury undergoing extended daily dialysis. J Antimicrob Chemother 2014;69(7):2008–10.
151. Leuppi-Taegtmeyer AB, Decosterd L, Osthoff M, et al. Multicenter population pharmacokinetic study of colistimethate sodium and colistin dosed as in normal renal function in patients on continuous renal replacement therapy. Antimicrob Agents Chemother 2019;63(2). e01957-18.
152. Lin YW, Zhou Q, Onufrak NJ, et al. Aerosolized polymyxin B for treatment of respiratory tract infections: determination of pharmacokinetic-pharmacodynamic indices for aerosolized polymyxin B against pseudomonas aeruginosa in a mouse lung infection model. Antimicrob Agents Chemother 2017;61(8). e00211-17.
153. Lakota EA, Landersdorfer CB, Nation RL, et al. Personalizing Polymyxin B dosing using an adaptive feedback control algorithm. Antimicrob Agents Chemother 2018;62(7). e00483-18.
154. Kwa AL, Lim TP, Low JG, et al. Pharmacokinetics of polymyxin B1 in patients with multidrug-resistant Gram-negative bacterial infections. Diagn Microbiol Infect Dis 2008;60(2):163–7.
155. Zavascki AP, Goldani LZ, Cao G, et al. Pharmacokinetics of intravenous polymyxin B in critically ill patients. Clin Infect Dis 2008;47(10):1298–304.
156. Sandri AM, Landersdorfer CB, Jacob J, et al. Population pharmacokinetics of intravenous polymyxin B in critically ill patients: implications for selection of dosage regimens. Clin Infect Dis 2013;57(4):524–31.
157. Thamlikitkul V, Dubrovskaya Y, Manchandani P, et al. Dosing and pharmacokinetics of polymyxin B in patients with renal insufficiency. Antimicrob Agents Chemother 2017;61(1). e01337-16.
158. Manchandani P, Thamlikitkul V, Dubrovskaya Y, et al. Population pharmacokinetics of polymyxin B. Clin Pharmacol Ther 2018;104(3):534–8.
159. Kubin CJ, Nelson BC, Miglis C, et al. Population pharmacokinetics of intravenous polymyxin B from Clinical Samples. Antimicrob Agents Chemother 2018; 62(3). e01493-17.

160. Miglis C, Rhodes NJ, Avedissian SN, et al. Population pharmacokinetics of polymyxin B in acutely ill adult patients. Antimicrob Agents Chemother 2018;62(3). e01475-17.
161. Kwa AL, Abdelraouf K, Low JG, et al. Pharmacokinetics of polymyxin B in a patient with renal insufficiency: a case report. Clin Infect Dis 2011;52(10):1280–1.
162. Sandri AM, Landersdorfer CB, Jacob J, et al. Pharmacokinetics of polymyxin B in patients on continuous venovenous haemodialysis. J Antimicrob Chemother 2013;68(3):674–7.
163. Baird JS. Polymyxin B and haemofiltration in an adolescent with leukaemia. J Antimicrob Chemother 2014;69(5):1434.
164. Oliveira MS, Prado GV, Costa SF, et al. Polymyxin B and colistimethate are comparable as to efficacy and renal toxicity. Diagn Microbiol Infect Dis 2009;65(4): 431–4.
165. Akajagbor DS, Wilson SL, Shere-Wolfe KD, et al. Higher incidence of acute kidney injury with intravenous colistimethate sodium compared with polymyxin B in critically ill patients at a tertiary care medical center. Clin Infect Dis 2013;57(9): 1300–3.
166. Phe K, Lee Y, McDaneld PM, et al. In vitro assessment and multicenter cohort study of comparative nephrotoxicity rates associated with colistimethate versus polymyxin B therapy. Antimicrob Agents Chemother 2014;58(5):2740–6.
167. Tuon FF, Rigatto MH, Lopes CK, et al. Risk factors for acute kidney injury in patients treated with polymyxin B or colistin methanesulfonate sodium. Int J Antimicrob Agents 2014;43(4):349–52.
168. Rigatto MH, Oliveira MS, Perdigao-Neto LV, et al. Multicenter prospective cohort study of renal failure in patients treated with colistin versus polymyxin B. Antimicrob Agents Chemother 2016;60(4):2443–9.
169. Vardakas KZ, Falagas ME. Colistin versus polymyxin B for the treatment of patients with multidrug-resistant Gram-negative infections: a systematic review and meta-analysis. Int J Antimicrob Agents 2017;49(2):233–8.
170. Crass RL, Rutter WC, Burgess DR, et al. Nephrotoxicity in patients with or without cystic fibrosis treated with polymyxin B compared to colistin. Antimicrob Agents Chemother 2017;61(4). e02329-16.
171. Lenhard JR, Nation RL, Tsuji BT. Synergistic combinations of polymyxins. Int J Antimicrob Agents 2016;48(6):607–13.
172. Bergen PJ, Li J, Nation RL, et al. Comparison of once-, twice- and thrice-daily dosing of colistin on antibacterial effect and emergence of resistance: studies with Pseudomonas aeruginosa in an in vitro pharmacodynamic model. J Antimicrob Chemother 2008;61(3):636–42.
173. Nation RL, Rigatto MHP, Falci DR, et al. Polymyxin acute kidney injury: dosing and other strategies to reduce toxicity. Antibiotics (Basel) 2019;8(1):24.
174. Turnidge J. Drug-drug combinations. In: Vinks A, Derendorf H, Mouton J, editors. Fundamentals of antimicrobial pharmacokinetics and pharmacodynamics. New York: Springer; 2014. p. 153–98.
175. Bergen PJ, Bulman ZP, Saju S, et al. Polymyxin combinations: pharmacokinetics and pharmacodynamics for rationale use. Pharmacotherapy 2015;35(1):34–42.
176. Zhang X, Guo F, Shao H, et al. Clinical translation of polymyxin-based combination therapy: facts, challenges and future opportunities. J Infect 2017;74(2): 118–30.
177. Bergen PJ, Smith NM, Bedard TB, et al. Rational combinations of polymyxins with other antibiotics. Adv Exp Med Biol 2019;1145:251–88.

178. Durante-Mangoni E, Signoriello G, Andini R, et al. Colistin and rifampicin compared with colistin alone for the treatment of serious infections due to extensively drug-resistant Acinetobacter baumannii: a multicenter, randomized clinical trial. Clin Infect Dis 2013;57(3):349–58.
179. Paul M, Daikos GL, Durante-Mangoni E, et al. Colistin alone versus colistin plus meropenem for treatment of severe infections caused by carbapenem-resistant Gram-negative bacteria: an open-label, randomised controlled trial. Lancet Infect Dis 2018;18(4):391–400.
180. Dickstein Y, Lellouche J, Schwartz D, et al. Colistin resistance development following colistin-meropenem combination therapy vs. colistin monotherapy in patients with infections caused by carbapenem-resistant organisms. Clin Infect Dis 2019. https://doi.org/10.1093/cid/ciz1146.
181. Wei W, Yang H, Liu Y, et al. In vitro synergy of colistin combinations against extensively drug-resistant Acinetobacter baumannii producing OXA-23 carbapenemase. J Chemother 2016;28(3):159–63.
182. Prevention CfD. Management of multidrug-resistant organisms in Healthcare settings 2006 2009. Available at: http://www.cdc.gov/hicpac/mdro/mdro_glossary.html. Accessed August 26, 2015.
183. Schwaber MJ, Lev B, Israeli A, et al. Containment of a country-wide outbreak of carbapenem-resistant Klebsiella pneumoniae in Israeli hospitals via a nationally implemented intervention. Clin Infect Dis 2011;52(7):848–55.
184. Hayden MK, Lin MY, Lolans K, et al. Prevention of colonization and infection by Klebsiella pneumoniae carbapenemase-producing enterobacteriaceae in long-term acute-care hospitals. Clin Infect Dis 2015;60(8):1153–61.
185. Schwaber MJ, Carmeli Y. An ongoing national intervention to contain the spread of carbapenem-resistant enterobacteriaceae. Clin Infect Dis 2014;58(5):697–703.
186. Goel G, Hmar L, Sarkar De M, et al. Colistin-resistant Klebsiella pneumoniae: report of a cluster of 24 cases from a new oncology center in eastern India. Infect Control Hosp Epidemiol 2014;35(8):1076–7.
187. Ben-Chetrit E, Wiener-Well Y, Lesho E, et al. An intervention to control an ICU outbreak of carbapenem-resistant Acinetobacter baumannii: long-term impact for the ICU and hospital. Crit Care 2018;22(1):319.
188. Wittekamp BH, Plantinga NL, Cooper BS, et al. Decontamination strategies and bloodstream infections with antibiotic-resistant microorganisms in ventilated patients: a randomized clinical trial. JAMA 2018;320(20):2087–98.
189. Pogue JM, Kaye KS, Cohen DA, et al. Appropriate antimicrobial therapy in the era of multidrug-resistant human pathogens. Clin Microbiol Infect 2015;21(4):302–12.
190. Kaye KS. Antimicrobial de-escalation strategies in hospitalized patients with pneumonia, intra-abdominal infections, and bacteremia. J Hosp Med 2012;7(Suppl 1):S13–21.

Resistance in Vancomycin-Resistant Enterococci

William R. Miller, MD[a,b], Barbara E. Murray, MD[a,b,c], Louis B. Rice, MD[d], Cesar A. Arias, MD, PhD[a,b,c,e,f,*]

KEYWORDS

- VRE • Vancomycin resistant enterococcus • VRE colonization
- Colonization resistance • Mechanisms of resistance

KEY POINTS

- Vancomycin-resistant enterococci are a leading cause of health care–associated infections.
- The emergence of resistance to most available antibiotics makes treatment a major clinical challenge.
- The sturdiness and genomic plasticity of vancomycin-resistant enterococci have led to the adaptation of a hospital-associated clade of *Enterococcus faecium* with multiple drug-resistance determinants.
- A healthy gastrointestinal microbiota can provide resistance to vancomycin-resistant enterococci colonization, but antibiotic use can disrupt this protective flora and leave vulnerable patients at risk for subsequent infection.
- New antibiotics with activity against vancomycin-resistant enterococci have entered clinical practice, but an understanding of the clinical role and mechanisms of resistance to these compounds is crucial to optimize their use.

INTRODUCTION

The genus *Enterococcus* consists of facultative gram-positive cocci that have been isolated from a variety of animals, plants, and environmental sources. Although 58 species have been described to date, *Enterococcus faecalis* and *Enterococcus faecium* are responsible for the majority of human infections.[1] These organisms are

[a] Department of Internal Medicine, Division of Infectious Diseases, University of Texas Health Science Center at Houston, McGovern Medical School, 6431 Fannin St. MSB 2.112, Houston, TX 77030, USA; [b] Center for Antimicrobial Resistance and Microbial Genomics (CARMiG); [c] Department of Microbiology and Molecular Genetics, 6431 Fannin St. MSB 2.112, Houston, TX 77030, USA; [d] Department of Internal Medicine, Brown University, 593 Eddy Street, Providence, RI 02903, USA; [e] University of Texas Health Science Center at Houston, School of Public Health, Houston, TX, USA; [f] Molecular Genetics and Antimicrobial Resistance Unit, International Center for Microbial Genomics, Universidad El Bosque, Bogota, Colombia
* Corresponding author. UTHealth McGovern Medical School, 6431 Fannin Street Room MSB 2.112, Houston, TX 77030.
E-mail address: Cesar.Arias@uth.tmc.edu

Infect Dis Clin N Am 34 (2020) 751–771
https://doi.org/10.1016/j.idc.2020.08.004
0891-5520/20/

frequently found as normal members of the gastrointestinal (GI) microbiota, but may become opportunistic pathogens, especially in the critically ill and immunocompromised patient population. Enterococci are known to cause a variety of infections, including skin and soft tissue infections, urinary tract infections, device infections, bloodstream infections, and infective endocarditis.[2] Taken together, from 2015 to 2017, enterococci were the second leading cause of health care–associated infections overall, as well as the leading cause of central line–associated bloodstream infections in long-term acute care hospitals and on oncology units.[3]

Complicating matters is the emergence of antibiotic resistance. Early experience in treating infective endocarditis with penicillin monotherapy revealed that a subset of streptococci (now known to be enterococci because the genus *Enterococcus* would not be formally established until 1984[4]) displayed an inherent tolerance to the action of this drug.[5] The advent of combination therapy with aminoglycosides improved cure rates from approximately 40% to 88%, at the cost of increased complexity and toxicity of the regimens.[6] As new therapies entered the clinical space, however, enterococci have responded with a diverse array of intrinsic and acquired resistance determinants that continue to present therapeutic dilemmas to physicians.

Vancomycin-resistant enterococci (VRE) have been identified by the Centers for Disease Control and Prevention as a serious threat, leading to at least 5400 estimated deaths and more than $500 million in excess health care costs annually, as of 2017.[7] Resistance to newer antibiotics, including daptomycin (DAP) and oxazolidinones, continues to emerge,[8] and microbiological and clinical data guiding the most effective use of these agents remains to be resolved.[9,10] Thus, an understanding of emergent mechanisms of resistance in enterococci can provide insights into the best treatment approaches for these opportunistic pathogens and help to guide the physician in making rational therapeutic decisions at the patient bedside.

FROM COMMENSAL TO A FORMIDABLE CLINICAL CHALLENGE

The origins of the enterococci can be traced back some 400 million years ago, to the appearance of the first terrestrial land animals.[11] It is likely that these ancestral enterococci emerged from the water in the GI tract of their hosts, because members of this genus are able to tolerate high concentrations of bile acids and possess a diverse set of genes involved in the metabolism of carbohydrates. To survive in this new environment, enterococci also developed a rugged adaptability, including a tolerance to elevated temperatures and high salt concentrations, and a resistance to killing by a variety of chemical disinfectants.[12] These same traits have enabled enterococci to colonize the human GI tract and survive in the modern hospital environment.

More recently, the beginning of the antibiotic era and the widespread use of antibiotics in clinical practice, animal husbandry, and agriculture has shaped the evolutionary trajectory of enterococci, particularly in relation to drug resistance. These factors have driven both the sequential emergence of *E faecalis* in the 1970s and then vancomycin-resistant *E faecium* in the late 1980s. Additionally, the selective antibiotic pressure has driven the continued evolution of resistance to newer antimicrobials.[13] Although β-lactam antibiotics have long been the backbone of therapy for serious enterococcal infections, it was observed that the minimum inhibitory concentrations (MICs) for these agents were at least an order of magnitude higher than those for streptococci, and combination therapy with aminoglycosides was needed to achieve a reliable bactericidal effect. Activity across classes of β-lactam antibiotics also varies, with the aminopenicillins (such as ampicillin) having the greatest potency, followed by ureidopenicillins, penicillin G, and imipenem.[14,15] Most cephalosporins, as monotherapy, have no activity. This intrinsic resistance can be traced, in part, to the penicillin-binding proteins (PBPs) which construct the peptidoglycan layer that surrounds the enterococcal cell. Functionally, PBPs can be divided into 2 classes. The type A bifunctional enzymes are capable of performing both the transglycosylation and transpeptidation reactions needed to elongate and crosslink peptidoglycan chains. In contrast, type B monofunctional transpeptidases catalyze only peptide crosslinking.[16] Both *E faecalis* and *E faecium* produce 6 PBPs, 3 class A and 3 class B, each of which have varying affinities for β-lactams.[17,18] The primary determinant of reduced susceptibility to β-lactam antibiotics is the low affinity class B enzyme PBP5 in *E faecium.*[19] This phenotype is conferred via a combination of factors, including alterations in PBP5 gene expression and a mosaic of changes in the amino acid sequence of the enzyme, which seem to influence the conformation of the active site and the resultant affinity for β-lactams.[20–22] The presence of the resistance alleles encoding PBP5 variants has been associated with hospital-adapted strains of *E faecium*, and may be one of several factors that allowed these isolates to thrive in the health care setting.[23]

The orthologue in *E faecalis* is PBP4, which is required for cephalosporin resistance but, in general, does not confer resistance to aminopenicillins.[17,24] Penicillin-resistant, ampicillin-susceptible *E faecalis*, as well as fully ampicillin-resistant isolates, have been described. The mechanistic basis for these resistance phenotypes seems to be related to amino acid substitutions, which remodel the PBP4 active site, and promoter mutations, which increase expression of the gene.[25,26] Ampicillin susceptibility may not reflect concomitant susceptibility to penicillin, piperacillin, or imipenem, and this assumption should be made with caution, especially when the latter compounds are used for treatment of deep-seated infections when isolates display elevated ampicillin MICs, although still within the susceptible range.[25,27]

Resistance to cephalosporins relies on the contribution of multiple proteins, though the full scope of this intrinsic resistance has not yet been elucidated. The presence of PBP4 (or PBP5 in *E faecium*) is necessary, but not sufficient, for elevated cephalosporin MICs, and the class B enzyme seems to work in concert with 1 of 2 class A PBPs (PonA or PbpF) to synthesize the cell wall in the presence of drug.[17] Additionally, 2 stress response systems, the CroRS 2 component system and IreK eukaryotic-like serine/threonine kinase, and MurAA (a cytosolic enzyme which catalyzes the first committed step in peptidoglycan biosynthesis) are required for cephalosporin resistance in *E faecalis*.[28–31]

Aminoglycosides are not usually active at generally achievable concentrations against enterococci as monotherapy, limited by poor uptake of the antibiotic into the cytoplasm. In addition, several commonly encoded aminoglycoside-modifying enzymes confer resistance to various clinically available aminoglycosides. These include the 6′-acetyltransferase AAC(6′)-Ii, which is an intrinsic property of *E faecium* and inactivates tobramycin, sisomicin, kanamycin, and netilmicin, and the acquired phosphotransferase APH(3′)-IIIa present in many clinical enterococcal isolates that mediates resistance to kanamycin and amikacin.[32,33] As a result, only gentamicin and streptomycin are reliably active for synergistic use with β-lactams, which became the standard of care for enterococcal endocarditis for many decades. The emergence of high-level resistance to the aminoglycosides gentamicin and streptomycin in the United States was first documented in 1983.[34] Isolates with high-level resistance, defined as growth in the presence of 500 μg/mL of gentamicin, or 2000 μg/mL of streptomycin, do not show synergism in combination with β-lactams. High-level resistance to gentamicin is most commonly mediated by acquisition of a bifunctional aminoglycoside-modifying enzymes, the AAC(6′)-Ie-APH(2″)Ia enzyme, although streptomycin retains synergistic activity in the presence of this enzyme.[35] In the case of streptomycin, inactivation by an adenyltransferase abolishes synergy, as do mutations in the 30S ribosomal subunit; the latter allow the translation of RNA despite extremely high concentrations (>128,000 μg/mL) of streptomycin.[36]

Given the differential binding affinities of the enterococcal PBPs to β-lactams, Mainardi and colleagues[37] noted that a combination of amoxicillin and cefotaxime was capable of saturating all major PBPs from *E faecalis* with a synergistic effect. Subsequent studies confirmed this synergism with the combination of ampicillin and ceftriaxone in vitro, and in a rabbit model of infective endocarditis.[38,39] These observations, and the increasing frequency with which high-level resistance to the aminoglycosides gentamicin and streptomycin was encountered in clinical isolates, eventually led to the clinical evaluation of dual β-lactam combinations for the treatment of *E faecalis* infections.[40] Of note, the limited in vitro data available for dual β-lactam combinations against ampicillin-sensitive *E faecium* indicated that only a few strains exhibited the synergistic phenotype (only 3 of 9 strains tested by time-kill curves).[41] Thus, the double β-lactam combination does not seems to be reliable for infections caused by *E faecium*. Further, some enterococcal isolates possessing a beta-lactamase have been described, and such strains may not be readily recognized by the clinical microbiology laboratory, because enterococci do not release enzyme into the extracellular environment, and resistance may only be apparent at high inoculum.[42]

As rates of high-level ampicillin resistance (>128 μg/mL) in *E faecium* became increasingly common, the glycopeptide vancomycin began to see increased use. Vancomycin binds to the terminal 2 D-alanine residues of the pentapeptide moiety of peptidoglycan, inhibiting the transglycosylation and transpeptidation reactions and leading to an arrest of cell wall synthesis.[43] Resistance arises via alteration of the terminal D-Ala-D-Ala, to either D-Ala-D-Ser (low-level resistance, 7-fold decrease in binding) or D-Ala-D-Lac (high-level resistance, 1000-fold decrease in binding).[44] The metabolic machinery needed to carry out this substitution are encoded on the *van* operons, named by convention after the gene encoding the amino acid ligase (eg, VanA, VanB). Intrinsic resistance among enterococci can be seen in *Enterococcus gallinarum* and *Enterococcus casseliflavus*, which carry the *vanC* operons (C1 and C2) on the chromosome and display low-level resistance to glycopeptides (MICs of 2–32 μg/mL).[45,46] Among clinical isolates, acquired vancomycin resistance owing to *vanA*, frequently found on the Tn*1546* transposon in association with plasmids, predominates. The *vanB*-mediated resistance has been associated with a different conjugative transposon (Tn*5382,* sometimes referred to as Tn*1549*), and is less common among clinical isolates of enterococci, although geographic variation of the circulating clones may influence local frequencies.[47–49]

Gene clusters coding for vancomycin resistance are common in nature, and the source of the *van* genes identified in current enterococcal isolates is likely a soil bacteria of the genus *Paenibacillus*.[50] The emergence of vancomycin resistance in clinical strains of enterococci was first reported in England in 1986, with resistance subsequently reported from other countries in Europe and the United States.[51] In Europe, VRE reservoirs were identified in livestock animals and in humans in the community. The niches of VRE were related to the widespread use of the glycopeptide avoparcin as a growth promoter in animal husbandry.[52] In the United States, avoparcin was not approved for agricultural use, and VRE were largely limited to the hospital setting, without widespread dissemination among healthy humans or livestock.[53] Subsequent to the ban of avoparcin use in 1995 in Europe, the frequency of VRE isolated from animals began to decrease, with data from Denmark showing a decrease in chickens from a peak of 72.7% at the time of the ban to 5.8% in 2000.[54] In contrast, in US hospitals, rates of vancomycin resistance have remained relatively stable, with approximately 80% and 7% to 10% of *E faecium* and *E faecalis* isolates reported as resistant, respectively, although the overall numbers of infections owing to VRE have decreases from 2012 to 2017, which is likely a result of infection control measures.[3,7]

MAPPING MULTIDRUG RESISTANCE

The advent of whole genome sequencing has led to further advances in the understanding of the population dynamics of enterococci and the spread of VRE. In *E faecalis*, older analyses using a multilocus sequence type–based strategy described a diversity of sequence types without a particular host specificity, because both human and animal isolates had a uniform distribution among the clonal complexes identified.[55] These studies also identified recombination as an important contributor to the evolution and population structure of *E faecalis*, and, unlike *E faecium*, did not point to the emergence of a specific hospital adapted lineage, although some hospital-associated clonal clusters were more likely to carry resistance determinants.[56,57] The initial genomic studies, although limited by the numbers of isolates studied, supported the observations that *E faecalis* lacks a distinct division into hospital adapted clades.[58] In contrast, a larger study of 515 isolates from primarily the UK and the United States identified 3 distinct lineages (termed L1, L2, and L3), which the authors postulated could represent hospital-associated lineages of *E faecalis*.[59] Approximately 90% of the vancomycin-resistant *E faecalis* identified in the study clustered into 1 of these 3 lineages, although the lineages themselves were a mix of vancomycin-resistant and -susceptible isolates. Strains belonging to L1 to L3 were also enriched for aminoglycoside, chloramphenicol, macrolide, and tetracycline resistance determinants, as compared with nonlineage isolates. Further studies, with a larger number of more geographically diverse isolates, will be needed to firmly establish the existence of hospital adapted lineages in *E faecalis*.

The population structure of *E faecium* is more clearly defined, likely owing to the importance of vancomycin-resistant *E faecium* as health care–associated pathogens and concomitant surveillance studies to track their spread. Typing of *E faecium* using multilocus sequence type suggested a number of strains from health care–associated infections formed a related group named clonal complex 17, although evolutionary relationships were difficult to resolve owing to high rates of recombination.[52] The initial genomic studies confirmed this broad division of *E faecium* into 2 distinct lineages, a hospital-adapted clade A and human commensal clade B.[60] Lebreton and colleagues[61] described a further split of clade A isolates into epidemic hospital isolates (clade A1) and strains of animal origin (clade A2), and using a molecular clock analysis placed the bifurcation of this line approximately 80 years ago, or around the time antibiotics were introduced into clinical practice. There is significant genetic diversity between clade A and clade B (average nucleotide identity of 93.9%–95.6%), suggesting that a speciation event may be ongoing, potentially driven by adaptation, and subsequent isolation, of clade A1 strains in the hospital environment.[58,62] Subsequent studies have continued to add isolates and refine the population structure, although the majority originate from the United States and Europe, and may not reflect the true global diversity of the species. A large study of clinical isolates from hospitals across the UK and Ireland, and a study from Latin America, were not able to resolve a distinct animal associated clade A2, suggesting that these isolates may have been early branching points of clade A whose distribution on the phylogenetic tree may be impacted by recombination events.[63,64] A subsequent study from the UK including more than 1400 *E faecium* genomes from livestock, wastewater, and human sources, supports the division into human commensal, animal-associated, and hospital-associated clades, and the authors noted limited transfer of genes and resistance determinants between strains of human and livestock origin.[65] Strains collected from wastewater treatment plants belonged to all 3 groups, highlighting the potential for strain to strain contact, and gene transfer, in this setting, and the need for effective sanitation in low-resource settings to combat the spread of resistance.

In addition to understanding the evolution of a multidrug-resistant pathogen, features of each clade may provide insight into GI colonization. Although strains from both clade A and clade B were able to establish persistent GI colonization when introduced individually in a mouse model, when given together, strains from the commensal clade B were able to outcompete those from the hospital-adapted clade A.[66] Thus, understanding the population structure and selective pressures driving the evolution of VRE can inform potential prevention and control strategies in the hospital setting.

VANCOMYCIN-RESISTANT ENTEROCOCCI AND THE MICROBIOME

The microbiota of the human GI tract consists of more than 100 cultivable species and many more that rely on symbiotic relationships with members of the larger microbial community or human host for growth.[67] Although well-adapted to the human GI tract, enterococci generally comprise a small fraction of the microbial diversity under normal conditions. These healthy microbial communities limit the ability of multidrug-resistant bacterial strains, such as VRE, to establish a foothold in the colon, a phenomenon known as colonization resistance.[68] Risk factors for VRE colonization include features that either directly or indirectly lead to disruption of the normal microbial flora, including antibiotic use, hospitalization, discharge to a long-term care facility, or dialysis.[69–71] Clinical studies evaluating the duration of carriage report a median time to VRE clearance after hospital discharge from 2 to 4 months, consistent with a reconstitution of the colonic flora, although prolonged carriage may result from continued perturbation.[71,72]

Recent investigations have begun to probe both the host and microbial mechanisms behind colonization resistance. From the host standpoint, defense of the GI tract relies on physical traits, such as stomach pH and the intestinal mucous barrier, as well as antimicrobial peptides (AMPs) of the innate immune system secreted into the luminal interior.[68,73] The GI tract of healthy individuals is largely composed of obligate anaerobes belonging to the *Firmicutes* and *Bacteroidetes*, which survive through the metabolism of carbohydrates from the host diet.[74] Restriction of this regular supply of dietary fibers, a situation that may occur in hospitalized or critically ill patients when enteral feeding is suspended or significantly altered, can induce the microbiota to turn to the host mucin layer for an energy source.[75] This phenomenon results in the thinning of an important GI-protective barrier, allowing pathogenic organisms to gain proximity to the host epithelium and potentially translocate into the bloodstream to cause disease. In the clinical setting, the loss of a diverse intestinal flora after antibiotic administration with subsequent domination by VRE was a precipitating event that predicted subsequent bacteremia in hospitalized patients with neutropenia.[76,77] The microbial community also influences immune mediated colonization resistance. AMPs such as RegIIIγ, an antibacterial lectin secreted by murine epithelial and Paneth cells with activity against gram-positive organisms including VRE, are produced via stimulation of Toll-like receptors by lipopolysaccharide from intestinal gram-negative bacteria.[78] In a murine GI colonization model, depletion of gram-negative commensals via the administration of broad-spectrum antibiotics promoted VRE colonization, a phenotype that could be rescued through exogenous administration of lipopolysaccharide.[79]

Microbial communities in the intestinal lumen can also provide protection against VRE colonization independent of the influence on host response. A high relative abundance of the genus *Barnesiella* was associated with a resistance to domination of the murine microbiota by VRE, even in mouse knockout strains deficient in the signaling mediators necessary for activation of the innate immune response and production of AMPs such as RegIIIγ.[80] Moreover, patients who developed VRE colonization after allogeneic-hematopoietic stem cell transplantation were more likely to have lower levels of anaerobic *Barnesiella* in the pretransplant microbiota, suggesting a role for this genus in preventing VRE domination in the clinical setting, although the specific mechanism of this effect is not known.[80] In addition, some members of the microbiota are able to produce compounds with a direct inhibitory effect on VRE. Bacteriocins are a class of bacterial derived AMPs that can have narrow or broad range activity against other bacterial species and may be involved in competition for resources in an ecological niche.[81] Commensal strains of *E faecalis* carrying a pheromone-responsive plasmid defective for conjugation encoding the enterococcal Bacteriocin-21 were able to colonize and clear the GI tract of mice dominated by VRE.[82]

Highlighting the complexity of the interactions leading to microbiota derived colonization resistance, the anaerobic commensal, *Blautia producta*, was found to produce a novel lantibiotic with similarities to nisin capable of killing VRE in vitro, but was unable to provide protection in the mouse intestine when given by itself.[83] A synergistic consortium of 4 different bacterial species was required to prevent VRE domination in the GI tract of ampicillin-treated mice.[84] Production of β-lactamases by the gram-negative anaerobes *Bacteroides sartorii* and *Parabacteroides distasonis* provided protection for the ampicillin-susceptible *B producta*, whereas *Clostridium bolteae* was associated with engraftment and persistence of *B producta* in the perturbed colonic flora. Thus, commensal members of the microbiota play a role in colonization resistance, but even small changes from the pressure of broad-spectrum antibiotics can alter the balance needed for protection.

Adaptations by enterococci that promote intestinal colonization may also be tied to antibiotic resistance. Upon exposure to certain bile acids present in the mammalian GI tract, *E faecium* was observed to undergo a morphotype switch from distinct diplococci to long chains.[85] This phenotype was associated with an increase in biofilm formation (dependent on the activity of the autolysin AtlA) and colonic aggregation seen in the GI tract of VRE colonized mice. In a serial passage experiment designed to identify the genes that contribute to this phenotype, mutations were observed in genes encoding proteins of the LiaFSR and YycFG stress response systems, which have been implicated in resistance to DAP (a lipopeptide antibiotic similar to AMPs) in clinical enterococcal isolates (the see section on DAP resistance).[86,87] It is conceivable that mutations in genes modulating the cell envelope stress response, which could allow for increased survival in the face of host-secreted and microbiota-derived AMPs, may also prime intestinal pathogens to resist attack by antibiotics with similar mechanisms or bacterial targets. Indeed, DAP resistance in enterococcal isolates from patients without exposure to the drug has been reported,[88,89] although more research is needed to identify if exposure to host-derived AMPs can induce cross-resistance to currently used therapeutics.

ANTIBIOTIC RESISTANCE IN THE NEW MILLENNIUM

The intrinsic and ever-expanding repertoire of acquired resistance determinants in enterococci have necessitated the progressive development of new strategies to meet clinical needs. Despite the introduction of novel compounds with VRE activity, enterococcal infections in the setting of multidrug resistance remain a clinical challenge. Here, we provide an overview of the mechanisms of resistance to newer agents that are often used in treating severe enterococcal infections.

Daptomycin

DAP is a lipopeptide antibiotic with in vitro bactericidal activity against vancomycin-resistant *E faecalis* and *E faecium*. Indeed, DAP has become first-line therapy for VRE, in particular for *E faecium*.[90] DAP was originally isolated as a mix of natural products from *Streptomyces roseosporus*, and consists of a 13 amino acid peptide core with a fatty acyl tail made by a nonribosomal peptide synthetase complex.[91] In the active form of the drug, this cyclic core binds a calcium ion, leading to an amphipathic molecule with a positively charged surface and a hydrophobic tail.[92] DAP is then able to insert into the gram-positive bacterial membrane in a phosphatidylglycerol-dependent manner, in which the positively charged surface interacts with the negatively charged phosphatidylglycerol headgroups, and the hydrophobic tail anchors among the lipid acyl chains.[93] The next steps in the mechanism of action are more poorly understood, but the DAP-calcium complex seems to equilibrate and oligomerize across the outer and inner membrane leaflets.[94] Initial studies found that DAP treatment led to membrane disruption and ion leakage suggesting pore formation,[95] but this seems to be a late phenomenon in DAP-treated cells and likely is not the primary mechanism of action. Müller and colleagues[96] have shown that DAP is capable of rigidifying the bacterial membrane, sequestering fluid lipids and leading to the dissociation of membrane bound enzymes that are important for cell envelope biogenesis and peptidoglycan synthesis. The exact membrane or cellular target by which DAP exerts its bactericidal action is an area of intensive research.

DAP resistance arises in both *E faecalis* and *E faecium*, and although the genetic pathways implicated in resistance share similarities between the strains, the molecular mechanisms that underlie resistance seem to have important differences.[90] The unifying features of resistance to DAP involve 2 sets of mutations that work in concert to bring about high-level resistance to the antibiotic. The first involves changes in 2 component signaling systems that activate the cell envelope stress response (inducing tolerance to the antibiotic), and the second alters enzymes important for phospholipid metabolism and result in a full resistance phenotype. In *E faecalis*, these changes lead to redistribution of membrane phospholipid microdomains away from the division septum, potentially as a diversion tactic to protect the sensitive biosynthetic machinery located at the septum where cell division occurs.[97] In *E faecium*, major changes in membrane architecture are not observed in DAP resistant strains.[87] Instead, DAP resistance-associated mutations seem to influence the cell surface charge similar to the repulsion mechanism proposed for *Staphylococcus aureus*.

Three major 2-component regulatory systems have been implicated in enterococcal DAP resistance to date, including LiaFSR, YycFG, and YxdJK.[86,87,98] Using whole genome sequencing across a variety of DAP-resistant *E faecium* strains of clinical origin, the LiaFSR (for *L*ipid II *I*nteracting *A*ntibiotics) operon was implicated as the major pathway associated with resistance.[87] This system is conserved among medically important members of the *Firmicutes*, and consists of a sensor histidine kinase (LiaS), its cognate response regulator (LiaR), and a predicted transmembrane regulatory protein (LiaF).[99] In the presence of cell membrane stress, LiaS activates the system by phosphorylating LiaR, which induces oligomerization and increases its DNA binding affinity upstream of target genes.[100] DAP resistance is tied to mutations leading to changes in LiaR, which mimic phosphorylation, or alterations of LiaF, which seem to activate the system.[101,102] Clinically, these changes can have important consequences, because they may lead to tolerance (lack of bacterial killing, even at 5× the MIC of DAP) despite only minor changes in MIC (eg, from 1 to 4 μg/mL, previously in the susceptible category).[103] Indeed, the clinical failures of DAP have been associated with this scenario,[101] and isolates with DAP MICs in the 3 to 4 μg/mL range are associated with mutations in the LiaFSR system.[104]

Critical among the genes regulated by LiaR is an operon encoding 3 proteins, LiaXYZ, of which LiaX sits at the fulcrum of the enterococcal stress response. LiaX possesses 2 predicted domains, an *N*-terminal α-helical domain capable of binding DAP and the human cathelicidin LL-37 (a cationic AMP of the innate immune system), and a C-terminal domain of β-pleated sheets that seems to function in a regulatory role.[105] A frameshift mutation resulting in premature truncation of the C-terminal domain of LiaX obtained from an experimental evolution model of DAP resistance in *E faecalis* was sufficient to activate the LiaFSR response, bring about redistribution of phospholipid microdomains, and increase virulence in a *C elegans* model related to resisting attack by host AMPs.[105,106] Further, the purified *N*-terminus of LiaX was able to confer protection to DAP susceptible *E faecalis* strains, but not to strains lacking the response regulator LiaR or *S aureus*, suggesting a specific role for LiaFSR signaling in enterococcal DAP resistance.

The YycFG 2 component system is an essential regulator of cell wall homeostasis, known to be active in modulating peptidoglycan synthesis, cell wall remodeling and autolysin expression.[107] It seems to be the second most frequent pathway to DAP resistance in *E faecium*, and it is important to note that isolates with mutations in *yycFG* do not seem to demonstrate the same synergistic interaction between DAP and β-lactams (the see-saw effect), as is seen in LiaFSR-mediated DAP resistance.[87]

YxdJK is a 2-component system that controls a network of ATP binding cassette transporters involved in bacitracin resistance.[108] In *E faecalis* strains lacking the LiaR response regulator, a putative activating mutation of the YxdK sensor kinase was associated with an increased DAP MIC. Indeed, deletion of the YxdJ response regulator was sufficient to revert strains to DAP susceptibility.[98] In *E faecium*, the YxdJK system (ChtRS) has been associated with modulation of tolerance to the cationic disinfectant chlorhexidine.[109]

Lipoglycopeptides

The lipoglycopeptide antibiotics are built around a glycopeptide core similar to vancomycin, with the addition of a hydrophobic substituent that serves to anchor the antibiotic molecule to the target cell. Telavancin, dalbavancin, and oritavancin are the currently available antibiotics in this class, and there are significant differences in their activity against VRE.[110] The glycopeptide core of telavancin and dalbavancin binds preferentially to peptidoglycan precursors ending in D-Ala-D-Ala, and, as a result, they do not exhibit clinically significant activity against enterococci with *vanA*-mediated vancomycin resistance.[111] These agents may test susceptible against *vanB*-mediated resistance in vitro, because, similar to teicoplanin, they do not seem to be inducers of expression the *vanB* gene cluster. However, mutations may arise that lead to constitutive activation of the *vanB* operon and expression of resistance against these compounds.[112,113]

Oritavancin, in contrast, retains in vitro activity against VRE exhibiting both *vanA* and *vanB* resistance. This compound has an expanded set of interactions with peptidoglycan precursors, extending to the L-lysine in the third position of both the pentadepsipeptide and amino acid cross-bridge, which seems to increase its affinity for D-Ala-D-Lac.[114] In addition, the 4′-chlorobiphenylmethyl side chain allows for an increased binding affinity to lipid II, disrupts the transglycosylation reaction needed for peptidoglycan extension, and can compromise the membrane integrity of target bacteria.[115] The multiplicity of the modes of action for this compound lead to potent bactericidal activity. Despite these potential advantages, the optimal setting and dosing strategy for the use of oritavancin against VRE in clinical practice, especially in the setting of DAP resistance or treatment failure, remains unclear. Reduced susceptibility to oritavancin upon serial passage in the laboratory has been documented in both vancomycin-susceptible and -resistant isolates of *E faecalis* and *E faecium*, with MIC increases from 4- to 32-fold.[116] The mechanistic bases behind these increases are not well understood. Overexpression of the *vanA* operon, with the exclusive production of D-Ala-D-Lac termini, was associated with a 16-fold increase in the MIC.[117] Expression of *vanZ*, a gene encoding a protein of unknown function also present in the *vanA* operon and known to mediate teicoplanin resistance, was also able to independently increase the MIC of oritavancin by 8-fold.[117] Cross-resistance to oritavancin was also found to develop in 2 clinical *E faecium* isolates exposed in vitro to simulated exposures of DAP at 12 mg/kg.[118] Whole genome sequencing revealed changes in LiaS, the sensor kinase of the LiaFSR system, in 1 isolate, and a mutation in a bacitracin resistance transporter gene in the second isolate. Although further work is needed to characterize the contributions of these systems to increasing oritavancin MICs, these results suggest caution is needed when using oritavancin as salvage therapy for DAP-resistant VRE infections.

Oxazolidinones

Linezolid and tedizolid are the 2 clinically available compounds in the oxazolidinone class, and linezolid is the only antibiotic with US Food and Drug Administration approval for the treatment of VRE bacteremia. These compounds act at the bacterial ribosome, binding to the A site and preventing the docking of the aminoacyl–transfer RNA complex, thus inhibiting the synthesis of the polypeptide chain.[119,120] Tedizolid exhibits greater potency than linezolid, with MICs from 4- to 8-fold lower, owing to a hydroxymethyl modification of the oxazolidinone ring and a fourth D-ring moiety not present in linezolid.[121] Mutational resistance arises from changes in the 23S ribosomal RNA (rRNA) (most commonly the substitutions G2505A and G2576U) that alter the binding site for both antibiotics, leading to decreased affinity for the drug and higher MICs. Enterococci possess multiple copies of each 23S rRNA gene; thus, the number of mutated alleles present in a strain determines the ultimate efficacy of the drug, as the bacteria will have a mixed population of sensitive and resistant ribosomes.[122] Under selective pressure, resistant alleles may recombine to replace wild-type alleles in the genome, leading to progressively fewer ribosomes susceptible to inhibition and a loss of drug activity.[123] In the setting of recombination, this gene–dosage effect can lead to the rapid emergence of resistance. In a comparison of an *E faecalis* laboratory strain and its recombination-deficient mutant under linezolid selection, emergence of the first 23S rRNA mutation did not differ between the strains.[124] Subsequent mutations at alternate alleles, however, occurred in the wild-type strain 6 passages before the recombination-deficient mutant. The potential for the emergence of resistance in this manner may be a consideration when using oxazolidinones for VRE infections with a high inoculum. Resistance related to mutations in the genes encoding the ribosomal proteins L3 and L4 has been described in enterococci, although the specific contribution to the resistance phenotype is not known.[125] In other gram-positive cocci, changes in ribosomal proteins occur concomitantly with 23S rRNA mutations, and may represent compensatory mutations which mitigate a potential fitness defect.[126]

Transmissible resistance to oxazolidinones is more worrisome, given the potential for horizontal gene transfer to lead to the wide dissemination of resistance. Two main transmissible determinants of oxazolidinone resistance have been characterized, *cfr* and *optrA*, with a third *poxtA* recently described in a clinical methicillin-resistant *S aureus* isolate and animal isolates of enterococci from China and Tunisia.[127,128] Cfr, for *c*hloramphenicol-*f*lorfenicol *r*esistance, is an enzyme that methylates the adenine nucleotide at position 2503 of the 23S rRNA and leads to resistance to oxazolidanones in addition to phenicols, pleuromutilins, and streptogramin A. The gene was first isolated in Germany from *Staphylococcus sciuri* recovered from a bovine mastitis infection, in association with a plasmid that was transferable to *S aureus* laboratory strains.[129] The first *cfr*-positive clinical isolate of *E faecalis* was described in 2012,[130] and the gene has since been reported from both animal and clinical isolates recovered across the globe.[131] Although tedizolid exhibits lower MICs than linezolid against *cfr* positive strains in vitro, tedizolid showed decreased efficacy in a mouse peritonitis model against a strain of *E faecium* with *cfr(B)*, as compared with either linezolid or DAP.[132] Both *optrA* (*o*xazolidinone *p*henicol *t*ransferable *r*esistance) and *poxtA* (*p*henicol *ox*azolidinone and *t*etracyclines) encode proteins with homology to the ATP binding subunit of ATP binding cassette transporters, and seem to be associated with IS*1216* mobile elements.[133–135] Initially thought to be a part of a drug efflux system, it was later shown that this class of ATP binding cassette-F family proteins confer resistance via a mechanism of ribosomal protection.[136] As is implied by their name, each determinant provides protection against a different spectrum of antibiotics active at the ribosome, and, in vitro, *optrA* is associated with a greater fold-change in MIC for oxazolidinones. These genes seem to be widespread among animal enterococcal isolates, potentially linked to phenicol use in veterinary medicine. Although the *optrA* gene was the most commonly identified transmissible oxazolidinone resistance determinant in *E faecalis* strains resistant to linezolid from a wide survey of clinical isolates, the overall resistance mediated by these genes remains low.[131]

New-Generation Tetracyclines

Resistance to the tetracycline class of antibiotics is common in enterococci and is primarily mediated through one of 2 mechanisms, drug efflux via efflux pumps typically carried on plasmids (*tet*(K), *tet*(L)) and target protection at the ribosome mediated by genes on mobile elements such as Tn*916* (*tet*(M), *tet*(O), *tet*(S)).[8] The newer compounds to enter the market, including the glycylcycline tigecycline, the aminomethylcycline omadacycline, and the synthetic eravacycline, were designed to retain activity in the setting of common tetracycline resistance determinants, and offer potential options for the treatment of VRE infections. The agent with the most clinical experience, tigecycline, is approved for use in intra-abdominal infections and skin and soft tissue infections for vancomycin-susceptible isolates of *E faecalis*, and shows in vitro activity against VRE of both species.[137,138] Owing to low serum concentrations, this antibiotic has typically been used only for intra-abdominal infections or as a part of combination therapy in recalcitrant enterococcal bacteremia and infective endocarditis.

Resistance to tigecycline has emerged with clinical use. The primary mechanism of resistance appears to involve mutations in the S10 protein of the 30S ribosomal subunit.[139] These mutations cluster into an extended loop of the protein, which protrudes near the tigecycline binding site on the 16S rRNA, potentially leading to decreased access or binding to the ribosome.[140] Although tigecycline is a less efficient substrate for both efflux pumps and ribosomal protection proteins, the presence of the genes encoding both the *tet*(L) efflux pump and *tet*(M) protection factor was associated with resistance in clinical isolates of *E faecium*.[141] An analysis of gene expression suggested that both increases in transcription and an expansion of gene copy number were responsible for the phenotype. Further, in an experimental evolution model performed with *E faecalis* under tigecycline exposure in a bioreactor, antibiotic exposure led to the excision and amplification of *tet*(M) in association with a Tn*916* transposon, leading to an expansion of gene copy number and inducing high rates of conjugative transfer of resistance, as well as increased expression of *tet*(M), with the concurrent emergence of S10 protein mutations.[142] Thus, the proliferation of traditional tetracycline resistance determinants may play a role in the emergence of tigecycline resistance. Mutations in the *rpsJ* gene encoding the S10 protein, or in the 16S rRNA itself, also seem to influence the susceptibility of eravacycline and omadacycline,[143,144] and the role of these agents in the clinical treatment of VRE infections remains to be defined.

SUMMARY

Since the emergence of VRE in the late 1980s, clinicians have faced major challenges when treating patients infected with these problematic pathogens. Despite possessing a relatively low virulence potential, the intrinsic tolerance to common broad-spectrum antimicrobials and an enduring ability to adapt have allowed enterococci to leave behind their roots as a commensal of the GI tract and evolve into a leading cause of health care–associated infections. Unfortunately, the factors predisposing to enterococcal infections often leave the most vulnerable patient populations at the greatest risk. Innovation has brought new therapeutics with activity against VRE to the patient bedside, but this has not slowed the emergence of novel mechanisms of resistance. Thus, new strategies are needed to win the evolutionary arms race against these organisms.

A deep understanding of the molecular mechanisms of resistance may offer insights into how to disarm VRE. The identification of the 2-component signaling systems responsible for activating the stress response may allow for the development of new compounds, which block the adaptive response and resensitize resistant bacteria, breathing new life into currently available therapeutics. Research into the complex interactions of the microbiome can lead to prebiotics or probiotics that prevent colonization or restore a colonization-resistant flora after antibiotic treatment. The emergence of phage therapy may also permit developing therapeutic interventions capable of evolving alongside the pathogen itself. Until these novel options enter the clinical arena, it will be up to physicians to make the most efficient use of currently available drugs against these multidrug-resistant organisms.

CLINICS CARE POINTS

- For infective endocarditis due to E. faecalis, the authors suggest ampicillin plus ceftriaxone based on observational studies indicating similar efficacy to aminoglycoside containing regimens without associated aminoglycoside toxicity.
- For infective endocarditis due to vancomycin resistant E. faecium, the authors suggest a daptomycin containing regimen, though comparative clinical data are limited. It should be noted that in 2020 the Clinical and Laboratory Standards Institute (CLSI) revised daptomycin breakpoints for enterococci, with all isolates

of E. faecium with an MIC of 4 μg/mL or less categorized as susceptible dose dependent based on daptomycin doses of 8–12 mg/kg/day.

- Ampicillin susceptibility may not reflect concomitant susceptibility to penicillin, piperacillin, or imipenem, and this assumption should be made with caution, especially when the latter compounds are used for treatment of deep-seated infections when isolates display elevated ampicillin MICs, although still within the susceptible range.
- Mutations in stress response pathways (such as LiaFSR) can result in daptomycin tolerance, or lack of bactericidal activity, with only minor changes in MIC (e.g., from 1 to 4 μg/mL).
- Cross resistance to oritavancin has been seen in *E. faecium* isolates exposed to daptomycin in vitro, suggesting caution is needed when using oritavancin as salvage therapy for daptomycin-resistant VRE infections.
- While tedizolid exhibits lower MICs than linezolid in vitro against *E. faecium* strains with Cfr mediated oxazolidinone resistance, animal studies suggest this lower MIC may not always translate to greater efficacy against some Cfr positive isolates.
- Tigecycline should only be used as part of a combination therapy regimen for serious VRE bacteremia or infective endocarditis given the low serum concentrations of the drug.

DISCLOSURE

Dr W.R. Miller has received grants from Merck and Entasis Therapeutics, and honoraria from Achaogen and Shionogi. Dr B.E. Murray has received grant support from Theravance Biopharma, Paratek, and Cubist/Merck, and has served as consultant for Paratek. Dr L.B. Rice has served on data safety monitoring boards for Zavante Pharmaceuticals and VenatoRx Pharmaceuticals. Dr C.A. Arias has received grant support from Merck, MeMed Diagnostics, and Entasis Therapeutics.

REFERENCES

1. García-Solache M, Rice LB. The enterococcus: a model of adaptability to its environment. Clin Microbiol Rev 2019;32:1–28.
2. Miller WR, Arias CA, Murray BE. Enterococcus species, *Streptococcus gallolyticus* group, and leuconostoc species. In: Bennett JE, Dolin R, Blaser MJ, editors. Mandell, Douglas, and Bennett's principles and practice of infectious diseases. 9th edition. Philadelphia: Elsevier; 2020. p. 2492–504.
3. Weiner-Lastinger LM, Abner S, Edwards JR, et al. Antimicrobial-resistant pathogens associated with adult healthcare-associated infections: summary of data reported to the National Healthcare Safety Network, 2015-2017. Infect Control Hosp Epidemiol 2020;41:1–18.
4. Schleifer KH, Kilpper-Bälz R. Transfer of *Streptococcus faecalis* and *Streptococcus faecium* to the Genus Enterococcus nom. rev. as *Enterococcus faecalis* comb. nov. and *Enterococcus faecium* comb. nov. Int J Syst Evol Microbiol 1984;34:31–4.
5. Williamson R, Calderwood SB, Moellering RC, et al. Studies on the mechanism of intrinsic resistance to beta-lactam antibiotics in group D streptococci. J Gen Microbiol 1983;129:813–22.
6. Robbins WC, Tompsett R. Treatment of enterococcal endocarditis and bacteremia; results of combined therapy with penicillin and streptomycin. Am J Med 1951;10:278–99.

7. CDC. Antibiotic resistance threats in the United States, 2019. Atlanta (GA): U.S. Department of Health and Human Services; 2019.
8. Miller WR, Munita JM, Arias CA. Mechanisms of antibiotic resistance in enterococci. Expert Rev Anti Infect Ther 2014;12:1221–36.
9. Satlin MJ, Nicolau DP, Humphries RM, et al, CLSI Subcommittee on Antimicrobial Susceptibility Testing and Ad Hoc Working Group on Revision of Daptomycin Enterococcal Breakpoints. Development of daptomycin susceptibility breakpoints for *Enterococcus faecium* and revision of the breakpoints for other Enterococcal species by the Clinical and Laboratory Standards Institute. Clin Infect Dis 2020;70(6):1240–6.
10. Contreras GA, Munita JM, Arias CA. Novel strategies for the management of vancomycin-resistant enterococcal infections. Curr Infect Dis Rep 2019;21:22.
11. Lebreton F, Manson AL, Saavedra JT, et al. Tracing the enterococci from paleozoic origins to the hospital. Cell 2017;169:849–61.e13.
12. Bradley CR, Fraise AP. Heat and chemical resistance of enterococci. J Hosp Infect 1996;34:191–6.
13. Arias CA, Murray BE. The rise of the Enterococcus: beyond vancomycin resistance. Nat Rev Microbiol 2012;10:266–78.
14. Fontana R, Amalfitano G, Rossi L, et al. Mechanisms of resistance to growth inhibition and killing by beta-lactam antibiotics in enterococci. Clin Infect Dis 1992;15:486–9.
15. Weinstein MP. Comparative evaluation of penicillin, ampicillin, and imipenem MICs and susceptibility breakpoints for vancomycin-susceptible and vancomycin-resistant *Enterococcus faecalis* and *Enterococcus faecium*. J Clin Microbiol 2001;39:2729–31.
16. Goffin C, Ghuysen JM. Multimodular penicillin-binding proteins: an enigmatic family of orthologs and paralogs. Microbiol Mol Biol Rev 1998;62:1079–93.
17. Arbeloa A, Segal H, Hugonnet J-E, et al. Role of class A penicillin-binding proteins in PBP5-mediated beta-lactam resistance in *Enterococcus faecalis*. J Bacteriol 2004;186:1221–8.
18. Rice LB, Carias LL, Rudin S, et al. Role of class A penicillin-binding proteins in the expression of β-lactam resistance in *Enterococcus faecium*. J Bacteriol 2009;191:3649–56.
19. Sifaoui F, Arthur M, Rice L. Role of Penicillin-Binding Protein 5 in Expression of Ampicillin Resistance and Peptidoglycan Structure in *Enterococcus faecium*. Antimicrob Agents Chemother 2001;45:1–5.
20. Rice LB, Bellais S, Carias LL, et al. Impact of specific *pbp5* mutations on expression of beta-lactam resistance in *Enterococcus faecium*. Antimicrob Agents Chemother 2004;48:3028–32.
21. Pietta E, Montealegre MC, Roh JH, et al. *Enterococcus faecium* PBP5-S/R, the missing link between PBP5-S and PBP5-R. Antimicrob Agents Chemother 2014;58:6978–81.
22. Montealegre MC, Roh JH, Rae M, et al. Differential penicillin-binding protein 5 (PBP5) levels in the *Enterococcus faecium* clades with different levels of ampicillin resistance. Antimicrob Agents Chemother 2017;61:1–10.
23. Galloway-Peña JR, Rice LB, Murray BE. Analysis of PBP5 of early U.S. isolates of *Enterococcus faecium*: sequence variation alone does not explain increasing ampicillin resistance over time. Antimicrob Agents Chemother 2011;55:3272–7.
24. Moon TM, D'Andréa ÉD, Lee CW, et al. The structures of penicillin-binding protein 4 (PBP4) and PBP5 from Enterococci provide structural insights into β-lactam resistance. J Biol Chem 2018;293:18574–84.

25. Conceição N, da Silva LEP, da Costa Darini AL, et al. Penicillin-resistant, ampicillin-susceptible *Enterococcus faecalis* of hospital origin: pbp4 gene polymorphism and genetic diversity. Infect Genet Evol 2014;28:289–95.
26. Rice LB, Desbonnet C, Tait-Kamradt A, et al. Structural and regulatory changes in PBP4 trigger decreased β-lactam susceptibility in *Enterococcus faecalis*. mBio 2018;9(2). e00361-18.
27. Metzidie E, Manolis EN, Pournaras S, et al. Spread of an unusual penicillin- and imipenem-resistant but ampicillin-susceptible phenotype among *Enterococcus faecalis* clinical isolates. J Antimicrob Chemother 2006;57:158–60.
28. Comenge Y, Quintiliani R Jr, Li L, et al. The CroRS two-component regulatory system is required for intrinsic beta-lactam resistance in *Enterococcus faecalis*. J Bacteriol 2003;185:7184–92.
29. Hall CL, Tschannen M, Worthey EA, et al. IreB, a Ser/Thr kinase substrate, influences antimicrobial resistance in *Enterococcus faecalis*. Antimicrob Agents Chemother 2013;57:6179–86.
30. Desbonnet C, Tait-Kamradt A, Garcia-Solache M, et al. Involvement of the eukaryote-like kinase-phosphatase system and a protein that interacts with penicillin-binding protein 5 in emergence of cephalosporin resistance in cephalosporin-sensitive class A penicillin-binding protein mutants in *Enterococcus faecium*. mBio 2016;7:1–10.
31. Vesić D, Kristich CJ. MurAA is required for intrinsic cephalosporin resistance of *Enterococcus faecalis*. Antimicrob Agents Chemother 2012;56:2443–51.
32. Costa Y, Galimand M, Leclercq R, et al. Characterization of the chromosomal *aac(6')-Ii* gene specific for *Enterococcus faecium*. Antimicrob Agents Chemother 1993;37:1896–903.
33. Krogstad DJ, Korfhagen TR, Moellering RC, et al. Aminoglycoside-inactivating enzymes in clinical isolates of *Streptococcus faecalis*. An explanation for resistance to antibiotic synergism. J Clin Invest 1978;62:480–6.
34. Mederski-Samoraj BD, Murray BE. High-level resistance to gentamicin in clinical isolates of enterococci. J Infect Dis 1983;147:751–7.
35. Courvalin P, Carlier C, Collatz E. Plasmid-mediated resistance to aminocyclitol antibiotics in group D streptococci. J Bacteriol 1980;143:541–51.
36. Eliopoulos GM, Farber BF, Murray BE, et al. Ribosomal resistance of clinical enterococcal to streptomycin isolates. Antimicrob Agents Chemother 1984;25: 398–9.
37. Mainardi JL, Gutmann L, Acar JF, et al. Synergistic effect of amoxicillin and cefotaxime against *Enterococcus faecalis*. Antimicrob Agents Chemother 1995;39: 1984–7.
38. Gavaldà J, Torres C, Tenorio C, et al. Efficacy of ampicillin plus ceftriaxone in treatment of experimental endocarditis due to *Enterococcus faecalis* strains highly resistant to aminoglycosides. Antimicrob Agents Chemother 1999;43: 639–46.
39. Gavaldá J, Onrubia PL, Gómez MTM, et al. Efficacy of ampicillin combined with ceftriaxone and gentamicin in the treatment of experimental endocarditis due to *Enterococcus faecalis* with no high-level resistance to aminoglycosides. J Antimicrob Chemother 2003;52:514–7.
40. Beganovic M, Luther MK, Rice LB, et al. A review of combination antimicrobial therapy for *Enterococcus faecalis* bloodstream infections and infective endocarditis. Clin Infect Dis 2018;67:303–9.

41. Lorenzo MP, Kidd JM, Jenkins SG, et al. In vitro activity of ampicillin and ceftriaxone against ampicillin-susceptible *Enterococcus faecium*. J Antimicrob Chemother 2019;74:2269–73.
42. Murray BE. Beta-lactamase-producing enterococci. Antimicrob Agents Chemother 1992;36:2355–9.
43. Courvalin P. Vancomycin resistance in gram-positive cocci. Clin Infect Dis 2006; 42(Suppl 1):S25–34.
44. Gold HS. Vancomycin-resistant enterococci: mechanisms and clinical observations. Clin Infect Dis 2001;33:210–9.
45. Leclercq R, Dutka-Malen S, Duval J, et al. Vancomycin resistance gene vanC is specific to *Enterococcus gallinarum*. Antimicrob Agents Chemother 1992;36: 2005–8.
46. Navarro F, Courvalin P. Analysis of genes encoding D-alanine-D-alanine ligase-related enzymes in *Enterococcus casseliflavus* and *Enterococcus flavescens*. Antimicrob Agents Chemother 1994;38:1788–93.
47. Arthur M, Molinas C, Depardieu F, et al. Characterization of Tn1546, a Tn3-related transposon conferring glycopeptide resistance by synthesis of depsipeptide peptidoglycan precursors in *Enterococcus faecium* BM4147. J Bacteriol 1993;175:117–27.
48. Carias LL, Rudin SD, Donskey CJ, et al. Genetic linkage and cotransfer of a novel, *vanB*-containing transposon (Tn*5382*) and a low-affinity penicillin-binding protein 5 gene in a clinical vancomycin-resistant *Enterococcus faecium* isolate. J Bacteriol 1998;180:4426–34.
49. Garnier F, Taourit S, Glaser P, et al. Characterization of transposon Tn*1549*, conferring VanB-type resistance in *Enterococcus spp.* Microbiology 2000;146: 1481–9.
50. Guardabassi L, Agersø Y. Genes homologous to glycopeptide resistance *vanA* are widespread in soil microbial communities. FEMS Microbiol Lett 2006;259: 221–5.
51. Uttley AH, Collins CH, Naidoo J, et al. Vancomycin-resistant enterococci. Lancet 1988;1:57–8.
52. Top J, Willems R, Bonten M. Emergence of CC17 *Enterococcus faecium*: from commensal to hospital-adapted pathogen. FEMS Immunol Med Microbiol 2008;52:297–308.
53. Wegener HC. Historical yearly usage of glycopeptides for animals and humans: the American-European paradox revisited. Antimicrob Agents Chemother 1998; 42:3049.
54. Aarestrup FM, Seyfarth AM, Emborg HD, et al. Effect of abolishment of the use of antimicrobial agents for growth promotion on occurrence of antimicrobial resistance in fecal enterococci from food animals in Denmark. Antimicrob Agents Chemother 2001;45:2054–9.
55. Ruiz-Garbajosa P, Bonten MJM, Robinson DA, et al. Multilocus sequence typing scheme for *Enterococcus faecalis* reveals hospital-adapted genetic complexes in a background of high rates of recombination. J Clin Microbiol 2006;44: 2220–8.
56. Tedim AP, Ruiz-Garbajosa P, Corander J, et al. Population biology of intestinal enterococcus isolates from hospitalized and nonhospitalized individuals in different age groups. Appl Environ Microbiol 2015;81:1820–31.
57. Guzman Prieto AM, van Schaik W, Rogers MRC, et al. Global emergence and dissemination of enterococci as nosocomial pathogens: attack of the clones? Front Microbiol 2016;7:788.

58. Palmer KL, Godfrey P, Griggs A, et al. Comparative genomics of enterococci: variation in *Enterococcus faecalis*, clade structure in *E. faecium*, and defining characteristics of *E. gallinarum* and *E. casseliflavus*. mBio 2012;3. e00318-11.
59. Raven KE, Reuter S, Gouliouris T, et al. Genome-based characterization of hospital-adapted *Enterococcus faecalis* lineages. Nat Microbiol 2016;1:15033.
60. Galloway-Peña J, Roh JH, Latorre M, et al. Genomic and SNP analyses demonstrate a distant separation of the hospital and community-associated clades of *Enterococcus faecium*. PLoS One 2012;7:e30187.
61. Lebreton F, Van Schaik W, Manson A. Emergence of epidemic multidrug-resistant *Enterococcus faecium*. mBio 2013;4:1–10.
62. Willems RJL, Top J, van Schaik W, et al. Restricted gene flow among hospital subpopulations of *Enterococcus faecium*. mBio 2012;3. e00151-12.
63. Raven KE, Reuter S, Reynolds R, et al. A decade of genomic history for healthcare-associated *Enterococcus faecium* in the United Kingdom and Ireland. Genome Res 2016;26:1388–96.
64. Rios R, Reyes J, Carvajal LP, et al. Genomic epidemiology of vancomycin-resistant *Enterococcus faecium* (VREfm) in Latin America: revisiting the global VRE population structure. Sci Rep 2020;10(1):5636.
65. Gouliouris T, Raven KE, Ludden C, et al. Genomic surveillance of *Enterococcus faecium* reveals limited sharing of strains and resistance genes between livestock and humans in the United Kingdom. mBio 2018;9(6). e01780-18.
66. Montealegre MC, Singh KV, Murray BE. Gastrointestinal tract colonization dynamics by different *Enterococcus faecium* clades. J Infect Dis 2016;213:1914–22.
67. Ley RE, Peterson DA, Gordon JI. Ecological and evolutionary forces shaping microbial diversity in the human intestine. Cell 2006;124:837–48.
68. Keith JW, Pamer EG. Enlisting commensal microbes to resist antibiotic-resistant pathogens. J Exp Med 2019;216:10–9.
69. Karki S, Land G, Aitchison S, et al. Long-term carriage of vancomycin-resistant enterococci in patients discharged from hospitals: a 12-year retrospective cohort study. J Clin Microbiol 2013;51:3374–9.
70. Yoon YK, Lee SE, Lee J, et al. Risk factors for prolonged carriage of vancomycin-resistant *Enterococcus faecium* among patients in intensive care units: a case-control study. J Antimicrob Chemother 2011;66:1831–8.
71. Sohn KM, Peck KR, Joo E-J, et al. Duration of colonization and risk factors for prolonged carriage of vancomycin-resistant enterococci after discharge from the hospital. Int J Infect Dis 2013;17:e240–6.
72. Byers KE, Anglim AM, Anneski CJ, et al. Duration of colonization with vancomycin-resistant Enterococcus. Infect Control Hosp Epidemiol 2002;23:207–11.
73. Stiefel U, Rao A, Pultz MJ, et al. Suppression of gastric acid production by proton pump inhibitor treatment facilitates colonization of the large intestine by vancomycin-resistant *Enterococcus spp.* and *Klebsiella pneumoniae* in clindamycin-treated mice. Antimicrob Agents Chemother 2006;50:3905–7.
74. Sonnenburg ED, Sonnenburg JL. Starving our microbial self: the deleterious consequences of a diet deficient in microbiota-accessible carbohydrates. Cell Metab 2014;20:779–86.
75. Desai MS, Seekatz AM, Koropatkin NM, et al. A dietary fiber-deprived gut microbiota degrades the colonic mucus barrier and enhances pathogen susceptibility. Cell 2016;167:1339–53.e21.

76. Ubeda C, Taur Y, Jenq RR, et al. Vancomycin-resistant Enterococcus domination of intestinal microbiota is enabled by antibiotic treatment in mice and precedes bloodstream invasion in humans. J Clin Invest 2010;120:4332–41.
77. Taur Y, Xavier JB, Lipuma L, et al. Intestinal domination and the risk of bacteremia in patients undergoing allogeneic hematopoietic stem cell transplantation. Clin Infect Dis 2012;55:905–14.
78. Cash HL, Whitham CV, Behrendt CL, et al. Symbiotic bacteria direct expression of an intestinal bactericidal lectin. Science 2006;313:1126–30.
79. Brandl K, Plitas G, Mihu CN, et al. Vancomycin-resistant enterococci exploit antibiotic-induced innate immune deficits. Nature 2008;455:804–7.
80. Ubeda C, Bucci V, Caballero S, et al. Intestinal microbiota containing Barnesiella species cures vancomycin-resistant *Enterococcus faecium* colonization. Infect Immun 2013;81:965–73.
81. Cotter PD, Ross RP, Hill C. Bacteriocins - a viable alternative to antibiotics? Nat Rev Microbiol 2013;11:95–105.
82. Kommineni S, Bretl DJ, Lam V, et al. Bacteriocin production augments niche competition by enterococci in the mammalian gastrointestinal tract. Nature 2015;526:719–22.
83. Kim SG, Becattini S, Moody TU, et al. Microbiota-derived lantibiotic restores resistance against vancomycin-resistant Enterococcus. Nature 2019;572:665–9.
84. Caballero S, Kim S, Carter RA, et al. Cooperating commensals restore colonization resistance to vancomycin-resistant Enterococcus faecium. Cell Host Microbe 2017;21:592–602.e4.
85. McKenney PT, Yan J, Vaubourgeix J, et al. Intestinal bile acids induce a morphotype switch in vancomycin-resistant enterococcus that facilitates intestinal colonization. Cell Host Microbe 2019;25:695–705.e5.
86. Arias CA, Panesso D, McGrath DM, et al. Genetic basis for in vivo daptomycin resistance in enterococci. N Engl J Med 2011;365:892–900.
87. Diaz L, Tran TT, Munita JM, et al. Whole-genome analyses of *Enterococcus faecium* isolates with diverse daptomycin MICs. Antimicrob Agents Chemother 2014;58:4527–34.
88. Kamboj M, Cohen N, Gilhuley K, et al. Emergence of daptomycin-resistant VRE: experience of a single institution. Infect Control Hosp Epidemiol 2011;32:391–4.
89. Douglas AP, Marshall C, Baines SL, et al. Utilizing genomic analyses to investigate the first outbreak of *vanA* vancomycin-resistant Enterococcus in Australia with emergence of daptomycin non-susceptibility. J Med Microbiol 2019;68:303–8.
90. Miller WR, Bayer AS, Arias CA. Mechanism of action and resistance to daptomycin in *Staphylococcus aureus* and Enterococci. Cold Spring Harb Perspect Med 2016;6:a026997.
91. Baltz RH. Daptomycin: mechanisms of action and resistance, and biosynthetic engineering. Curr Opin Chem Biol 2009;13:144–51.
92. Ho SW, Jung D, Calhoun JR, et al. Effect of divalent cations on the structure of the antibiotic daptomycin. Eur Biophys J 2008;37:421–33.
93. Jung D, Rozek A, Okon M, et al. Structural transitions as determinants of the action of the calcium-dependent antibiotic daptomycin. Chem Biol 2004;11:949–57.
94. Muraih JK, Harris J, Taylor SD, et al. Characterization of daptomycin oligomerization with perylene excimer fluorescence: stoichiometric binding of phosphatidylglycerol triggers oligomer formation. Biochim Biophys Acta 2012;1818:673–8.

95. Silverman JA, Perlmutter NG, Shapiro HM. Correlation of daptomycin bactericidal activity and membrane depolarization in *Staphylococcus aureus*. Antimicrob Agents Chemother 2003;47:2538–44.
96. Müller A, Wenzel M, Strahl H, et al. Daptomycin inhibits cell envelope synthesis by interfering with fluid membrane microdomains. Proc Natl Acad Sci U S A 2016;113:E7077–86.
97. Tran TT, Panesso D, Mishra NN, et al. Daptomycin-resistant *Enterococcus faecalis* diverts the antibiotic molecule from the division septum and remodels cell membrane phospholipids. mBio 2013;4:1–10.
98. Miller WR, Tran TT, Diaz L, et al. LiaR-independent pathways to daptomycin resistance in *Enterococcus faecalis* reveal a multilayer defense against cell envelope antibiotics. Mol Microbiol 2019;111:811–24.
99. Tran TT, Munita JM, Arias CA. Mechanisms of drug resistance: daptomycin resistance. Ann N Y Acad Sci 2015;1354:32–53.
100. Davlieva M, Shi Y, Leonard PG, et al. A variable DNA recognition site organization establishes the LiaR-mediated cell envelope stress response of enterococci to daptomycin. Nucleic Acids Res 2015;43:4758–73.
101. Munita JM, Tran TT, Diaz L, et al. A *liaF* codon deletion abolishes daptomycin bactericidal activity against vancomycin-resistant *Enterococcus faecalis*. Antimicrob Agents Chemother 2013;57:2831–3.
102. Davlieva M, Tovar-Yanez A, DeBruler K, et al. An adaptive mutation in *Enterococcus faecium* LiaR associated with antimicrobial peptide resistance mimics phosphorylation and stabilizes LiaR in an activated state. J Mol Biol 2016;428:4503–19.
103. Munita JM, Panesso D, Diaz L, et al. Correlation between mutations in *liaFSR* of *Enterococcus faecium* and MIC of daptomycin: revisiting daptomycin breakpoints. Antimicrob Agents Chemother 2012;56:4354–9.
104. Shukla BS, Shelburne S, Reyes K, et al. Influence of minimum inhibitory concentration in clinical outcomes of *Enterococcus faecium* bacteremia treated with daptomycin: is it time to change the breakpoint? Clin Infect Dis 2016;62:1514–20.
105. Khan A, Davlieva M, Panesso D, et al. Antimicrobial sensing coupled with cell membrane remodeling mediates antibiotic resistance and virulence in *Enterococcus* faecalis. Proc Natl Acad Sci U S A 2019;116(52):26925–32.
106. Miller C, Kong J, Tran TT, et al. Adaptation of *Enterococcus faecalis* to daptomycin reveals an ordered progression to resistance. Antimicrob Agents Chemother 2013;57:5373–83.
107. Dubrac S, Bisicchia P, Devine KM, et al. A matter of life and death: cell wall homeostasis and the WalKR (YycGF) essential signal transduction pathway. Mol Microbiol 2008;70:1307–22.
108. Gebhard S, Fang C, Shaaly A, et al. Identification and characterization of a bacitracin resistance network in *Enterococcus faecalis*. Antimicrob Agents Chemother 2014;58:1425–33.
109. Guzmán Prieto AM, Wijngaarden J, Braat JC, et al. The two-component system ChtRS contributes to chlorhexidine tolerance in *Enterococcus faecium*. Antimicrob Agents Chemother 2017;61. e02122-16.
110. Zhanel GG, Calic D, Schweizer F, et al. New lipoglycopeptides: a comparative review of dalbavancin, oritavancin and telavancin. Drugs 2010;70:859–86.
111. Zhanel GG, Trapp S, Gin AS, et al. Dalbavancin and telavancin: novel lipoglycopeptides for the treatment of Gram-positive infections. Expert Rev Anti Infect Ther 2008;6:67–81.

112. Smith JR, Roberts KD, Rybak MJ. Dalbavancin: a novel lipoglycopeptide antibiotic with extended activity against gram-positive infections. Infect Dis Ther 2015;4:245–58.
113. Hayden MK, Trenholme GM, Schultz JE, et al. In vivo development of teicoplanin resistance in a VanB *Enterococcus faecium* isolate. J Infect Dis 1993;167:1224–7.
114. Zhanel GG, Schweizer F, Karlowsky JA. Oritavancin: mechanism of action. Clin Infect Dis 2012;54:214–9.
115. Belley A, McKay GA, Arhin FF, et al. Oritavancin disrupts membrane integrity of *Staphylococcus aureus* and vancomycin-resistant enterococci to effect rapid bacterial killing. Antimicrob Agents Chemother 2010;54:5369–71.
116. Arhin FF, Seguin DL, Belley A, et al. In vitro stepwise selection of reduced susceptibility to lipoglycopeptides in enterococci. Diagn Microbiol Infect Dis 2017;89:168–71.
117. Arthur M, Depardieu F, Reynolds P, et al. Moderate-level resistance to glycopeptide LY333328 mediated by genes of the vanA and vanB clusters in enterococci. Antimicrob Agents Chemother 1999;43:1875–80.
118. Belley A, Arhin FF, Moeck G. Evaluation of oritavancin dosing strategies against vancomycin-resistant *Enterococcus faecium* isolates with or without reduced susceptibility to daptomycin in an in vitro pharmacokinetic/pharmacodynamic model. Antimicrob Agents Chemother 2018;62. e01873-17.
119. Shinabarger DL, Marotti KR, Murray RW, et al. Mechanism of action of oxazolidinones: effects of linezolid and eperezolid on translation reactions. Antimicrob Agents Chemother 1997;41:2132–6.
120. Leach KL, Swaney SM, Colca JR, et al. The site of action of oxazolidinone antibiotics in living bacteria and in human mitochondria. Mol Cell 2007;26:393–402.
121. Shaw KJ, Poppe S, Schaadt R, et al. In vitro activity of TR-700, the antibacterial moiety of the prodrug TR-701, against linezolid-resistant strains. Antimicrob Agents Chemother 2008;52:4442–7.
122. Marshall SH, Donskey CJ, Hutton-Thomas R, et al. Gene dosage and linezolid resistance in *Enterococcus faecium* and *Enterococcus faecalis*. Antimicrob Agents Chemother 2002;46:3334–6.
123. Bourgeois-Nicolaos N, Massias L, Couson B, et al. Dose dependence of emergence of resistance to linezolid in *Enterococcus faecalis* in vivo. J Infect Dis 2007;195:1480–8.
124. Boumghar-Bourtchaï L, Dhalluin A, Malbruny B, et al. Influence of recombination on development of mutational resistance to linezolid in *Enterococcus faecalis* JH2-2. Antimicrob Agents Chemother 2009;53:4007–9.
125. Chen H, Wu W, Ni M, et al. Linezolid-resistant clinical isolates of enterococci and *Staphylococcus cohnii* from a multicentre study in China: molecular epidemiology and resistance mechanisms. Int J Antimicrob Agents 2013;42:317–21.
126. Billal DS, Feng J, Leprohon P, et al. Whole genome analysis of linezolid resistance in *Streptococcus pneumoniae* reveals resistance and compensatory mutations. BMC Genomics 2011;12:512.
127. Lei C-W, Kang Z-Z, Wu S-K, et al. Detection of the phenicol-oxazolidinone-tetracycline resistance gene *poxtA* in *Enterococcus faecium* and *Enterococcus faecalis* of food-producing animal origin in China. J Antimicrob Chemother 2019;74:2459–61.
128. Elghaieb H, Freitas AR, Abbassi MS, et al. Dispersal of linezolid-resistant enterococci carrying *poxtA* or *optrA* in retail meat and food-producing animals from Tunisia. J Antimicrob Chemother 2019;74:2865–9.

129. Schwarz S, Werckenthin C, Kehrenberg C. Identification of a plasmid-borne chloramphenicol-florfenicol resistance gene in *Staphylococcus sciuri.* Antimicrob Agents Chemother 2000;44:2530–3.
130. Diaz L, Kiratisin P, Mendes RE, et al. Transferable plasmid-mediated resistance to linezolid due to *cfr* in a human clinical isolate of *Enterococcus faecalis.* Antimicrob Agents Chemother 2012;56:3917–22.
131. Deshpande LM, Castanheira M, Flamm RK, et al. Evolving oxazolidinone resistance mechanisms in a worldwide collection of enterococcal clinical isolates: results from the SENTRY Antimicrobial Surveillance Program. J Antimicrob Chemother 2018;73:2314–22.
132. Singh KV, Arias CA, Murray BE. Efficacy of Tedizolid against Enterococci and Staphylococci, Including *cfr*+ Strains, in a Mouse Peritonitis Model. Antimicrob Agents Chemother 2019;63. e02627-18.
133. Wang Y, Lv Y, Cai J, et al. A novel gene, *optrA*, that confers transferable resistance to oxazolidinones and phenicols and its presence in *Enterococcus faecalis* and *Enterococcus faecium* of human and animal origin. J Antimicrob Chemother 2015;70:2182–90.
134. Antonelli A, D'Andrea MM, Brenciani A, et al. Characterization of *poxtA*, a novel phenicol-oxazolidinone-tetracycline resistance gene from an MRSA of clinical origin. J Antimicrob Chemother 2018;73:1763–9.
135. Chen H, Wang X, Yin Y, et al. Molecular characteristics of oxazolidinone resistance in enterococci from a multicenter study in China. BMC Microbiol 2019; 19:162.
136. Sharkey LKR, Edwards TA, O'Neill AJ. ABC-F proteins mediate antibiotic resistance through ribosomal protection. mBio 2016;7:e01975.
137. Kresken M, Leitner E, Seifert H, et al. Susceptibility of clinical isolates of frequently encountered bacterial species to tigecycline one year after the introduction of this new class of antibiotics: results of the second multicentre surveillance trial in Germany (G-TEST II, 2007). Eur J Clin Microbiol Infect Dis 2009;28: 1007–11.
138. Namdari H, Tan TY, Dowzicky MJ. Activity of tigecycline and comparators against skin and skin structure pathogens: global results of the tigecycline evaluation and surveillance trial, 2004-2009. Int J Infect Dis 2012;16:e60–6.
139. Cattoir V, Isnard C, Cosquer T, et al. Genomic analysis of reduced susceptibility to Tigecycline in *Enterococcus faecium.* Antimicrob Agents Chemother 2015;59: 239–44.
140. Beabout K, Hammerstrom TG, Perez AM, et al. The ribosomal S10 protein is a general target for decreased tigecycline susceptibility. Antimicrob Agents Chemother 2015;59:5561–6.
141. Fiedler S, Bender JK, Klare I, et al. Tigecycline resistance in clinical isolates of *Enterococcus faecium* is mediated by an upregulation of plasmid-encoded tetracycline determinants *tet*(L) and *tet*(M). J Antimicrob Chemother 2016;71: 871–81.
142. Beabout K, Hammerstrom TG, Wang TT, et al. Rampant parasexuality evolves in a hospital pathogen during antibiotic selection. Mol Biol Evol 2015;32:2585–97.
143. Scott LJ. Eravacycline: a review in complicated intra-abdominal infections. Drugs 2019;79:315–24.
144. Barber KE, Bell AM, Wingler MJB, et al. Omadacycline enters the ring: a new antimicrobial contender. Pharmacotherapy 2018;38:1194–204.

Resistance to Novel β-Lactam–β-Lactamase Inhibitor Combinations

The "Price of Progress"

Krisztina M. Papp-Wallace, PhD*[,1], Andrew R. Mack, BS[1], Magdalena A. Taracila, MS, Robert A. Bonomo, MD*

KEYWORDS

- β-Lactamase • β-Lactamase inhibitor • Ceftolozane • Avibactam • Vaborbactam • Relebactam • Resistance

KEY POINTS

- The novel β-lactam–β-lactamase inhibitor combinations (ceftazidime-avibactam, ceftolozane-tazobactam, meropenem-vaborbactam, and imipenem-relebactam) are a significant advance in the therapeutic armamentarium against multidrug-resistant gram-negative pathogens. Unfortunately, resistance to these very powerful agents is emerging rapidly in clinics.
- Resistance to ceftolozane-tazobactam is mediated largely by amino acid substitutions, insertions, and/or deletions in the chromosomal AmpC, *Pseudomonas*-derived cephalosporinase (PDC), of *P aeruginosa*; many of these changes also confer cross-resistance to ceftazidime-avibactam.
- Mutations in bla_{KPC} are the source of most reports of ceftazidime-avibactam resistance in gram negatives.
- The cephalosporin partners in ceftolozane-tazobactam and ceftazidime-avibactam are the major evolutionary drivers toward resistance in these combinations.
- Permeability and efflux are the primary basis for resistance to meropenem-vaborbactam and imipenem-relebactam.

Funded by: NIAID. *Grant number(s):* R01AI063517; R01AI072219; R01AI100560. 1I01BX002872 (K.M. Papp-Wallace) and 1I01BX001974 (R.A. Bonomo).

Research Service, Louis Stokes Cleveland Department of Veterans Affairs, 151W, 10701 East Boulevard, Cleveland, OH 44106, USA

[1] Contributed equally to this work.

* Corresponding authors.

E-mail addresses: kmp12@case.edu; krisztina.papp@va.gov (K.M.P.-W.); robert.bonomo@va.gov (R.A.B.)

Infect Dis Clin N Am 34 (2020) 773–819
https://doi.org/10.1016/j.idc.2020.05.001
0891-5520/20/Published by Elsevier Inc.

INTRODUCTION

As a class, the β-lactams are the most commonly prescribed and clinically dependable antimicrobials in the United States, representing more than 65% of injected antibiotic prescriptions from 2004 to 2014[1] and 45% of oral antibiotic prescriptions in 2016.[2] Given their effectiveness, the development of resistance to β-lactam antibiotics creates a major concern for physicians, scientists, and policymakers around the world. This review focuses on the emergence of resistance to the 4 novel β-lactam–β-lactamase inhibitor combinations approved between 2014 and 2019 in the United States: ceftolozane-tazobactam, ceftazidime-avibactam, meropenem-vaborbactam, and imipenem-relebactam (**Fig. 1**). The resistance mechanisms that have been reported at the time of this writing are summarized and the implications of these findings highlighted.

MECHANISM OF ACTION OF β-LACTAM ANTIBIOTICS

Cell wall biosynthesis is critical to bacterial cell division, and most bacteria require a cell wall for survival.[3] Cell walls are made of peptidoglycan, long polymers of *N*-acetylglucosamine (NAG) and *N*-acetylmuramic acid (NAM) joined in alternating order by β-1,4 glycosidic linkages. Each NAM subunit is attached a short pentapeptide, which is cross-linked between peptidoglycan strands to create a meshlike structure that provides strength to the cell wall. These linkages, which occur between the penultimate D-alanine of 1 peptide and the lysine or diaminopimelic acid of another, are catalyzed by DD-transpeptidases, known as penicillin-binding proteins (PBPs).[4,5]

β-Lactam antibiotics enter the transpeptidase active site of PBPs and stereochemically mimic the terminal D-alanine residues of the peptide.[5] When the active site serine of the PBP attacks the β-lactam ring rather than a peptide bond, it forms a covalent acyl-enzyme complex that deacylates very slowly, crippling the PBP and preventing the final step of cell wall biosynthesis.[1] This leads to potentially endless cycles of futile synthesis and degradation of nonfunctional peptidoglycan, depleting cellular stores of precursors and amplifying cytotoxicity in the process by permitting the entry of water into the cell.[6]

β-LACTAMASES

β-Lactamases are bacterial enzymes that hydrolyze the β-lactam bonds in β-lactam antibiotics, rendering them nonfunctional. β-Lactamases are divided into 4 molecular classes by mechanism, conserved residues, and sequence homology. Class A, C, and D β-lactamases use a conserved serine-based mechanism to hydrolyze the β-lactam bond. Class B metallo-β-lactamases catalyze the hydrolysis of the β-lactam bond using a Zn^{2+}-based mechanism.[7] For purposes of this review, alterations to class A and class C β-lactamases are discussed using the standardized numbering scheme of Ambler and colleagues[8] and Structural Alignment-based Numbering of class C β-lactamases, respectively.[9]

The basic mechanism used by class A and class C serine β-lactamases involves binding, acylation, and deacylation phases with 2 transition states (**Fig. 2**). Binding occurs when a substrate associates with the enzyme to form a reversible Michaelis complex. In the acylation phase of a class A or class C serine β-lactamase mechanism, a general base deprotonates the catalytic serine residue, permitting nucleophilic attack of the carbonyl carbon of the β-lactam ring, forming a high-energy transition state, which quickly collapses into the acyl-enzyme complex. Deacylation occurs when a water molecule is deprotonated and nucleophilically attacks the same carbon atom,

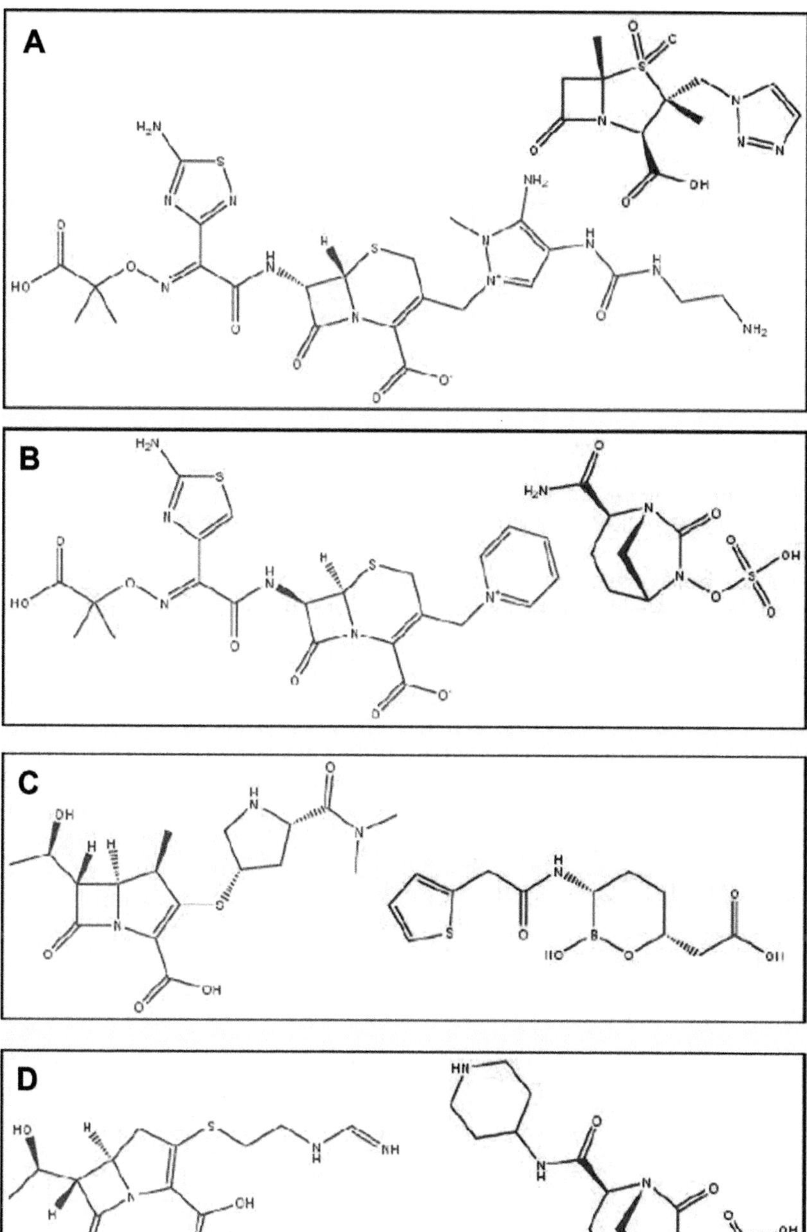

Fig. 1. Structures of (*A*) ceftolozane-tazobactam, (*B*) ceftazidime-avibactam, (*C*) meropenem-vaborbactam, and (*D*) imipenem-relebactam. In all panels, the β-lactamase inhibitor (*red*) is located to the right of the β-lactam partner (*blue*).

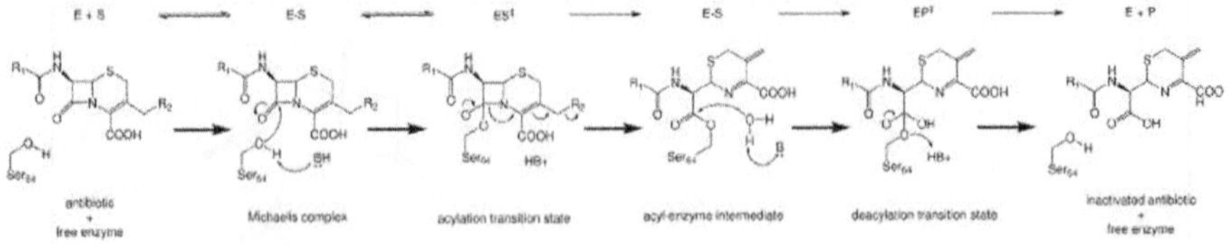

E + S → ES → ES‡ → E-S → EP‡ → E + P

antibiotic + free enzyme → Michaelis complex → acylation transition state → acyl-enzyme intermediate → deacylation transition state → inactivated antibiotic + free enzyme

Fig. 2. The class A and class C serine β-lactamase mechanism involves acylation and deacylation through high-energy tetrahedral transition states. In this example with a class C enzyme, B and HB^+ represent a generic base and conjugate acid, respectively. The identity of the bases may vary by class, enzyme, and substrate.

creating a second high-energy transition state that collapses to restore the serine and release an inactive β-lactam (see **Fig. 2**).[10–13]

THE Ω-LOOP OF β-LACTAMASES

Named for its structural resemblance to the Greek letter Ω, the Ω-loop is a highly mobile and dynamic region in β-lactamases[14] and is roughly defined as encompassing residues 164 to 179 in class A enzymes (15 amino acids), residues 188 through 221 (33 amino acids) in class C enzymes, and residues 143 through 173 (30 amino acids) in class D enzymes, although exact designations vary by research group and by family within a class (**Fig. 3**). The Ω-loop forms the floor of the active site and creates a wall that binds and positions the R1 group of β-lactams, helping to determine substrate specificity.[15] In class A β-lactamases, the Ω-loop is believed to be rigid (rather than flexible) due to hydrogen bonding but remains mobile and able to move as a unit. Simulations suggest class C β-lactamases have a more balanced Ω-loop with both flexible and rigid characteristics and the ability to serve as a mechanical switch, meaning it is able to alternate between more flexible and more rigid states based on changes in the hydrogen bonding network.[14] Amino acid substitutions in the Ω-loop of class A and class C β-lactamases were shown to expand the substrate spectrum of these enzymes toward oxyimino-cephalosporins.[16–19] The precise details and mechanisms by which this enhanced ability to hydrolyze these novel cephalosporins with complex R1 side chains occurs still are uncertain.

β-LACTAMASE INHIBITORS

An established approach to overcoming β-lactam resistance is to reduce the activity of β-lactamases, thus preserving the efficacy of penicillins, cephalosporins,

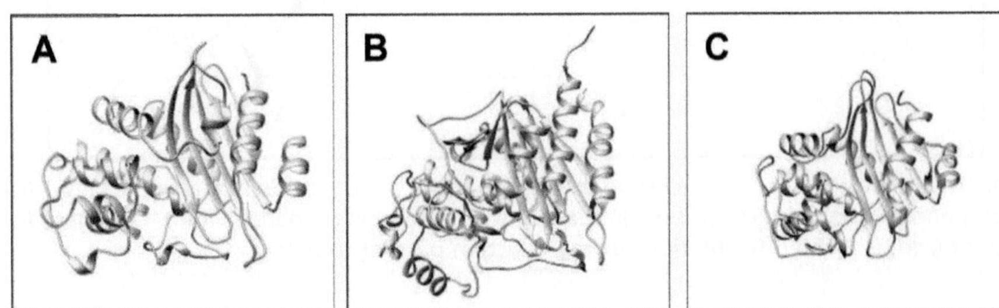

Fig. 3. The location of the Ω-loop (*blue*) in (*A*) KPC-2 (PDB#: 2OV5), (*B*) PDC-1 (PDB#: 4GZB), and (*C*) OXA-48 (PDB#: 4S2P).

monobactams, and carbapenem antibiotics. Two approaches to inhibition have targeted β-lactamases successfully, using (1) a suicide, or mechanism-based, inhibitor, and (2) a reversible inhibitor. Suicide inhibitors (including clavulanic acid, sulbactam, and tazobactam) form stable acyl-enzyme complexes, which can undergo postacylation chemistry and fragment or deacylate very slowly. In some cases, these inhibitors permanently inactivate the enzyme in the process. In contrast, reversible inhibitors (including diazabicyclooctanes [DBOs] and boronates) are able to deacylate from the β-lactamase without being modified and proceed to inhibit another β-lactamase molecule.[20–22] Current β-lactamase inhibitors fall into 1 of 3 chemical classes: the suicide inhibitors, which contain β-lactam rings but are less readily hydrolyzed (eg, clavulanic acid, sulbactam and tazobactam); the DBOs, which consist of an 8-membered ring partially analogous to the β-lactam bond (avibactam and relebactam); and the boronic acid transition state inhibitors, which mimic transition states (vaborbactam).[20,23]

NEWER β-LACTAM AND β-LACTAMASE INHIBITOR COMBINATIONS: CEFTOLOZANE-TAZOBACTAM

Approved by the US Food and Drug Administration (FDA) in 2014, ceftolozane-tazobactam is indicated for use in complicated intra-abdominal infections (cIAIs), complicated urinary tract infections (cUTIs), hospital-acquired bacterial pneumonia (HABP), and ventilator-associated bacterial pneumonia (VABP) in adults.[24] Ceftolozane-tazobactam additionally is being or has been investigated for use in adult patients with burns (NCT03002506), indwelling external ventricular drains (NCT03309657), and multidrug-resistant *Pseudomonas aeruginosa* infections (NCT03510351), and in pediatric patients for gram-negative infections or as perioperative prophylaxis (NCT02266706), for cUTIs (NCT03230838), and for cIAIs (NCT03217136). Ceftolozane-tazobactam is clinically effective against a wide variety of common gram-negative bacteria and some gram-positive xxxs (**Table 1**).[24]

Limitations for the combination against indicated organisms include *P aeruginosa* or Enterobacterales that carry class A and class B carbapenemases (eg, KPC, VIM, NDM, and IMP) or class A, class C, and class D extended-spectrum β-lactamases (ESBLs) (eg, GES-6, PER-1, FOX-4, and OXA-539) that are not readily inhibited by tazobactam.[30–34] *E coli*–producing class A ESBLs are more susceptible to ceftolozane-tazobactam than *K pneumoniae*-expressing or *Enterobacter cloacae*–expressing class A ESBLs.[35–38] Chromosomal and acquired bla_{AmpC}s likely contribute to the former phenotype, because the hyperproduction of AmpCs or class A ESBLs was shown to reduce efficacy of ceftolozane-tazobactam.[33,36,39–41]

Ceftolozane is an expanded-spectrum cephalosporin that was developed with the intention of creating a novel, antipseudomonal β-lactam antibiotic that targets PBP3.[42] Ceftolozane is modeled on the success of the closely related cephalosporin, ceftazidime, which is a first-line treatment of *P aeruginosa* infections. Specifically, ceftolozane was designed to be stable to the presence of *Pseudomonas*-derived cephalosporinase (PDC),[43] the class C or AmpC β-lactamase of *P aeruginosa*.[44] Unfortunately, as with other oxyimino-cephalosporins, ceftolozane is susceptible to hydrolysis by certain ESBLs (eg, PER-1) and carbapenemases (eg, KPCs) that often occur in conjunction with other ceftolozane-susceptible enzymes and overexpression of class C enzymes reduces its potency.[45] Moreover, ceftolozane is readily hydrolyzed by class B metallo-β-lactamases (eg, VIM, IMP, and NDM) and activity against bacteria producing class D OXA β-lactamases is variable.[46]

Table 1
Clinical indications for the use of ceftolozane-tazobactam

Indication	Indicated Bacteria	Patient Population	Clinical Trial
cIAIs	*Enterobacter cloacae, Escherichia coli, K oxytoca, K pneumoniae, Proteus mirabilis, P aeruginosa, Bacteroides fragilis, Streptococcus anginosus, Streptococcus constellatus,* and *Streptococcus salivarius*	Adults	ASPECT-cIAI[25] NCT01445665 NCT01445678 NCT02739997[26]
cUTIs, including pyelonephritis	*E coli, K pneumoniae, Proteus mirabilis,* and *P aeruginosa*	Adults	ASPECT-cUTI[27] NCT01345929 NCT01345955 NCT02728089[28]
HABP/VABP	*Enterobacter cloacae, E coli, Haemophilus influenzae, K oxytoca, K pneumoniae, Proteus mirabilis, P aeruginosa,* and *S marcescens*	Adults	ASPECT-NP[29] NCT02070757

Data from Merck & Co., Inc. ZERBAXA (Ceftolozane and Tazobactam) for Injection, for Intravenous Use. Whitehouse Station, NJ 08889 USA; 2019.

Tazobactam is a penicillin-based sulfone derivative developed as a β-lactamase inhibitor[47] that inactivates most class A β-lactamases. Tazobactam demonstrates variable activity against bacteria producing class A carbapenemases, class C β-lactamases, and class D β-lactamases.[48,49] By using tazobactam in this combination, the goal was to inhibit class A ESBLs (eg, CTX-M) and tazobactam-susceptible class C β-lactamases (eg, CMY), thus extending the usefulness of the combination.[33,35,45]

REPORTS AND MECHANISMS OF RESISTANCE: CEFTOLOZANE-TAZOBACTAM

In **Table 2**, the reports of resistance to ceftolozane-tazobactam available at the time of this writing are summarized. The most frequently reported cause of ceftolozane-tazobactam resistance in isolates for which it is indicated is alterations in PDC, the chromosomally encoded class C β-lactamase of *P aeruginosa*. Amino acid substitutions, insertions, and deletions in PDC were found in broad survey studies, individual case reports, and laboratory selection experiments, suggesting they can emerge in a variety of ways. Additional mechanisms including acquisition of rare class A β-lactamases as well as amino acid substitutions in OXA enzymes are described herein (see also above).

Pseudomonas-Derived Cephalosporinase Variants that Confer Ceftolozane-Tazobactam Resistance

Not surprisingly, given the role it plays in β-lactamase function, the Ω-loop of PDC appears to be an important region for amino acid substitutions leading to ceftolozane-tazobactam resistance when these β-lactamases are expressed in bacteria, with V211A,[50,51] G214R,[51] E219G,[51] E219K,[51,52] and Y221H[51] leading to varying levels of resistance (minimum inhibitory concentrations [MICs] range for clinical isolates: 32–256 μg/mL) even as single amino acid substitutions (see **Fig. 3**, **Table 2**).[53] Several of these substitutions also occur in tandem with others, including

Table 2
Mechanisms of resistance to ceftolozane-tazobactam

Type	Organism	Mechanism(s)	Relevant Amino Acid Substitutions in β-Lactamase	Minimum Inhibitory Concentration of Isolate[a]	Minimum Inhibitory Concentration in a Susceptible Background[b]	Reference
Case report	*P aeruginosa*	PDC	G156D	≥64	≥64	57
Case report	*P aeruginosa*	Overexpression of PDC, loss of *oprD*	T96I	>32	32	52
Case report	*P aeruginosa*	Overexpression of PDC, loss of *oprD*	E219K	>32	16	52
Case report	*P aeruginosa*	Overexpression of PDC, loss of *oprD*	ΔG202-E219	32	32	52
Case report	*P aeruginosa*	Overexpression of PDC, loss of *oprD*, mutations in *mexD, mexT, mexI* and *mexR*	R52Q, T79 A, G156D	≥256	N/A	61
Case report	*P aeruginosa*	Overexpression of PDC	V211A	64	N/A	50
Case report	*P aeruginosa*	PDC, mutation in *mexR*	ΔP208-G214	>128	N/A	50
Case report	*P aeruginosa*	PDC, loss of *oprD*	G156D	32–48	N/A	60
Laboratory strain	*P aeruginosa*	Overexpression of PDC	G156D	64	32	55
Laboratory strain	*P aeruginosa*	Overexpression of PDC	E219K, V329I	32	64	55
Laboratory strain	*P aeruginosa*	Overexpression of PDC	F121L, Q130R, E219K, V329I	128	128	55
Survey	*P aeruginosa*	Overexpression of PDC, loss of *oprD*	Q128R, V211T, S279T	256	N/A	54
Survey	*P aeruginosa*	PDC, loss of *oprD* and mutations in *mexT*	A5V, V211A, G214R, G220S	12	N/A	54
Survey	*P aeruginosa*	Overexpression of PDC, loss of *oprD*	Q128R, V211A, G220S	256	N/A	54

(continued on next page)

Table 2 (*continued*)

Type	Organism	Mechanism(s)	Relevant Amino Acid Substitutions in β-Lactamase	Minimum Inhibitory Concentration of Isolate[a]	Minimum Inhibitory Concentration in a Susceptible Background[b]	Reference
Survey	*P aeruginosa*	Overexpression of PDC, loss of *oprD*	V211A	256	N/A	54
Survey	*P aeruginosa*	PDC	P153L	N/A	8	51
Survey	*P aeruginosa*	PDC	G214R	N/A	8	51
Survey	*P aeruginosa*	PDC	N346I	N/A	4–8	51
Survey	*P aeruginosa*	PDC	R100H, G214R	N/A	16	51
Survey	*P aeruginosa*	PDC	E219K	N/A	64 to >64	51
Survey	*P aeruginosa*	PDC	E219G	N/A	32	51
Survey	*P aeruginosa*	PDC	F121L, M174L	N/A	16	51
Survey	*P aeruginosa*	PDC	V211A, N346I	N/A	16	51
Survey	*P aeruginosa*	PDC	ΔT289-M291	N/A	4–8	51
Survey	*P aeruginosa*	PDC	ΔT289-A292	N/A	16	51
Case report	*P aeruginosa*	Overexpression of PDC, loss of *oprD*	ΔG202-E219	32	N/A	56
Survey	*P aeruginosa*	Overexpression of PDC and/or MexAB-OprM or MexXY-OprM and/or loss of *oprD*		8–16	N/A	68
Case report	*P aeruginosa*	PAC-1		>128	>128	74
Case report	*P aeruginosa*	FOX-4		16	16	34
Laboratory strain	*P aeruginosa*	GES-1		N/A	32	34
Laboratory strain	*P aeruginosa*	GES-2	G170N	N/A	16	34
Laboratory strain	*P aeruginosa*	GES-5	G170S	N/A	8	34

Laboratory Strain	*P aeruginosa*	GES-6	E104K, G170S	N/A	32	[34]
Case report	*P aeruginosa*	GES-6	E104K, G170S	32	64	[75]
Laboratory strain	*P aeruginosa*	PER-1		N/A	512	[34]
Laboratory strain	*P aeruginosa*	BEL-1		N/A	8	[34]
Laboratory strain	*P aeruginosa*	BEL-2		N/A	32	[34]
Survey	*P aeruginosa*	BEL-3	P160S	16	N/A	[80]
Laboratory strain	*P aeruginosa*	VEB-1		N/A	64	[34]
Case report	*P aeruginosa*	OXA-2, loss of *oprD*	Duplication D149	>32	16	[78]
Case report	*P aeruginosa*	OXA-2, VIM-20, mutation of *mexZ* *mexX,* and *mexB,* loss of *oprD*	ΔI159 + E160 K in OXA-2	>32	32	[79]
Survey	*P aeruginosa*	OXA-2	W159R	16–32	16	[68,80]
Survey	*P aeruginosa*	OXA-10	N73S	64	N/A	[80]
Survey	*P aeruginosa*	OXA-101		32	N/A	[80]
Case report	*P aeruginosa*	OXA-10, loss of *oprD*	N146S	32	N/A	[52]
Laboratory strain	*E coli*	GES-1		N/A	8	[31]
Laboratory strain	*E coli*	GES-5	G170S	N/A	8	[31]
Laboratory strain	*E coli*	GES-6	E104K, G170S	N/A	64	[31]
Case report	*E coli*	GES-19, GES-26		N/A	48	[77]
Laboratory strain	*E coli*	PER-1		N/A	128	[31]
Laboratory strain	*E coli*	BEL-1		N/A	4	[31]
Laboratory strain	*E coli*	BEL-2		N/A	8	[31]

Tazobactam is maintained at 4 μg/mL when in combination with ceftolozane.[81]

P aeruginosa breakpoints: intermediate = 8 μg/mL; resistant ≥16 μg/mL.

Enterobacterales breakpoints: intermediate = 4 μg/mL; resistant ≥8 μg/mL.

Abbreviation: NA, not available.

[a] The MIC values for the isolate represent the MIC values obtained for either a clinical isolate obtained from a patient in a case study or part of a surveillance study or a laboratory-selected strain.

[b] The MIC values in a susceptible background represent the MIC value after the *bla* gene for the β-lactamase of interest was cloned and expressed in a susceptible strain.

Data from Clinical and Laboratory Standards Institute (CLSI). *M100: Performance Standards for Antimicrobial Susceptibility Testing*. 30th ed.; 2020.

Q128R V211T S279T,[54] A5V V211A G214R G220S,[54] Q128R V211A G220S,[54] E219K V329I,[55] F121L Q130R E219K V329I,[55] R100H G214R,[51] and V211A N346I[51] (see **Fig. 3**). Of these Ω-loop substitutions, the V211A, E219K, and E219G variants of PDC surfaced alone and E219K in conjunction with G154R substitution during treatment of patients.[50,52,56]

Outside the Ω-loop, substitutions are found in several regions of the enzyme but do not seem to cluster in a specific area. These substitutions include T96I,[57,58] F121L,[56,59] G156D[55,57,60] and G156D in combination with R52Q and T79A,[61] P154L,[51] L293P, N346I,[51] and F121L M174L[51] (**Fig. 4**). At this writing, it is unknown if these substitutions outside the Ω loop serve to stabilize the protein (serve as a global suppressor) or specifically enhance catalytic activity. The T96I, F121L, and G156D variants of PDC emerged during treatment of patients for infections caused by *P aeruginosa* and ceftolozane-tazobactam MICs were elevated from 1 μg/mL to 4 μg/mL at the start of treatment to 32 μg/mL to 64 μg/mL during treatment.[52,56,57,60,61] Moreover, multiple amino acid deletions leading to ceftolozane-tazobactam resistance were reported in PDC and are found both in the Ω-loop, deleting residues P208-G214,[50,58,61] G202-E219,[53,56] and G204-Y221[58] as well as the R2 loop, deleting residues T289-P290, T289-M291, T289-A292, and L293-Q294.[51] The R2 loop deletions tend to be associated with relatively low-level resistance when expressed in *P aeruginosa* 4098 (MIC range: 4–16 μg/mL)[51] (see **Fig. 4**, **Table 2**). Of these loop deletions, at the time of this writing, only Ω-loop deletion variants of PDC in *P aeruginosa* were reported to have surfaced in the clinic during treatment and resulted in ceftolozane-tazobactam MICs of 32 μg/mL to 256 μg/mL.[50,52,56,58]

The Molecular Basis of the Resistance Phenotype: PDC E219K, an Ω-Loop Variant

Among the best-characterized β-lactamase variants conferring ceftolozane-tazobactam resistance is the E219K variant of PDC. When the negatively charged glutamic acid (E) residue at 219 is changed to a positively charged lysine (K) and expressed in *P aeruginosa* PAO1 Δbla_{PDC}, the ceftolozane-tazobactam MIC increases from 0.5 μg/mL to 16 μg/mL.[52] Steady-state kinetic characterization of the purified PDC-3 E219K variant with ceftolozane revealed a K_m of 341 μM ± 64 μM and a k_{cat} of 10 s^{-1} ± 1 s^{-1} compared with the wild-type PDC-3

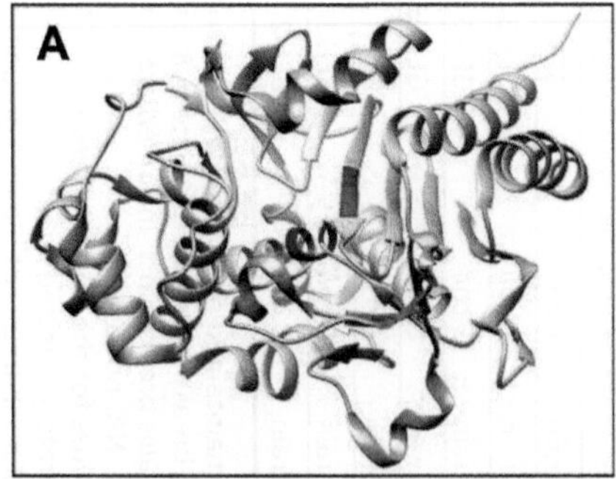

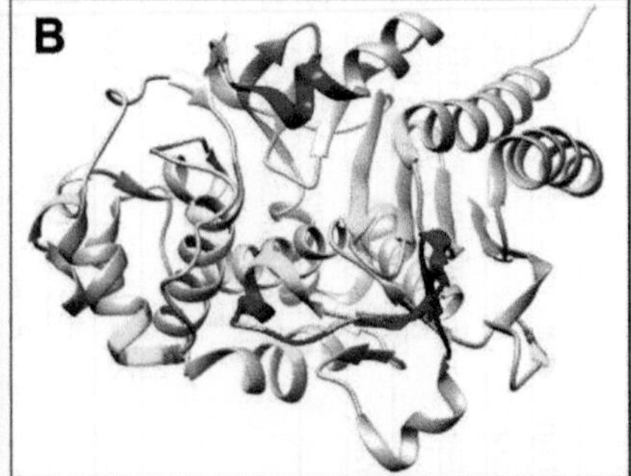

Fig. 4. PDC crystal structure highlighting the major active site motifs (*blue*: Ω-loop; *magenta*: $S_{64}X_{65}X_{66}K_{67}$ motif; *dark green*: $K_{315}T_{316}G_{316}$ motif; *light green*: $Y_{150}X_{151}K_{152}$ motif; and *pink*: R2 loop) (A) and the location of the amino acid substitutions, insertions, and deletions (*red*: deletion; *yellow*: substitution; and *orange*: deletion or substitution) that confer ceftolozane-tazobactam resistance (B).

enzyme, which had undetectable hydrolysis of ceftolozane and interacted with ceftolozane very poorly with a $K_{i\ app}$ of 1300 μM.[62] Moreover, electrospray-ionization mass spectrometry used to capture β-lactamase–ceftolozane adducts supported the kinetic observations, because, true to its design, ceftolozane was not detected bound to the wild-type *Pseudomonas* AmpC (PDC-3); conversely, ceftolozane was hydrolyzed by the PDC-3 E219K variant and acyl-enzyme complexes were not detected.[62] Thermal stability assays revealed that the PDC-3 E219K variant possessed a lower T_m of 45°C compared with 52°C for PDC-3; these data suggest that the PDC-3 E219K variant is less stable.

The molecular mechanism that allows the PDC-3 E219K variant to hydrolyze ceftolozane is perhaps best revealed by using classic atomistic molecular dynamics and well-tempered metadynamic simulations that model the interactions between the enzyme and substrate. The metadynamic simulations uncovered that the PDC-3 E219K variant was more conformationally flexible than the wild-type PDC-3. Moreover, the molecular dynamics showed that the flexibility of the PDC-3 E219K variant allows the nearby Y221 residue to rotate perpendicular to its usual position and open a hidden cavity adjacent to the active site (**Fig. 5**). This cavity is better able to accommodate the R1 group of ceftolozane (which normally faces a steric clash with Y221), allowing for better positioning of ceftolozane within the active site of the PDC-3 E219K variant to facilitate hydrolysis.

Other Contributing Resistance Factors in Pseudomonas aeruginosa

Variants of PDC that result in ceftolozane-tazobactam resistance are found in strains that also have decreased expression of *oprD* and/or up-regulation of *mexAB-oprM* or *mexXY-oprM* efflux pumps and/or de-repression of bla_{PDC} expression, which is

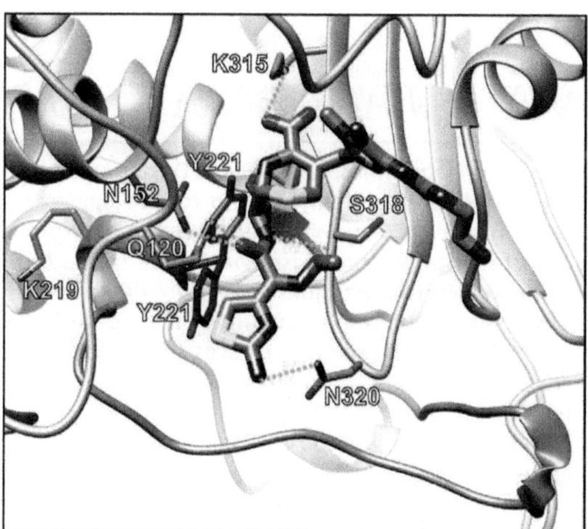

Fig. 5. Ceftolozane (*pink*) docked in the active site of the PDC-3 E219K variant. Hydrogen bonds between ceftolozane and residues are indicated with green dashed lines, the catalytic S64 is in cyan, and the Ω-loop in blue. Two conformations of Y221 showcase the increased flexibility of the variant: purple represents a conformation found in both PDC-3 and the PDC-3 E219K variant whereas green represents a conformation found only in the PDC-3 E219K variant, the E219K substitution enables the movement between these conformations, allowing ceftolozane to enter the active site and bind while maintaining residues in catalytically favorable conformations.

normally expressed at a low basal level and induced by the presence of β-lactam antibiotics(**Fig. 6**, see **Table 2**).[63–67] Regarding ceftolozane-tazobactam resistance, OprD does not appear to be necessary for entry of either compound and neither component is greatly impacted by hyperexpression of efflux pumps.[43,68] Controlled (eg, Δ*ampD* and Δ*dacB*) de-repression of wild-type *bla*$_{PDC-1}$ in a *P aeruginosa* PAO1 background revealed that ceftolozane MICs are not impacted by hyperexpression of *bla*$_{PDC-1}$.[69] In conjunction with other factors (eg, *bla*$_{PDC}$ mutants and other *bla* genes), however, de-

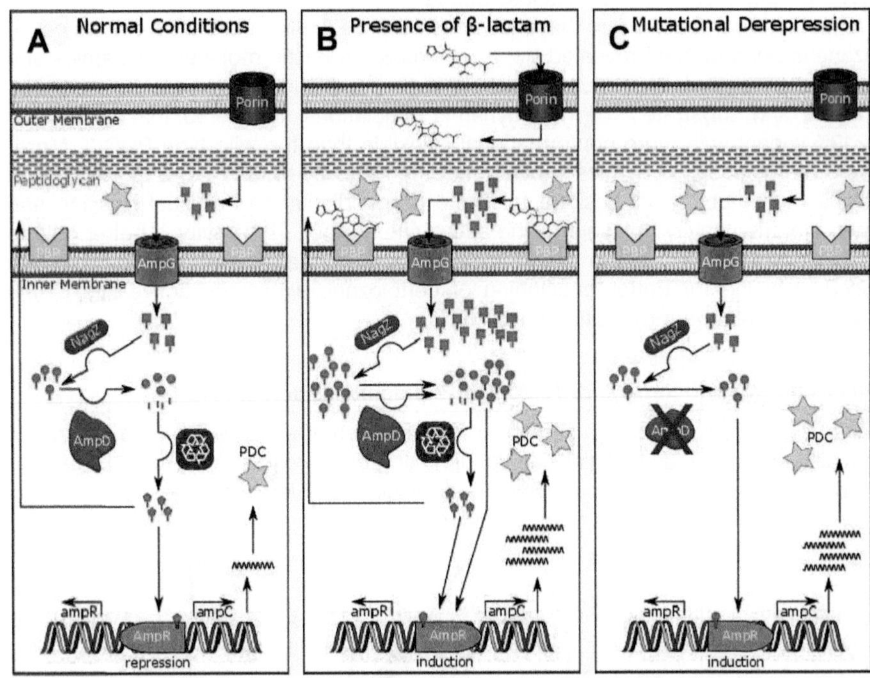

Fig. 6. Regulation of *bla*$_{PDC}$ in *P aeruginosa* (64–67). (*A*) During normal cell growth, bacteria degrade approximately half their peptidoglycan and recycle approximately 90% of these degradation products or Glc-NAc-1,6-anhydro-MurNAc-peptides (*green rectangular lollipops*), which are transported into the cytoplasm via AmpG. In the cytosol, NagZ catalyzes the formation of 1,6-anhydro-MurNAc-peptides (*green circular lollipops*) that are activating peptides of AmpR, a LysR-type transcriptional regulator that controls expression of *bla*$_{ampC}$. AmpD, an N-acetylmuramyl-L-alanine amidase, cleaves the peptide (*green stick*) from the 1,6-anhydro-MurNAc (*green circle*) and the components enter the recycling pathway, keeping the cytoplasmic levels of activating 1,6-anhydro-MurNAc-peptides low and producing UDP-MurNAc-pentapeptides (*green pentagonal lollipops*) that are suppressing peptides that bind AmpR to repress the transcription of *bla*$_{PDC}$. (*B*) In the presence of β-lactam antibiotics, the low molecular mass PBP4 (DacB) is inhibited (along with other PBPs), leading to an increase and shift in the composition of the Glc-NAc-1,6-anhydro-MurNAc-peptides entering the cytoplasm. This increase ultimately overpowers the capacity of AmpD to cleave the peptide from 1,6-anhydro-MurNAc, leading to a buildup of 1,6-anhydro-MurNAc-peptide in the cell. The 1,6-anhydro-MurNAc-peptide is then able to bind AmpR, activating transcription of *bla*$_{ampC}$. The AmpC β-lactamases are exported to the periplasm where they inactivate β-lactams. (*C*) Mutations in *ampD* are the most common cause of derepressed *bla*$_{ampC}$ by severely crippling the production and/or activity of AmpD, levels of 1,6-anhydro-MurNAc-peptides greatly increase within the cell, bind to AmpR, and induce the production of high levels of *bla*$_{ampC}$.

repression of bla_{PDC} (eg, mutations in *ampR*, *dacB*, *ampG*, and *ampD*) was shown to elevate ceftolozane-tazobactam MICs.[30,52,55] Importantly, high-level resistance due to overexpression of bla_{PDC} variants was associated with the hypermutator background of *P aeruginosa*.[55] Other potential contributors toward ceftolozane-tazobactam resistance in *P aeruginosa* are single amino acid substitutions in PBP3 (R504 C and F533 L); this may be an emerging phenotype due to selective pressure.[30,59]

The Impact of Other AmpCs

Resistance to ceftolozane-tazobactam in class C β-lactamases other than PDC is reported or studied much less frequently, but the Y221H substitution in CMY-2 was also shown to result in an elevated ceftolozane-tazobactam MIC (2.5 μg/mL).[70] Other Ω-loop substitutions leading to ceftolozane-tazobactam resistance in *P aeruginosa* have been reported in other species producing class C β-lactamases, but in the context of nonsusceptibility to different substrates (eg, ceftazidime), including E219K in *Citrobacter freundii* AmpC[71] and V211A combined with L239S in CMY-95.[72]

Additionally, SRT-1 of *Serratia marcescens* has lysine in the 219 position and exhibits better hydrolysis of several cephalosporins (eg, ceftazidime) than the closely related SST-1 with glutamic acid at 219.[73] Additionally, 4 cases of *P aeruginosa* harboring bla_{PAC-1} were reported in patients repatriated from Mauritius and Afghanistan.[74] PAC-1 is a unique class C β-lactamase with 47% sequence identity to PDC-1 and confers ceftolozane-tazobactam resistance; the introduction of bla_{PAC-1} into *P aeruginosa* PAO1 increased the ceftolozane-tazobactam MIC from less than or equal to 0.5 μg/mL to greater than 128 μg/mL. Recently, the FOX-4 cephamycinase was found responsible for elevated ceftolozane-tazobactam MICs (16 μg/mL) in a *P aeruginosa* clinical isolate.[34] Much remains to be explored with non-PDC AmpCs and their involvement in ceftolozane-tazobactam resistance.

Uncommon Class A β-Lactamases

The acquisition of several different class A β-lactamases (eg, GES, PER-1, BEL-1, BEL-2, and VEB-1) has been associated with the emergence of ceftolozane-tazobactam resistance.[31,36,53,59,75,76] Depending on the strain background in which these β-lactamases are produced, *P aeruginosa* versus *E coli*, the ceftolozane-tazobactam MICs vary (eg, *P aeruginosa* with bla_{GES-1} MIC = 32 μg/mL vs *E coli* with bla_{GES-1} MIC = 8 μg/mL)[31] (see **Table 4**). When the combination of bla_{GES-19} and bla_{GES-26} was expressed in *E coli* TG1, the MIC values for ceftolozane-tazobactam increased to 48 μg/mL compared with an MIC of greater than 256 μg/mL when in *P aeruginosa*.[77] The production of PER-1 in *P aeruginosa* PA01 resulted in high level ceftolozane-tazobactam resistance (MIC: 512 μg/mL).[31] Except for GES β-lactamases, rare class A carbapenemases (eg, IMI and SME) are poor cephalosporinases; thus, when expressed, these strains usually are susceptible to ceftolozane-tazobactam.[36]

Resistance Observed in Class D β-Lactamases

Ceftolozane-tazobactam–resistant OXA variants (eg, OXA-14) also were identified in surveillance studies and have emerged during treatment of infections due to *P aeruginosa*[52,56,68,78–80] (see **Table 2**). Many of these OXA variants acquired a single amino acid substitution, such as a strain of *P aeruginosa* producing the OXA-10 N146S variant possessed a ceftolozane-tazobactam MIC of 64 μg/mL.[52] The continued evolution of narrow-spectrum oxacillinases in *P aeruginosa* (such as OXA-14) to ceftolozane-tazobactam resistant variants may represent an emerging challenge when using ceftolozane-tazobactam.

NEWER β-LACTAM AND β-LACTAMASE INHIBITOR COMBINATIONS: CEFTAZIDIME-AVIBACTAM

Ceftazidime-avibactam was approved by the FDA in 2015 for adult and pediatric use in cIAIs (with metronidazole) and cUTIs, including pyelonephritis, and for adult use in HABP and VABP.[82] Ceftazidime-avibactam is being actively investigated for use in adult cystic fibrosis patients (NCT02504827), for nosocomial pneumonia in pediatric patients (NCT04040621), and in neonates and infants with gram-negative infections (NCT04126031).

Ceftazidime-avibactam is effective against a variety of gram-negative bacteria (**Table 3**).[82] Limitations for the combination against indicated organisms include *P aeruginosa* or Enterobacterales that carry class B carbapenemases (eg, VIM, NDM, and IMP)[83,84] and non–OXA-48–like class D β-lactamases with ESBL activity (eg, OXA-2 variants).[78,79,85,86]

Why is this combination so important? Ceftazidime is a broad-spectrum amino-thiazolyl cephalosporin originally approved by the FDA in July 1985. Ceftazidime demonstrates potent activity against a wide variety of gram-negative bacteria and some gram-positive bacteria, with particular strengths against *P aeruginosa* and Enterobacterales, including strains expressing many important β-lactamases.[93,94] Unfortunately, resistance to ceftazidime rapidly emerged (presence of ESBLs in many enteric bacilli, such as *E coli* and *K pneumoniae* and the overexpression of class C β-lactamases among other mechanisms) and the drug became less attractive and use was heavily monitored.[20,95,96] Ceftazidime-avibactam helped fill an important gap in the spectrum of other β-lactamases known and evolving at the time with its potent activity against *P aeruginosa* and ESBLs. In fact, an early article went so far as to describe ceftazidime as "the most effective antibiotic thus far known against *P. aeruginosa*."[94]

Table 3
Clinical indications for the use of ceftazidime-avibactam

Indication	Indicated Bacteria	Patient Population	
cIAI (with metronidazole)	*E coli, K pneumoniae, Proteus mirabilis, Enterobacter cloacae, K oxytoca, C freundii* complex, and *P aeruginosa*	Adult and pediatric (≥3 mo)	RECLAIM 1 and 2[87] NCT01499290 NCT01500239 REPRISE[88] NCT01644643 NCT02475733[89]
cUTI, including pyelonephritis	*E coli, K pneumoniae, Enterobacter cloacae, C freundii* complex, *Proteus mirabilis*, and *P aeruginosa*	Adult and pediatric (≥3 mo)	RECAPTURE[90] NCT01595438 NCT01599806 REPRISE[88] NCT01644643 NCT02497781
HABP/VABP	*K pneumoniae, Enterobacter cloacae, E coli, S marcescens, Proteus mirabilis, P aeruginosa*, and *Haemophilus influenzae*	Adult	REPROVE[91] NCT01808092[92]

Data from Allergan USA, Inc. AVYCAZ (Ceftazidime and Avibactam) for Injection, for Intravenous Use. Madison, NJ 07940 USA.; 2019.

Avibactam is the first of a novel class of β-lactamase inhibitors known as the DBOs and has a wide spectrum of activity against class A, class C, and some class D β-lactamases. Unique among previously available β-lactamase inhibitors (clavulanic acid, tazobactam, and sulbactam), the DBOs do not contain a β-lactam group. Inhibition is accomplished by the formation of a covalent acyl-enzyme complex between the active-site serine of the β-lactamase and the 8-membered cyclooctane ring of the DBO. Interestingly, deacylation typically occurs through a reversible mechanism that regenerates an intact molecule of avibactam, allowing for inhibition of further enzymes.[22,97,98] KPC-2 and metallo-β-lactamases possess the ability to hydrolyze avibactam; however, the rate of hydrolysis is very slow.[85,99]

REPORTS AND MECHANISMS OF RESISTANCE: CEFTAZIDIME-AVIBACTAM

Table 4 lists the existing reports of resistance to ceftazidime-avibactam described at the time of this writing. Phenotypic resistance to ceftazidime-avibactam appears to be driven largely by amino acid substitutions and deletions to the KPC carbapenemase found in Enterobacterales. These changes were reported mostly in case studies and laboratory selection experiments. Alarmingly, the first case report of ceftazidime-avibactam resistance in a *K pneumoniae* strain with $bla_{KPC\text{-}3}$ was in the same year that ceftazidime-avibactam was released.[100,101]

Ceftazidime-Avibactam–Resistant KPC Variants

Substitutions in KPC that lead to ceftazidime-avibactam resistance tend to cluster into 1 of 2 regions of the enzyme: substitutions, insertions, and deletions in the Ω-loop, residues 164 to 179 in class A β-lactamases, or insertions in the B3-4 β-strands and adjacent helices (**Fig. 7**, see **Table 4**). The importance of the Ω-loop of KPC in ceftazidime-avibactam resistance was revealed first in the summer of 2015 shortly after the release of the combination.[102] By exploiting the knowledge that evolution of the Ω-loop in β-lactamases is the Achilles heel for ceftazidime's antimicrobial activity,[16–19] several Ω-loop variants (R164A, R164P, D179A, D179Q, and D179N) of KPC-2 were tested and found resistant to ceftazidime-avibactam (MIC range: 16–64 μg/mL). Additionally, in vitro selection experiments conducted using KPC-3-producing Enterobacterales resulted in the selection of the D179Y variant of KPC-3 among other alterations (see **Table 4**) that led to ceftazidime-avibactam resistance, further exposing the Ω-loop as a weakness for this combination.[103] Subsequently, reports of ceftazidime-avibactam resistance began to emerge during treatment of patients with infections caused by carbapenem-resistant Enterobacterales carrying the D179Y variant of KPC-3, which elevated the ceftazidime-avibactam MICs from 2 μg/mL to 4 μg/mL prior to the start of treatment up to 64 μg/mL to greater than 256 μg/mL after treatment[104,105] (see **Table 4**). Concomitant with the development of ceftazidime-avibactam resistance, bacteria producing the D179Y variant lose carbapenem resistance. Importantly, the tyrosine substitution at 179 was shown to revert back to aspartic acid when grown in the presence of a carbapenem; thus, KPC regains its ability to hydrolyze carbapenems when exposed to a carbapenem.[106–109]

Another group found this reversion phenotype with other Ω-loop amino acid substitutions (D176Y, P174L, and R164S) in KPC that also caused elevated ceftazidime-avibactam MICs.[110] In 1 case, the 179 substitution reverted to aspartic acid and ceftazidime-avibactam resistance was maintained (MIC: 12 μg/mL) through amplification of $bla_{KPC\text{-}2}$ and loss of OmpK35 and OmpK36 when treating the patient with meropenem/polymyxin B.[108] Moreover, the addition of a polymyxin, colistin, to

Table 4
Mechanisms of resistance to ceftazidime-avibactam

Type	Organism	Mechanism(s)	Relevant Amino Acid Substitutions in β-Lactamase	Minimum Inhibitory Concentration of Isolate[a]	Minimum Inhibitory Concentration in a Susceptible Background[b]	Reference
Laboratory	*E coli*	KPC-2	R164A	N/A	16	102
Laboratory	*E coli*	KPC-2	R164P	N/A	64	102
Laboratory	*E coli*	KPC-2	D179A	N/A	64	102
Laboratory	*E coli*	KPC-2	D179Q	N/A	32	102
Laboratory	*E coli*	KPC-2	D179N	N/A	32	102
Laboratory	*E coli*	KPC-2	D179Y	N/A	32	106
Survey	*K pneumoniae*	KPC-2, SHV-12, TEM-1, and loss of *ompK35*, *ompk36*, and *ompK37*		16	N/A	166
Survey	*E coli*	KPC-2, TEM-1, 344_ins_TIPY_345_PBP3		8	N/A	153
Case	*K pneumoniae*	Overexpression of KPC-2, loss of *ompK35* and *ompK36*		12	N/A	108
Laboratory	*C freundii*	KPC-2, overexpression of *acrA*, loss of *ompF*	D176Y	32	8	110
Laboratory	*C freundii*	KPC-2, overexpression of *acrA*, loss of *ompF*	R146S, P147L	64	8	110
Laboratory	*C freundii*	KPC-2, overexpression of *acrA*, loss of *ompF*	D179Y	64	8	110
Case	*K pneumoniae*	KPC-2, SHV-11, SHV-12, TEM-1, loss of *ompK35*, *ompK36*, and *ompK37*	D179Y	>256		120

Survey	*K pneumoniae*	KPC-2	E166_ins_EL_L167, V278_ins_ SEAV_A281	128	64	117
Case	*K pneumoniae*	KPC-2	L169P	16	4	125
Case	*K pneumoniae*	KPC-2, SHV-11	L259_ins_ AVYTRAPNKDDKHSE_V260	>16		127
Laboratory	*E coli*	KPC-2	ΔG242-T243	N/A	24	126
Laboratory	*K pneumoniae*	KPC-3	S181_ins_S_S182	64		103
Laboratory	*K pneumoniae*	KPC-3	D179Y	8–64		103
Laboratory	*K pneumoniae*	KPC-3	D163G	32		103
Laboratory	*Enterobacter cloacae*	KPC-3	S181_ins_SS_S182	32		103
Laboratory	*Enterobacter cloacae*	KPC-3	P174L	8–16		103
Laboratory	*Enterobacter cloacae*	KPC-3	T243P	32		103
Laboratory	*Enterobacter cloacae*	KPC-3	T265_ins_AR_R266	16		103
Laboratory	*Enterobacter cloacae*	KPC-3	P183_ins-RAVTTSSP_R184	128		103
Case	*K pneumoniae*	KPC-3, SHV-11, TEM-1, OXA-9 and loss of *ompk36*	D179Y	64–256	8	104
Case	*K pneumoniae*	KPC-3, SHV-11, TEM-1, OXA-9 and loss of *ompk36*	D179Y, T243M	256	64	104
Case	*K pneumoniae*	KPC-3, SHV-11, TEM-1, OXA-9	V240G	32	2	104
Case	*K pneumoniae*	KPC-3, SHV-11, TEM-1, OXA-9 and loss of *ompk35*	A177E, D179Y	128	N/A	107
Case	*K pneumoniae*	Overexpression of KPC-3, loss of *ompk35* and *ompk35*, SHV-11, SHV-12		32		145
Survey	*K pneumoniae*	KPC-3	ΔE166-L167	16–32	8–16	117
Survey	*K pneumoniae*	KPC-3	L7P, D179Y, T243M	256	N/A	117

(*continued on next page*)

Table 4 (*continued*)

Type	Organism	Mechanism(s)	Relevant Amino Acid Substitutions in β-Lactamase	Minimum Inhibitory Concentration of Isolate[a]	Minimum Inhibitory Concentration in a Susceptible Background[b]	Reference
Case	*K pneumoniae*	KPC-3, SHV-11, TEM-1A, OXA-9 loss of *ompK35* and *ompK36*	V240A	16	N/A	118
Laboratory	*E coli*	KPC-3	ΔG242-T243	N/A	12	126
Laboratory	*K pneumoniae*	KPC-3	D163G	32	N/A	109
Laboratory	*K pneumoniae*	KPC-3	R164S	64	N/A	109
Laboratory	*K pneumoniae*	KPC-3	E168_ins_EL_L169	32	N/A	109
Laboratory	*K pneumoniae*	KPC-3	L169_ins-KL_N170	64	N/A	109
Laboratory	*K pneumoniae*	KPC-3	N170D	32	N/A	109
Laboratory	*K pneumoniae*	KPC-3	N170D + ΔS171	>256	N/A	109
Laboratory	*K pneumoniae*	KPC-3	A172S	64	N/A	109
Laboratory	*K pneumoniae*	KPC-3	A172T + T243A	64	N/A	109
Laboratory	*K pneumoniae*	KPC-3	A172P	64	N/A	109
Laboratory	*K pneumoniae*	KPC-3	P174L	64	N/A	109
Laboratory	*K pneumoniae*	KPC-3	P174_ins_PGDARD_D179	64	N/A	109
Laboratory	*K pneumoniae*	KPC-3	G175V	64	N/A	109
Laboratory	*K pneumoniae*	KPC-3	D176Y	32	N/A	109
Laboratory	*K pneumoniae*	KPC-3	D179A	>256	N/A	109
Laboratory	*K pneumoniae*	KPC-3	D179H	>256	N/A	109
Laboratory	*K pneumoniae*	KPC-3	D179N	32	N/A	109
Laboratory	*K pneumoniae*	KPC-3	D179Y	>256	N/A	109
Laboratory	*K pneumoniae*	KPC-3	ΔV240	128	N/A	109

Laboratory	*K pneumoniae*	KPC-3	Y241N	64	N/A	109
Laboratory	*K pneumoniae*	KPC-3	T243M	32	N/A	109
Laboratory	*K pneumoniae*	KPC-3	Y263_ins_YTRAPN_N269	>256	N/A	109
Laboratory	*K pneumoniae*	KPC-3	Y263_ins_ YTRAPNKDDKYSEAV_V278	>256	N/A	109
Laboratory	*K pneumoniae*	KPC-3	R266_ins_RAS_P268	>256	N/A	109
Laboratory	*K pneumoniae*	KPC-3	R266_ins_RAPNKDDKYS_S275	>256	N/A	109
Laboratory	*K pneumoniae*	KPC-3	P268_ins_PN_N269	64	N/A	109
Laboratory	*K pneumoniae*	KPC-3	K270_ins_ KD_D271	128	N/A	109
Case	*K pneumoniae*	KPC-3	K270_PNK_D271	>128	128	128
Case	*K pneumoniae*	KPC-3	L169P, A172T	>16		122
Case	*K pneumoniae*	KPC-3	A172T, T243A	>16		122
Case	*K pneumoniae*	KPC-3	A172T	>16		122
Survey	*K oxytoca*	SHV-12, TEM-1		16		134
Laboratory	*E coli*	CTX-M-15	S130G, L169Q	N/A	16	133
Case	*K pneumoniae*	CTX-M-14, OXA-48	CTX-M-14: P167S, T264I	32		132
Laboratory	*E coli*	GES-5		N/A	0.5	31
Laboratory	*E coli*	PER-1		N/A	8	31
Laboratory	*E coli*	GES-19, GES-26		N/A	256	77
Case	*K pneumoniae*	VEB-1, TEM-1, OXA-10	K234R	32–128		138
Survey	*E coli*	CMY-42, CTX-M-15, OXA-1, 333_ins_YRIK_334_PBP3		8	N/A	154
Survey	*E coli*	CMY-42, CMY-2, OXA-1, OXA-9, TEM-1, 333_ins_YRIK_334_PBP3		8	N/A	154
Survey	*K pneumoniae*	DHA-1, loss of *ompK35* and *ompK36*		16	N/A	41
Survey	*Enterobacter cloacae*	AmpC	ΔS289-A294	64	N/A	140

(*continued on next page*)

Table 4
(continued)

Type	Organism	Mechanism(s)	Relevant Amino Acid Substitutions in β-Lactamase	Minimum Inhibitory Concentration of Isolate[a]	Minimum Inhibitory Concentration in a Susceptible Background[b]	Reference
Laboratory	*Enterobacter cloacae*	AmpC	G156R	64	N/A	139
Laboratory	*Enterobacter cloacae*	AmpC	G156D	16	N/A	139
Laboratory	*C freundii*	AmpC	N346Y	16	N/A	139
Laboratory	*C freundii*	AmpC	R148P	16	N/A	139
Laboratory	*C freundii*	AmpC	R148H	32	N/A	139
Survey	*K pneumoniae*	OXA-48, SHV		16	N/A	161
Survey	*S marcescens*	OXA-48, CTX-M-22, SHV		64	N/A	161
Survey	*P aeruginosa*	GES-5		16	N/A	31
Case	*P aeruginosa*	GES-19, GES-26		128 to >256	N/A	77
Survey	*P aeruginosa*	PER-1		64	N/A	31
Laboratory	*P aeruginosa*	PDC	ΔR210-E219	64–256	N/A	141
Laboratory	*P aeruginosa*	PDC	ΔK204a-G222	64	N/A	141
Laboratory	*P aeruginosa*	PDC	ΔD217-Y221	256	N/A	141
Laboratory/Case	*P aeruginosa*	PDC	G156D	128	>32	57,60,141,142
Case	*P aeruginosa*	Overexpression of PDC, loss of *oprD*	T96I	16–32	8	52

Case	*P aeruginosa*	Overexpression of PDC, loss of *oprD*	E219K	>32	16	52
Case	*P aeruginosa*	Overexpression of PDC, loss of *oprD*	ΔG202-E219	32	16	52
Survey	*P aeruginosa*	Overexpression of PDC and MexAB-OprM, loss of *oprD*		512	N/A	52
Case	*P aeruginosa*	Overexpression of PDC	V211A	>64	N/A	50
Case	*P aeruginosa*	PDC, mutation in *mexR*	ΔP208-G214	>64	N/A	50
Survey	*P aeruginosa*	Overexpression of PDC, loss of *oprD*	Q128R, V211T, S279T	256	N/A	54
Survey	*P aeruginosa*	Overexpression of PDC, loss of *oprD*	Q128R, V211A, G220S	256	N/A	54
Survey	*P aeruginosa*	Overexpression of PDC, loss of *oprD*	V211A	256	N/A	54
Case	*P aeruginosa*	PAC-1		>128	>128	74
Case	*P aeruginosa*	FOX-4		32	32	34
Case	*P aeruginosa*	OXA-2, loss of *oprD*	Duplication D149	>32	32	78
Case	*P aeruginosa*	OXA-10, loss of *oprD*	N146S	32	N/A	52
Case	*P aeruginosa*	OXA-2, VIM-20, mutation of *mexZ mexX*, and *mexB*, loss of *oprD*	ΔI159 + E160K in OXA-2	32	32	79

Avibactam is maintained at 4 μg/mL when in combination with ceftazidime.[81]

P aeruginosa breakpoint: resistant >8 μg/mL.

Enterobacterales breakpoint: resistant >8 μg/mL.

Abbreviation: NA, not available.

[a] The MIC values for the isolate represent the MIC values obtained for either a clinical isolate obtained from a patient in a case study or part of a surveillance study or a laboratory-selected strain.

[b] The MIC values in a clean background represent the MIC value after the *bla* gene for the β-lactamase of interest was cloned and expressed in a susceptible strain.

Data from Clinical and Laboratory Standards Institute (CLSI). *M100: Performance Standards for Antimicrobial Susceptibility Testing*. 30th ed.; 2020.

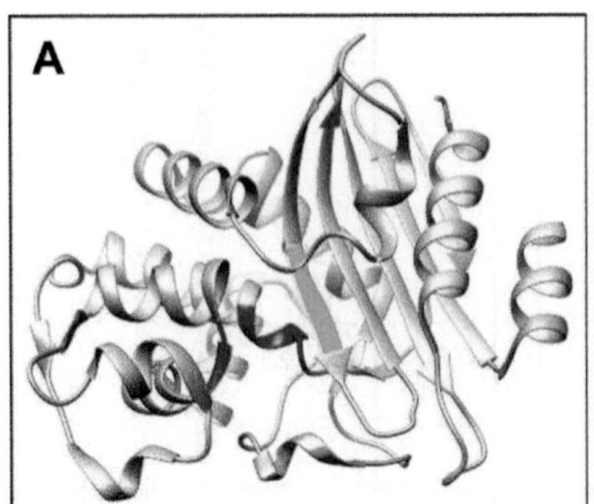

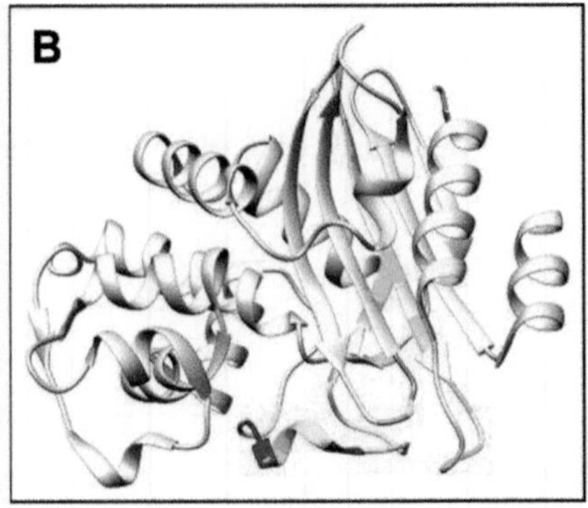

Fig. 7. KPC-2 crystal structure highlighting the major active site motifs (*blue*: Ω-loop, R_{164}-D_{179}; *magenta*: $S_{70}X_{71}X_{72}K_{73}$ motif; *dark green*: $S_{130}D_{131}N_{132}$ loop; and *bright green*: $K_{234}T_{235}G_{236}$ motif) (A) and the location of the amino acid substitutions, insertions, and deletions (*cyan*: insertion after residue; *yellow*: substitution; *orange*: deletion or substitution; *red*: deletion; *green*: insertion or substitution; and *purple* deletion or insertion) that confer ceftazidime-avibactam resistance (B).

ceftazidime-avibactam does not prevent the emergence of resistance to ceftazidime-avibactam by KPC-producing Enterobacterales.[111] Another study assessed population diversity and found that wild-type KPC-3 and KPC-3 D179Y coexisted as a mixed population.[112] Based on these observations, a case can be made that carbapenem monotherapy should not be considered as a therapeutic regimen against ceftazidime-avibactam–resistant KPC-producing Enterobacterales despite their carbapenem-susceptible phenotype.[113] The clinical risk factors associated with the potential for KPC-producing Enterobacterales to acquire ceftazidime-avibactam resistance during treatment include pneumonia and renal replacement therapy.[114] Likely, the concentration of the drug combination at the infection site does not remain above the MIC for a sufficient time and resistant variants are selected; therapeutic drug monitoring and proper dosage selection may be helpful in these cases.[115,116] This leads to speculation that perhaps the dosing of ceftazidime avibactam should be modified in certain cases.

In addition to the D179Y variant of KPC-3, other variants, D179Y T243M, V240G, A177E D179Y, Δ166-167, L7P D179Y T243M, and V240A, also began to emerge in the clinic.[104,117,118] The D179Y variant,[103,104,106,109,110,117,119–123] however, continues to be the most commonly reported substitution leading to ceftazidime-avibactam resistance and also has emerged in KPC-2.[108] The KPC-2 D179Y variant also was identified in a *P aeruginosa* strain in Chile, where ceftazidime-avibactam was never used.[124] Importantly, this study was evaluating a rapid immunochromatographic test for detection of KPC and the variant was not identified by this test or Carba-NP testing.[124] Also, in the Ω-loop, L169P occurred in KPC-2 during the treatment of a patient for VABP; the cloned KPC-2 L169P variant expressed in *E coli* DH5α possessed an MIC of 4 μg/mL, while the parent clinical strain's MIC was 16 μg/mL.[125] Subsequently, another L169P variant in conjunction with an A172T substitution emerged in KPC-3 during the treatment of an IAI caused by *K pneumoniae*; in the same study, the patient also was infected with 2 ceftazidime-avibactam–resistant *K pneumoniae* carrying the KPC-3 D179Y variant and a KPC-3 A172T variant and became colonized by a fourth ceftazidime-avibactam–resistant KPC-3 A172T T243A variant.[122] The rapidly converting and changing phenotypes of these KPC-3 variants is concerning.

Other KPC-2 variants that surfaced during treatment, include 1 that acquired 2 insertions (E and L) between Ω-loop residues 166-167 and S-E-A-V between the C-terminal α-helix residues 278-281 that resulted in a ceftazidime-avibactam MIC of 128 μg/mL.[117] A deletion of residues G242-T243 in the B4 β-strand of KPC-2 and KPC-3 (KPC-14 and KPC-28, respectively) resulted in low-level resistance to ceftazidime-avibactam (MICs: 12–24 μg/mL) due to increased catalytic efficiency toward ceftazidime mediated by lower K_m values; inhibition kinetics revealed that avibactam possessed similar IC_{50} values (range: 107–586 nM) against all variants tested.[126]

Two laboratory studies selected for ceftazidime-avibactam–resistant mutants using various Enterobacterales parent strains producing KPC-3 and found many substitutions that conferred resistance to ceftazidime-avibactam.[103,109] The D179Y, D163G (a location before the Ω loop), and P174L substitutions were identified in both studies; however, only D179Y emerged in the clinic. One study further examined if imipenem susceptibility was affected by the acquisition of ceftazidime-avibactam resistance.[109] The KPC-3 D163G, R164S, N170D, A172S, A172T, A172P, P174L, G175V, Y241N, and T243M variants, along with a KPC-3 ΔV240 variant, and several KPC-3 variants with different insertions in the B5 β-strand and subsequent loop residues (263–278) maintained imipenem resistance (MICs: ≥32 μg/mL), while correspondingly acquiring ceftazidime-avibactam resistance (range: 32 to >256 μg/mL).[109] These data further exemplify the need to screen KPC-producers against carbapenems and ceftazidime-avibactam.

Unfortunately, these gain-of-function observations were not limited to the laboratory. The B5 β-strand seems capable of absorbing large changes leading to increases in ceftazidime-avibactam MICs, with an insertion of NH_2-A-V-Y-T-R-A-P-N-K-D-D-K-H-S-E-CO_2 in the B5 β-strand between residues 261 and 262 of KPC-2 raising MICs from 1 μg/mL to greater than 16 μg/mL; this KPC-2 variant surfaced during treatment of a patient for bacteremia due to *K pneumoniae*.[127] In addition, another insertion in the B5 β-strand of PNK between K270 and D271 of KPC-3 in a *K pneumoniae* strain was obtained from a rectal swab of a patient and resulted in a ceftazidime-avibactam MIC of greater than 128 μg/mL.[128] This KPC-3 variant was purified for kinetic characterization and the results implicated a lower K_d for the variant with ceftazidime as the primary driver for resistance, as conversely the K_i for avibactam increased 6-fold from KPC-3.[128]

The Mechanism Behind the Resistance: KPC D179N, an Ω-Loop Variant

Among the most-studied β-lactamase variants leading ceftazidime-avibactam resistance is the D179N variant of KPC-2. The D179 residue forms a salt bridge with R164 in wild-type KPC-2 (**Fig. 8**). When the negatively charged aspartic acid residue at 179 (D) is changed to a polar asparagine (N) and expressed in *E coli* DH10 B, the ceftazidime-avibactam MIC increases from 1 μg/mL to 16 μg/mL.[129] Steady-state kinetic characterization of the purified KPC-2 D179N variant revealed that ceftazidime is hydrolyzed at a slower rate with the variant compared with wild-type KPC-2. The apparent K_m value for ceftazidime with the KPC-2 D179N variant, however, was 130 μM compared with 3500 μM with wild-type KPC-2. These kinetic observations suggest that the KPC-2 D179N variant forms more favorable interactions with ceftazidime than wild-type KPC-2 does. The inhibition by avibactam of the KPC-2 D179N variant was not significantly altered compared with wild-type KPC-2 (acylation rates: 38,000 $M^{-1}s^{-1}$ vs 17,000 $M^{-1}s^{-1}$, respectively).[102] Electrospray-ionization mass spectrometry used to capture β-lactamase adducts revealed the unique trapping phenotype of the KPC-2 D179N variant. Acyl-enzyme adducts were detected when all β-lactams (eg, ceftazidime, ceftolozane, and imipenem) were incubated with the KPC-2 D179N variant but not with wild-type KPC-2, which presumably hydrolyzed

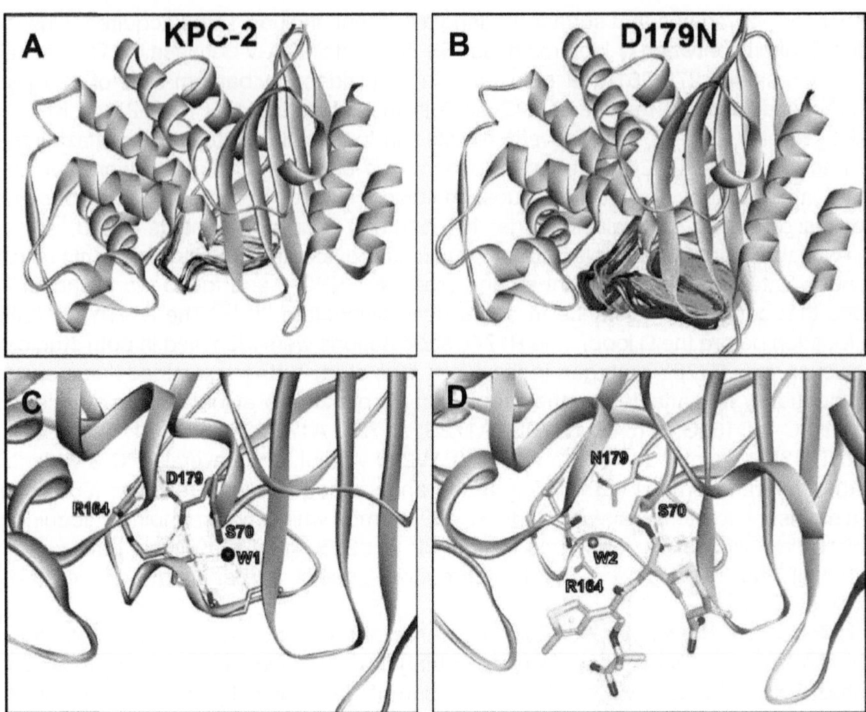

Fig. 8. Molecular modeling and 500-ns molecular dynamic simulation revealed the flexibility and mobility of the Ω-loop was increased in the (*B*) KPC-2 D179N variant due to disruption of the salt bridge with R164; mobility is RMSD of (*A*) 2 Å in KPC-2 versus (*B*) 10 Å for D179N variant. (*C*) In KPC-2, the R164 residue forms a salt bridge with D179 and hydrogen bonding network with a water molecule (W1). (*D*) The substitution D179N disrupts the salt bridge, and the nucleophilic S70 and the general base, E166 are repositioned, which results in the repositioning of the catalytic water (W2) and the formation of a longer-lasting acyl-enzyme complex with the variant and ceftazidime. RMSD, root-mean-square deviation.

these substrates. Moreover, when the β-lactamases were incubated with equimolar concentrations of β-lactam and avibactam, the KPC-2 D179N variant preferentially bound the β-lactam, whereas KPC-2 favored avibactam. Molecular modeling revealed that the flexibility and mobility of the Ω-loop were increased in the KPC-2 D179N variant due to disruption of the salt bridge with R164; this mobility likely allows ceftazidime to interact more favorably with the active site of the variant (see **Fig. 8**A, B). In addition, the catalytic residue S70 and the general base E166 were repositioned, thus allowing for a longer-lasting acyl-enzyme complex with the variant and the observed trapping phenotype (see **Fig. 8**C, D).[129]

In addition to the analysis of the KPC-2 D179N variant, the KPC-2 D179Y variant was investigated by another group and they found the variant to have a greater than 43-fold decrease in K_m toward ceftazidime and a greater than 1000-fold decrease in k_{cat} compared with wild-type KPC-2.[106] These data suggest that the variant can form favorable interactions with ceftazidime more readily than wild-type but is not able to hydrolyze ceftazidime; this is similar to the observation with the KPC-2 D179N variant.[106] Conversely, the acylation rate of avibactam toward the KPC-2 D179Y variant was decreased significantly compared with wild-type (0.4 $M^{-1}s^{-1}$ vs

29,000 $M^{-1}s^{-1}$, respectively). The KPC-2 D179Y variant also appears to trap ceftazidime but is not effectively inhibited by avibactam.

Avibactam-Resistant Variants of KPC

Oxapenem, sulfone, and DBO β-lactamase inhibitors follow a similar reaction pathway toward acyl-enzyme formation. Indeed, substitutions (eg, S130G, K234R, and R220M) that have an impact on inhibition by traditional inhibitors, such as clavulanic acid, also effect the ability of avibactam to inhibit β-lactamases.[130] The S130G substitution in KPC-2 resulted in the inability of avibactam to effectively acylate the enzyme. A subsequent report revealed the importance of the N132 residue in KPC-2 for acylation by avibactam; the N132G mutant was also unable to be acylated by avibactam.[131] Fortunately, these substitutions also reduced KPC-2's hydrolysis of β-lactams; thus, the contribution toward ceftazidime-avibactam resistance was limited. As KPC enzymes continue to evolve, however, the impact of these inhibitor-resistant substitutions may emerge.

Contributions of Other Class A Enzymes

Amino acid substitution of P167S in the Ω-loop of CTX-M-14 occurring in combination with T264I and OXA-48 resulted in a ceftazidime-avibactam MIC of 32 μg/mL for *K pneumoniae*.[132] The role of the Ω-loop in expanding the spectrum of CTX-M-15 enzymes against ceftazidime-avibactam was assessed and the combination of L169Q (Ω-loop) and S130G (SDN loop) in CTX-M-15 resulted in an MIC of 16 μg/mL, when expressed in *E coli*; the purified CTX-M-15 S130 G L169Q variant hydrolyzed ceftazidime efficiently and was not inhibited by avibactam (IC_{50} >50 mM).[133] *K oxytoca* with bla_{TEM-1} and bla_{SHV-12} tested nonsusceptible to ceftazidime-avibactam in a large surveillance study.[134] In other large surveillance studies, *P aeruginosa* isolates producing class A PER, GES, or VEB β-lactamases demonstrated reduced susceptibility to ceftazidime-avibactam[76,135–137]; however, some of these isolates were not evaluated for other potentially contributing mechanisms.[135] Another study found that the production of GES-5 and PER-1 in *P aeruginosa* did result in ceftazidime-avibactam resistance; however, when these *bla* genes were cloned and expressed in *E coli* TOP10, the MICs were lowered to 0.5 μg/mL and 16 μg/mL, respectively.[31] Similarly, the *P aeruginosa* background causes elevated MICs against these agents, as was seen with ceftolozane-tazobactam. Low-level resistance in *E coli* is amplified when both GES-19 and GES-26 are introduced in *E coli* TG1; the ceftazidime-avibactam MIC increased from 0.5 μg/mL to 256 μg/mL, which was comparable to the parent *P aeruginosa* MICs of 128 to greater than 256 μg/mL.[77] Recently, 2 different patients in Greece acquired *K pneumoniae* producing a VEB-1 K234R variant that demonstrated resistance to ceftazidime-avibactam (MICs: 32–128 μg/mL).[138]

Resistance in Enterobacterales AmpCs

Enterobacterales AmpCs can acquire resistance to ceftazidime-avibactam. Single amino acid substitutions were selected for in *Enterobacter cloacae* AmpC (G156R and G156D) and *C freundii* AmpC (R148H, R148P, and N346Y) that raised MICs to ceftazidime-avibactam from 0.5 μg/mL for the parent strains to 16 μg/mL to 32 μg/mL for the selected isolates.[139] Moreover, a deletion of 289-294 in the *Enterobacter cloacae* AmpC resulted in a ceftazidime-avibactam MIC of 64 μg/mL.[140] Evidence suggests that deletions in the vicinity of residue 290 are the result of enlargement in the R2 binding pocket allowing for β-lactams with larger R2 groups, such as ceftazidime, to be better accommodated.[140]

Ceftazidime-Avibactam Resistance of Pseudomonas-Derived Cephalosporinase Variants

Laboratory selection experiments in *P aeruginosa* identified several changes in PDC (ΔR210-E219, ΔK204a-G222, and ΔD217-Y221) that resulted in ceftazidime-avibactam resistance.[141] The ΔD217-Y221 in PDC increased the baseline MIC from 8 μg/mL to 256 μg/mL for ceftazidime-avibactam when expressed in *P aeruginosa*.[141] Purification of the wild-type and variant PDCs revealed that the ΔD217-Y221 variant's k_{cat} for ceftazidime increased by 650-fold and IC_{50} value for avibactam increased by 25-fold. Thus, resistance in this variant was due to increased turnover of ceftazidime as well as reduced inhibition by avibactam. Subsequently, during the selection of ceftolozane-tazobactam–resistant variants, cross-resistance to ceftazidime-avibactam was revealed. Several of the same substitutions in PDC including T96I,[52] G156D,[57,60,141,142] Ω-loop substitutions V211A[50,54] and E219K,[52] combinations Q128R V211T S279T, and Q128R V211A G220S,[54] and ΔP208-G214[50] and ΔG202-E219,[52] that result in resistance to ceftolozane-tazobactam have been reported to also lead to ceftazidime-avibactam resistance in *P aeruginosa*. Cross-resistance in *P aeruginosa* to ceftazidime-avibactam and ceftolozane-tazobactam is highly alarming. A large surveillance study also revealed many PDC variants present in *P aeruginosa* led to resistance to ceftazidime-avibactam; however, the contribution of these variants toward this resistance was not validated.[136] Acquisition of novel non-PDC AmpCs in *P aeruginosa*, PAC-1, or FOX-4 also resulted in resistance to ceftazidime-avibactam.[34,74] Moreover, the ability of *P aeruginosa* to become ceftazidime-avibactam–resistant was found more pronounced in a hypermutator background.[142]

Other Considerations

In Enterobacterales, loss of outer membrane proteins (porins) did not result in resistance to ceftazidime-avibactam even in KPC-producing, AmpC-producing, and/or ESBL-producing strains.[143,144] Strains carrying KPC-2, ESBLs (ie, TEM, SHV, or CTX-M), and *ompK36* porin mutations, however, demonstrated statistically significant higher MICs toward ceftazidime-avibactam.[143] Moreover, overexpression of bla_{KPC} in conjunction with loss of OmpK35 and OmpK36 and/or production of ESBLs has been reported to contribute to ceftazidime-avibactam resistance[119,123,145–148]; in a patient who failed on ceftazidime-avibactam treatment, the ceftazidime-avibactam MICs increased from 4 μg/mL to 32 μg/mL after therapy. Loss of OmpK35 and OmpK36 in concurrence with the production of the DHA-1 class C β-lactamase in *K pneumoniae* also elevated ceftazidime-avibactam MICs to 16 μg/mL,[41] as did loss of porins and production of CTX-M-15 and OXA-1 in *K pneumoniae*.[149]

In 3 large surveillance studies of 10,998 *Klebsiella* species, 6209 Enterobacterales, and 36,380 Enterobacterales, small subsets of isolates (n = 16, n = 5, and n = 14, respectively) were resistant to ceftazidime-avibactam and the mechanisms for most of these resistant strains could not be determined.[150–152] The investigators of 1 study proposed that potentially these isolates may have novel modifications of β-lactamases or PBP sequences or changes in drug efflux levels.[150] Indeed, 2 different 4–amino acid insertions in PBP3 found in 3 different *E coli* isolates carrying various *bla* genes possessed elevated ceftazidime-avibactam MICs of 8 μg/mL.[153,154] Contrary to Enterobacterales, out of 7062 *P aeruginosa* tested in a surveillance study, 272 isolates were resistant to ceftazidime-avibactam also with undefined resistance mechanisms; thus, a higher proportion of *P aeruginosa* are resistant to ceftazidime-avibactam compared with Enterobacterales.[155] In *P aeruginosa*, overexpression of bla_{PDC} as well as efflux and permeability of ceftazidime-avibactam appear to play a role in resistance to the combination.[63,136,156–159] In a *P aeruginosa* PAO1 background, however, controlled (eg, Δ*ampD* and Δ*dacB*) de-repression of wildtype bla_{PDC-1}, loss of *oprD*, and/or hyperexpression of efflux pumps (eg, Δ*mexR* and Δ*mexZ*) did not have a a significant impact on ceftazidime-avibactam MICs (range: 1–4 μg/mL).[156] In vitro selection experiments using *P aeruginosa* strain PA14 revealed the mutations in *dnaJ*, *pepA*, *ctpA*, *glnD*, *flgF*, *pcm*, *spoT*, and genes encoding an unidentified 2-component system and efflux pump component also effected resistance to ceftazidime-avibactam (MICs: ≥256 μg/mL); the exact mechanisms are not well understood.[160]

The Impact of Class D Oxacillinases

Except for OXA-48, most class D β-lactamases are not inhibited well by avibactam; however, as long as these enzymes are poor ceftazidimases, ceftazidime-avibactam will restore susceptibility, with ceftazidime doing the heavy lifting. Mutations in genes encoding OXA enzymes that extend their profile to ceftazidime have been reported to cause ceftazidime-avibactam resistance.[52,78,79] When the D149 residue in OXA-2 was duplicated, the ceftazidime-avibactam MIC for *P aeruginosa* PAO1 expressing OXA-2 versus the variant enzyme increased from 1 μg/mL to 32 μg/mL.[78] The expression of other *bla* genes (eg, bla_{SHV} and bla_{CTX-M}) also has been shown to result in elevated ceftazidime-avibactam MICs (16–64 μg/mL) in Enterobacterales producing OXA-48.[161] In vitro laboratory selection on ceftazidime-avibactam using *E coli* MG1655 expressing bla_{OXA-48} revealed that substitutions of P68A and Y211S in OXA-48 elevated ceftazidime-MICs and the OXA-48 P68A Y211S variant possessed an approximately 6-fold increase in K_i for avibactam.[162]

Overcoming the Limitation Incurred from Class B Metallo-β-Lactamases

Not surprising, given that they fall outside the target activity of avibactam, the class B metallo-β-lactamases commonly are associated with high-level resistance to ceftazidime-avibactam. Notably, clinical case reports[77] and laboratory testing[163–165] suggest that the addition of aztreonam to ceftazidime-avibactam may be able to overcome resistance caused by the coproduction of metallo-β-lactamases and serine β-lactamases.

NEWER β-LACTAM AND β-LACTAMASE INHIBITOR COMBINATIONS: MEROPENEM-VABORBACTAM

In 2017, the FDA approved meropenem-vaborbactam (vaborbactam previously was known as RPX-7009) for the treatment of adult patients with cUTI, including pyelonephritis.[167] The combination also is undergoing clinical testing for use in pediatric patients with severe infections (NCT02687906) as well as in patients with HABP/VABP (NCT03006679).

Meropenem-vaborbactam demonstrates antimicrobial activity against *E coli*, *K pneumoniae*, and *Enterobacter cloacae* complex (**Table 5**).[167] Limitations for this combination against indicated organisms include those that carry class B metallo-carbapenemases (eg, VIM, NDM, and IMP) and/or class D OXA β-lactamases that are not susceptible to inhibition by meropenem or vaborbactam.

Meropenem has been in use in the United States since 1996 and is a carbapenem β-lactam antibiotic noted for its stability in the presence of human dehydropeptidase I (an enzyme which quickly metabolizes imipenem).[169] Unfortunately, meropenem is susceptible to hydrolysis by class A carbapenemases, such as KPC; class B metallo-β-lactamases, such as NDM, VIM, and IMP; and class D OXA carbapenemases (eg, OXA-48). In addition, loss of outer membrane proteins (eg, OmpK35 and

Table 5
Clinical indications for the use of meropenem-vaborbactam

Indication	Indicated Bacteria	Patient Population	Clinical Trials
cUTI, including pyelonephritis	*E coli, K pneumoniae,* and *Enterobacter cloacae* species complex	Adult	TANGO I[168] NCT02166476

Data from Melinta Therapeutics, Inc. *VABOMERE (Meropenem and Vaborbactam) for Injection, for Intravenous Use.* Lincolnshire, IL 60069 USA; 2019.

OmpK36 in *K pneumoniae*) and increases in efflux pump production (eg, AcrAB-TolC) effect its penetration.[170]

Vaborbactam is a cyclic boronate-based β-lactamase inhibitor designed to be selective for β-lactamases over other serine hydrolase enzymes. Intended to have a carbapenem partner from early development, the focus was placed on inhibiting the class A carbapenemase, KPC.[171] Vaborbactam is a potent inhibitor of KPC ($K_{i\ app}$ = 69 nM) and other class A β-lactamases (CTX-M, SHV, and TEM) as well as class C β-lactamases (eg, CMY-2, P99) but not class D serine or class B metallo-β-lactamases.[172]

REPORTS AND MECHANISMS OF RESISTANCE: MEROPENEM-VABORBACTAM

In **Table 6**, the reports of resistance to meropenem-vaborbactam available at the time of this writing are presented. Despite 2 years on the market, clinical case reports of meropenem-vaborbactam resistance remain elusive in the literature. Whether this is indicative of the properties of the combination itself or the result of limited use and careful screening for susceptibility on the part of clinicians remains to be seen.

Enterobacterales Resistant to Meropenem-Vaborbactam

Unlike ceftolozane-tazobactam and ceftazidime-avibactam, reports of strains resistant to meropenem-vaborbactam are only now beginning to be reported. Moreover, meropenem-vaborbactam was shown to be effective against a case of bacteremia caused by a ceftazidime-avibactam–resistant *K pneumoniae* producing a KPC-2 D179Y variant.[120] Likely, the change from a cephalosporin β-lactam partner to a carbapenem β-lactam partner is a significant factor for the differences observed in the resistance patterns. The use of a carbapenem partner in a β-lactam–β-lactamase inhibitor combination, however, also presents its own challenges as resistance due to increased efflux and decreased permeability of carbapenems is more problematic than with cephalosporins in gram negatives.[170] In addition to carbapenems using porins for bacterial cell entry, vaborbactam also was found to traverse OmpK35 and OmpK36 in *K pneumoniae*.[172] Thus, permeability is likely the largest hurdle for meropenem-vaborbactam efficacy. Resistance to meropenem-vaborbactam largely was reported in strains of *K pneumoniae* producing KPC with loss of expression of OmpK35, OmpK36, and/or OmpK37—mutations in porin genes that result in the production of partially functioning porins (eg, duplication of GD at positions 134 and 135 in OmpK36) also elevated meropenem-vaborbactam MICs.[123,173–178] Increased expression of *acrAB* and/or bla_{KPC} additionally was reported.[123,176,177] In vitro selection of *K pneumoniae* producing KPC-2 on meropenem-vaborbactam revealed that the primary resistance mechanisms toward meropenem-vaborbactam were loss of OmpK36 as well as increased copy number of bla_{KPC}.[173] One report revealed that the emergence of meropenem-vaborbactam nonsusceptibility (MIC: 8 μg/mL) due to loss of *ompK36*

Table 6
Mechanisms of resistance to meropenem-vaborbactam

Type	Organism	Mechanism(s)	Minimum Inhibitory Concentraiton of Isolate[a]	Reference
Survey	*K pneumoniae*	KPC, loss of *ompK37* and up-regulation of AcrAB-TolC	16	177
Survey	*K pneumoniae*	KPC-2, TEM-181, SHV-11, loss of *ompK35* and *ompK36*	16	173
Survey	*K pneumoniae*	KPC-2, TEM-1, SHV-11, SHV-12, loss of *ompK35* and *ompK36*	32	173
Survey	*K pneumoniae*	KPC, loss of *ompK35* and *ompK36*	32	174
Survey	*K pneumoniae*	KPC-2, SHV, TEM, OXA-10, loss of *ompK35* and *ompK36*	64	178
Survey	*K pneumoniae*	KPC-3, SHV-11, SHV-12, loss of *ompK35* and *ompK36*	16	178
Survey	*K pneumoniae*	KPC-3, SHV-11, loss of *ompK35*, *ompK36*, and *ompK37*	256	123
Survey	*K pneumoniae*	KPC-3, SHV-11, TEM1a, OXA-9, loss of *ompK35*, *ompK36*, and *ompK37*	256	123

Vaborbactam is maintained at 8 μg/mL when in combination with meropenem
E coli, *K pneumoniae*, and *Enterobacter cloacae* complex breakpoint: resistant ≥16 μg/mL.[81]
[a] The MIC values for the isolate represent the MIC values obtained for either a clinical isolate obtained from a patient in a case study or part of a surveillance study or a laboratory-selected strain.
Data from Clinical and Laboratory Standards Institute (CLSI). *M100: Performance Standards for Antimicrobial Susceptibility Testing*. 30th ed.; 2020.

during treatment of a patient for bacteremia due to *K pneumoniae* producing KPC-3.[179] On a promising note, at least 1 study demonstrated synergy between meropenem-vaborbactam and aztreonam in the treatment of Enterobacterales carrying a metallo-β-lactamases.[165]

NEWER β-LACTAM AND β-LACTAMASE INHIBITOR COMBINATIONS: IMIPENEM-CILASTATIN-RELEBACTAM

Approved by the FDA in 2019, imipenem-cilastatin-relebactam is indicated for adult use in treating cIAIs and cUTIs, including pyelonephritis. The combination also is being evaluated for use in severe gram-negative infections in pediatric patients (NCT03969901 and NCT03230916) and for HABP/VABP in adults (NCT03583333) and was studied for bacterial pneumonia more broadly (NCT02493764). The combination demonstrates antimicrobial activity against a variety of gram-negative pathogens, including the anaerobes *Bacteroides* spp (**Table 7**).[180] Limitations of imipenem-cilastatin-relebactam against organisms for which it is approved to treat include

Enterobacterales or *P aeruginosa* that carry class B metallo-carbapenemases (eg, VIM, NDM, and IMP) or class D OXA β-lactamases that are not susceptible to inhibition by imipenem or relebactam.[181]

Imipenem-cilastatin originally approved by the FDA in November 1985 and was the first carbapenem in clinical use. The combination brings together a potent carbapenem antibiotic with an inhibitor of human renal dehydropeptidase (cilastatin), reducing renal metabolism of imipenem.[180] Unfortunately, imipenem is susceptible to hydrolysis by class A carbapenemases (KPC), class B metallo-β-lactamases (eg, VIM, NDM, and IMP), and class D carbapenemases (OXA-48). Moreover, decreased permeability due to loss of outer membrane porins (OmpK35, OmpK36, and OprD) and/or increases in efflux pump production (AcrAB-TolC and MexAB-OprM) effect its activity.[170]

Relebactam is a DBO β-lactamase inhibitor that was chosen from among many similar candidate compounds in a search for inhibitors to potentiate imipenem activity. It was selected for having particularly strong inhibitory activity against both class A and class C β-lactamases, demonstrating highly compatible pharmacokinetics with imipenem, effectiveness in mouse models of imipenem-resistant *P aeruginosa* and *K pneumoniae* strains, and favorable results in safety testing.[183]

REPORTS AND MECHANISMS OF RESISTANCE: IMIPENEM-RELEBACTAM

Table 8 lists all the reports of resistance to imipenem-relebactam described at the time of this writing. On the market in the United States for less than 6 months at the time of this writing, clinical case reports of resistance to imipenem-cilastatin-relebactam are not present in the literature. As with meropenem-vaborbactam, reports of strains producing β-lactamase variants resistant to imipenem-relebactam have not been described. Moreover, the carbapenem partner, imipenem is susceptible to the same mechanisms of resistance as meropenem; thus, increased efflux and decreased permeability are major barriers for carbapenem activity.[170] Being new to the market, a

Table 7
Clinical indications for the use of imipenem-cilastatin-relebactam

Indication	Indicated Bacteria	Patient Population	Clinical Trials
cIAI	*Enterobacter cloacae, E coli, K aerogenes, K pneumoniae, and P aeruginosa*	Adult	RESTORE-IMI 1[182] NCT02452047
cUTI, including pyelonephritis	*Bacteroides caccae, Bacteroides fragilis, Bacteroides ovatus, Bacteroides stercoris, Bacteroides thetaiotaomicron, Bacteroides uniformis, Bacteroides vulgatus, C freundii, Enterobacter cloacae, E coli, Fusobacterium nucleatum, K aerogenes, K oxytoca, K pneumoniae, Parabacteroides distasonis, and P aeruginosa*	Adult	RESTORE-IMI 1[182] NCT02452047

Data from Merck & Co., Inc. RECARBRIO (Imipenem, Cilastatin, and Relebactam) for Injection, for Intravenous Use. Whitehouse Station, NJ 08889 USA.; 2019.

Table 8
Mechanisms of resistance to imipenem-relebactam

Type	Organism	Mechanism(s)	Minimum Inhibitory Concentration of Isolate[a]	Reference
Survey	*K pneumoniae*	KPC, loss of *ompK36*	8	184
Survey	*K pneumoniae*	Overexpression of KPC-2, TEM-1, SHV-12, loss of *ompK35* and *ompK36*	512	186
Survey	*K pneumoniae*	KPC-3 TEM-1/SHV-11, loss of *ompK35* and *ompK36*	8	186
Survey	*S marcescens*	SME-1	4	190
Survey	*P aeruginosa*	PDC, loss of *oprD*	8	184
Survey	*P aeruginosa*	Hyperexpression of PDC, loss of *oprD*	8	184
Survey	*P aeruginosa*	GES-5	>8	53

Relebactam is maintained at 4 μg/mL when in combination with imipenem.[81]

P aeruginosa breakpoint: resistant ≥8 μg/mL.

Enterobacterales breakpoint: resistant ≥4 μg/mL.

[a] The MIC values for the isolate represent the MIC values obtained for either a clinical isolate obtained from a patient in a case study or part of a surveillance study or a laboratory-selected strain.

Data from Clinical and Laboratory Standards Institute (CLSI). *M100: Performance Standards for Antimicrobial Susceptibility Testing*. 30th ed.; 2020.

reasonable assumption is that further studies of resistance mechanisms and clinical case reports of emerging resistance and treatment failure of imipenem-relebactam will begin to emerge in the coming year, but until that time, data remains sparse and care should be taken to not draw any speculative conclusions.

Enterobacterales Resistant to Imipenem-Relebactam

Resistance to imipenem-relebactam was reported mostly in Enterobacterales due to loss of OmpK35/OmpF and OmpK36/OmpC as well as hyperexpression of bla_{KPC}.[184–188] For β-lactamase–mediated resistance, at the time of this writing 1 isolate of *K pneumoniae* was resistant to imipenem-relebactam and produced a GES-20,[189] whereas 2 isolates of *S marcescens* with SME also were reported as resistant.[32,190] The contribution (eg, lack of inhibition by relebactam vs enhanced hydrolysis of imipenem) of these β-lactamases toward imipenem-relebactam resistance remains to be established.

Pseudomonas aeruginosa Resistant to Imipenem-Relebactam

Contrary to Enterobacterales, most *oprD* mutants in *P aeruginosa* were more susceptible to imipenem-relebactam, despite imipenem using OprD for entry into *P aeruginosa*.[181,191,192] A previous study revealed that when *oprD* is not expressed, bla_{PDC} must be expressed,[193] and because bla_{PDC} is inhibited by relebactam the imipenem-relebactam combination is effective against many *oprD* mutants even when bla_{PDC} is overexpressed.[53,183,194] Some *P aeruginosa* strains with decreased expression of *oprD* and either wild-type or overexpressed levels of PDC, however, were resistant to imipenem-relebactam (MIC: 8 μg/mL).[184] These somewhat contradictory data may be due to the fact that the baseline MICs of *oprD* mutants toward imipenem and imipenem-relebactam were higher compared with wild-type *P aeruginosa* strains[181,184]; thus, a fine line between susceptibility and resistance exists in these *oprD* mutants. Efflux was found to not have an impact on the activity of imipenem-relebactam; an *oprD* mutant strain of *P aeruginosa* overexpressing MexAB, MexCD, MexXY, and MexJK possessed imipenem-relebactam MICs between 0.125 μg/mL and 1 μg/mL.[53,195] In 2 surveillance studies, of 17 of 589 and 5 of 42, *P aeruginosa* were found resistant to imipenem-relebactam (MIC range: 8–32 μg/mL) and the mechanism was not defined.[194,196] As with Enterobacterales, the presence of GES carbapenemases (eg, GES-5 and GES-6) in *P aeruginosa* was found to result in resistance to imipenem-relebactam.[197,198] Indeed, 11% of imipenem-relebactam–resistant *P aeruginosa* isolates carried GES β-lactamases; imipenem-relebactam MICs ranged from 8 μg/mL to 32 μg/mL for these isolates.[195]

SUMMARY

Although the combination therapies covered in this review are highly effective against large collections of clinical isolates, none is perfect, and all have shortcomings. KPC and PDC, the major resistant determinants in Enterobacterales and *P aeruginosa*, respectively, are evolving at an unprecedented rate. Perhaps the most important take-away from this review on the development of resistance to some of the most promising advancements in β-lactam antibiotics from the past decade is a reminder: humanity is locked in a constant battle with bacteria that have a huge evolutionary advantage in the fight. Although every new antibiotic or inhibitor that makes it to market provides new tools for physicians to treat otherwise untreatable infections, resistance seemingly remains inevitable. The release of promising new drugs should be heralded, but everyone from doctors and scientists to pharmaceutical companies to policymakers and to the general public needs to realize and remember to not become complacent and that continued research into resistance mechanisms, stewardship and conservation of existing drugs, and development of novel treatments remain essential in the great war between humans and "microbes" Judicious use and extensive laboratory testing are needed to prevent further spread especially as new agents enter the armamentarium.

ACKNOWLEDGMENTS

Research reported in this publication was supported by the National Institute of Allergy and Infectious Diseases of the National Institutes of Health (NIH) to R.A. Bonomo under Award Numbers R01AI100560, R01AI063517, and R01AI072219. This study also was supported in part by funds and/or facilities provided by the Cleveland Department of Veterans Affairs, Award Numbers 1I01BX002872 to K.M. Papp-Wallace and 1I01BX001974 to R.A. Bonomo from the Biomedical Laboratory Research & Development Service of the VA Office of Research and Development, and from the Geriatric Research Education and Clinical Center VISN 10. The content is solely the responsibility of the authors and does not necessarily represent the official views of the NIH or the Department of Veterans Affairs.

DISCLOSURE

K.M. Papp-Wallace and R.A. Bonomo are funded in part by research grants from Venatorx, Entasis, and Merck. K.M. Papp-Wallace and R.A. Bonomo are participating or have participated in collaborative research projects with Allecra, Allergan, Entasis, Merck, Roche, Venatorx, and Wockhardt.

REFERENCES

1. Bush K, Bradford PA. β-lactams and β-lactamase inhibitors: an overview. Cold Spring Harb Perspect Med 2016;6(8):a025247.
2. Centers for Disease Control and Prevention. Outpatient Antibiotic prescriptions — United States, 2016 2018. Available at: https://www.cdc.gov/antibiotic-use/community/programs-measurement/state-local-activities/outpatient-antibiotic-prescriptions-US-2016.html. Accessed November 25, 2018.
3. Errington J. L-form bacteria, cell walls and the origins of life. Open Biol 2013; 3(1):120143.
4. Osborn MJ. Structure and Biosynthesis of the Bacterial Cell Wall. Annu Rev Biochem 1969;38(1):501–38.
5. Tipper DJ, Strominger JL. Mechanism of action of penicillins: a proposal based on their structural similarity to acyl-D-alanyl-D-alanine. Proc Natl Acad Sci U S A 1965;54(4):1133–41.
6. Cho H, Uehara T, Bernhardt TG. Beta-lactam antibiotics induce a lethal malfunctioning of the bacterial cell wall synthesis machinery. Cell 2014;159(6):1300–11.
7. Bush K. The ABCD's of β-lactamase nomenclature. J Infect Chemother 2013; 19(4):549–59.
8. Ambler RP, Coulson AF, Frère JM, et al. A standard numbering scheme for the class A β-lactamases. Biochem J 1991;276(Pt 1):269–70.
9. Mack AR, Barnes MD, Taracila MA, et al. A standard numbering scheme for class C β-lactamases. Antimicrob Agents Chemother 2019. https://doi.org/10.1128/AAC.01841-19.

10. Oefner C, D'Arcy A, Daly JJ, et al. Refined crystal structure of β-lactamase from *Citrobacter freundii* indicates a mechanism for β-lactam hydrolysis. Nature 1990;343(6255):284–8.
11. Galleni M, Lamotte-Brasseur J, Raquet X, et al. The enigmatic catalytic mechanism of active-site serine β-lactamases. Biochem Pharmacol 1995;49(9): 1171–8.
12. Beadle BM, Trehan I, Focia PJ, et al. Structural milestones in the reaction pathway of an amide hydrolase: substrate, acyl, and product complexes of cephalothin with ampc β-lactamase. Structure 2002;10(3):413–24.
13. Chen Y, McReynolds A, Shoichet BK. Re-examining the role of Lys67 in class C β-lactamase catalysis. Protein Sci 2009. https://doi.org/10.1002/pro.60.
14. Brown JR, Livesay DR. Flexibility correlation between active site regions is conserved across four AmpC β-lactamase enzymes. PLoS One 2015;10(5): e0125832.
15. Jacoby GA. AmpC β-lactamases. Clin Microbiol Rev 2009;22(1):161–82.
16. Palzkill T, Le Q-Q, Venkatachalam KV, et al. Evolution of antibiotic resistance: several different amino acid substitutions in an active site loop alter the substrate profile of β-lactamase. Mol Microbiol 1994;12(2):217–29.
17. Banerjee S, Pieper U, Kapadia G, et al. Role of the Ω-loop in the activity, substrate specificity, and structure of class A β-lactamase. Biochemistry 1998; 37(10):3286–96.
18. Nukaga M, Taniguchi K, Washio Y, et al. Effect of an amino acid insertion into the omega loop region of a class C β-lactamase on its substrate specificity. Biochemistry 1998;37(29):10461–8.
19. Crichlow GV, Kuzin AP, Nukaga M, et al. Structure of the extended-spectrum class C β-Lactamase of *Enterobacter cloacae* GC1, a natural mutant with a tandem tripeptide insertion. Biochemistry 1999;38(32):10256–61.
20. Drawz SM, Bonomo RA. Three decades of β-lactamase inhibitors. Clin Microbiol Rev 2010;23(1):160–201.
21. Bush K. β-lactamase inhibitors from laboratory to clinic. Clin Microbiol Rev 1988; 1(1):109–23.
22. Ehmann DE, Jahić H, Ross PL, et al. Avibactam is a covalent, reversible, non–β-lactam β-lactamase inhibitor. Proc Natl Acad Sci U S A 2012;109(29):11663–8.
23. Papp-Wallace KM, Bonomo RA. New β-lactamase inhibitors in the clinic. Infect Dis Clin North Am 2016;30(2):441–64.
24. Merck & Co., Inc. ZERBAXA (Ceftolozane and Tazobactam) for injection, for intravenous use. Whitehouse Station (NJ); 2019.
25. Solomkin J, Hershberger E, Miller B, et al. Ceftolozane/tazobactam plus metronidazole for complicated intra-abdominal infections in an era of multidrug resistance: results from a randomized, double-blind, phase 3 trial (ASPECT-cIAI). Clin Infect Dis 2015;60(10):1462–71.
26. Mikamo H, Monden K, Miyasaka Y, et al. The efficacy and safety of tazobactam/ceftolozane in combination with metronidazole in Japanese patients with complicated intra-abdominal infections. J Infect Chemother 2019;25(2):111–6.
27. Huntington JA, Sakoulas G, Umeh O, et al. Efficacy of ceftolozane/tazobactam versus levofloxacin in the treatment of complicated urinary tract infections (cUTIs) caused by levofloxacin-resistant pathogens: results from the ASPECT-cUTI trial. J Antimicrob Chemother 2016;71(7):2014–21.
28. Arakawa S, Kawahara K, Kawahara M, et al. The efficacy and safety of tazobactam/ceftolozane in Japanese patients with uncomplicated pyelonephritis and complicated urinary tract infection. J Infect Chemother 2019;25(2):104–10.

29. Kollef MH, Nováček M, Kivistik Ü, et al. Ceftolozane-tazobactam versus meropenem for treatment of nosocomial pneumonia (ASPECT-NP): a randomised, controlled, double-blind, phase 3, non-inferiority trial. Lancet Infect Dis 2019; 19(12):1299–311.
30. Del Barrio-Tofiño E, López-Causapé C, Cabot G, et al. Genomics and susceptibility profiles of extensively drug-resistant *Pseudomonas aeruginosa* Isolates from Spain. Antimicrob Agents Chemother 2017;61(11). https://doi.org/10.1128/AAC.01589-17.
31. Ortiz de la Rosa J-M, Nordmann P, Poirel L. ESBLs and resistance to ceftazidime/avibactam and ceftolozane/tazobactam combinations in *Escherichia coli* and *Pseudomonas aeruginosa*. J Antimicrob Chemother 2019;74(7):1934–9.
32. Senchyna F, Gaur RL, Sandlund J, et al. Diversity of resistance mechanisms in carbapenem-resistant Enterobacteriaceae at a health care system in Northern California, from 2013 to 2016. Diagn Microbiol Infect Dis 2019;93(3):250–7.
33. Schmidt-Malan SM, Mishra AJ, Mushtaq A, et al. In vitro activity of imipenem-relebactam and ceftolozane-tazobactam against resistant gram-negative bacilli. Antimicrob Agents Chemother 2018;62(8). https://doi.org/10.1128/AAC.00533-18.
34. Fraile-Ribot PA, Del Rosario-Quintana C, López-Causapé C, et al. Emergence of resistance to novel β-lactam-β-lactamase inhibitor combinations due to horizontally acquired AmpC (FOX-4) in *Pseudomonas aeruginosa* Sequence Type 308. Antimicrob Agents Chemother 2019;64(1). https://doi.org/10.1128/AAC.02112-19.
35. Castanheira M, Doyle TB, Mendes RE, et al. Comparative activities of ceftazidime-avibactam and ceftolozane-tazobactam against enterobacteriaceae isolates producing extended-spectrum β-lactamases from U.S. Hospitals. Antimicrob Agents Chemother 2019;63(7). https://doi.org/10.1128/AAC.00160-19.
36. Livermore DM, Mushtaq S, Meunier D, et al. Activity of ceftolozane/tazobactam against surveillance and “problem” Enterobacteriaceae, *Pseudomonas aeruginosa* and non-fermenters from the British Isles. J Antimicrob Chemother 2017; 72(8):2278–89.
37. Farrell DJ, Flamm RK, Sader HS, et al. Antimicrobial activity of ceftolozane-tazobactam tested against Enterobacteriaceae and Pseudomonas aeruginosa with various resistance patterns isolated in U.S. Hospitals (2011-2012). Antimicrob Agents Chemother 2013;57(12):6305–10.
38. Tato M, García-Castillo M, Bofarull AM, et al, CENIT Study Group. In vitro activity of ceftolozane/tazobactam against clinical isolates of Pseudomonas aeruginosa and Enterobacteriaceae recovered in Spanish medical centres: Results of the CENIT study. Int J Antimicrob Agents 2015;46(5):502–10.
39. Castanheira M, Duncan LR, Mendes RE, et al. Activity of Ceftolozane-Tazobactam against Pseudomonas aeruginosa and Enterobacteriaceae Isolates Collected from Respiratory Tract Specimens of Hospitalized Patients in the United States during 2013 to 2015. Antimicrob Agents Chemother 2018; 62(3). https://doi.org/10.1128/AAC.02125-17.
40. Robin F, Auzou M, Bonnet R, et al. In Vitro activity of ceftolozane-tazobactam against enterobacter cloacae complex clinical isolates with different β-lactam resistance phenotypes. Antimicrob Agents Chemother 2018;62(9). https://doi.org/10.1128/AAC.00675-18.

41. Nicolas-Chanoine M-H, Mayer N, Guyot K, et al. Interplay between membrane permeability and enzymatic barrier leads to antibiotic-dependent resistance in *Klebsiella Pneumoniae.* Front Microbiol 2018;9:1422.
42. Moyá B, Beceiro A, Cabot G, et al. Pan-β-lactam resistance development in Pseudomonas aeruginosa clinical strains: molecular mechanisms, penicillin-binding protein profiles, and binding affinities. Antimicrob Agents Chemother 2012;56(9):4771–8.
43. Takeda S, Nakai T, Wakai Y, et al. In vi*tro* and *in vivo* activities of a new cephalosporin, FR264205, against *Pseudomonas aeruginosa.* Antimicrob Agents Chemother 2007;51(3):826–30.
44. Rodríguez-Martínez J-M, Poirel L, Nordmann P. Extended-spectrum cephalosporinases in *Pseudomonas aeruginosa.* Antimicrob Agents Chemother 2009; 53(5):1766–71.
45. Livermore DM, Mushtaq S, Ge Y. Chequerboard titration of cephalosporin CXA-101 (FR264205) and tazobactam versus β-lactamase-producing Enterobacteriaceae. J Antimicrob Chemother 2010;65(9):1972–4.
46. Giacobbe DR, Bassetti M, De Rosa FG, et al. Ceftolozane/tazobactam: place in therapy. Expert Rev Anti Infect Ther 2018;16(4):307–20.
47. Aronoff SC, Jacobs MR, Johenning S, et al. Comparative activities of the β-lactamase inhibitors YTR 830, sodium clavulanate, and sulbactam combined with amoxicillin or ampicillin. Antimicrob Agents Chemother 1984;26(4):580–2.
48. Bush K, Jacoby GA. Updated functional classification of β-lactamases. Antimicrob Agents Chemother 2010;54(3):969–76.
49. Bush K, Macalintal C, Rasmussen BA, et al. Kinetic interactions of tazobactam with β-lactamases from all major structural classes. Antimicrob Agents Chemother 1993;37(4):851–8.
50. Skoglund E, Abodakpi H, Rios R, et al. In Vivo resistance to ceftolozane/tazobactam in *Pseudomonas aeruginosa* Arising by AmpC- and Non-AmpC-mediated pathways. Case Rep Infect Dis 2018. https://doi.org/10.1155/2018/9095203.
51. Berrazeg M, Jeannot K, Enguéné VYN, et al. Mutations in β-lactamase AmpC increase resistance of *Pseudomonas aeruginosa* isolates to antipseudomonal cephalosporins. Antimicrob Agents Chemother 2015;59(10):6248–55.
52. Fraile-Ribot PA, Cabot G, Mulet X, et al. Mechanisms leading to *in vivo* ceftolozane/tazobactam resistance development during the treatment of infections caused by MDR *Pseudomonas aeruginosa.* J Antimicrob Chemother 2018; 73(3):658–63.
53. Fraile-Ribot P, Zamorano L, Orellana R, et al. Activity of imipenem/relebactam against a large collection of *Pseudomonas aeruginosa* clinical isolates and isogenic β-lactam resistant mutants. Antimicrob Agents Chemother 2019. https://doi.org/10.1128/AAC.02165-19.
54. Zamudio R, Hijazi K, Joshi C, et al. Phylogenetic analysis of resistance to ceftazidime/avibactam, ceftolozane/tazobactam and carbapenems in piperacillin/tazobactam-resistant *Pseudomonas aeruginosa* from cystic fibrosis patients. Int J Antimicrob Agents 2019;53(6):774–80.
55. Cabot G, Bruchmann S, Mulet X, et al. *Pseudomonas aeruginosa* ceftolozane-tazobactam resistance development requires multiple Mutations leading to overexpression and structural modification of AmpC. Antimicrob Agents Chemother 2014;58(6):3091–9.

56. Díaz-Cañestro M, Periañez L, Mulet X, et al. Ceftolozane/tazobactam for the treatment of multidrug resistant *Pseudomonas aeruginosa*: experience from the Balearic Islands. Eur J Clin Microbiol Infect Dis 2018;37(11):2191–200.
57. MacVane SH, Pandey R, Steed LL, et al. Emergence of ceftolozane-tazobactam-resistant *Pseudomonas aeruginosa* during treatment is mediated by a single AmpC structural mutation. Antimicrob Agents Chemother 2017; 61(12). e01183-17.
58. Haidar G, Philips NJ, Shields RK, et al. Ceftolozane-tazobactam for the treatment of multidrug-resistant *Pseudomonas aeruginosa* infections: clinical effectiveness and evolution of resistance. Clin Infect Dis 2017;65(1):110–20.
59. Del Barrio-Tofiño E, Zamorano L, Cortes-Lara S, et al. Spanish nationwide survey on *Pseudomonas aeruginosa* antimicrobial resistance mechanisms and epidemiology. J Antimicrob Chemother 2019;74(7):1825–35.
60. Boulant T, Jousset AB, Bonnin RA, et al. A 2.5-years within-patient evolution of a *Pseudomonas aeruginosa* with *in vivo* acquisition of ceftolozane-tazobactam and ceftazidime-avibactam resistance upon treatment. Antimicrob Agents Chemother 2019. https://doi.org/10.1128/AAC.01637-19.
61. So W, Shurko J, Galega R, et al. Mechanisms of high-level ceftolozane/tazobactam resistance in *Pseudomonas aeruginosa* from a severely neutropenic patient and treatment success from synergy with tobramycin. J Antimicrob Chemother 2019. https://doi.org/10.1093/jac/dky393.
62. Barnes MD, Taracila MA, Rutter JD, et al. Deciphering the Evolution of Cephalosporin Resistance to Ceftolozane-Tazobactam in Pseudomonas aeruginosa. mBio 2018;9(6). https://doi.org/10.1128/mBio.02085-18.
63. Wi YM, Greenwood-Quaintance KE, Schuetz AN, et al. Activity of ceftolozane-tazobactam against carbapenem-resistant, non-carbapenemase-producing *Pseudomonas aeruginosa* and associated resistance mechanisms. Antimicrob Agents Chemother 2018;62(1). https://doi.org/10.1128/AAC.01970-17.
64. Lister PD, Wolter DJ, Hanson ND. Antibacterial-resistant *Pseudomonas aeruginosa*: clinical impact and complex regulation of chromosomally encoded resistance mechanisms. Clin Microbiol Rev 2009;22(4):582–610.
65. Juan C, Torrens G, González-Nicolau M, et al. Diversity and regulation of intrinsic β-lactamases from non-fermenting and other Gram-negative opportunistic pathogens. FEMS Microbiol Rev 2017;41(6):781–815.
66. Johnson JW, Fisher JF, Mobashery S. Bacterial cell-wall recycling. Ann N Y Acad Sci 2013;1277:54–75.
67. Dik DA, Fisher JF, Mobashery S. Cell-wall recycling of the gram-negative bacteria and the nexus to antibiotic resistance. Chem Rev 2018;118(12):5952–84.
68. Castanheira M, Mills JC, Farrell DJ, et al. Mutation-driven β-lactam resistance mechanisms among contemporary ceftazidime-nonsusceptible *Pseudomonas aeruginosa* isolates from U.S. hospitals. Antimicrob Agents Chemother 2014; 58(11):6844–50.
69. Moya B, Zamorano L, Juan C, et al. Activity of a new cephalosporin, CXA-101 (FR264205), against β-lactam-resistant *Pseudomonas aeruginosa* mutants selected *in vitro* and after antipseudomonal treatment of intensive care unit patients. Antimicrob Agents Chemother 2010;54(3):1213–7.
70. Zavala A, Retailleau P, Elisée E, et al. Genetic, biochemical, and structural characterization of CMY-136 β-lactamase, a peculiar CMY-2 variant. ACS Infect Dis 2019;5(4):528–38.

71. Tsukamoto K, Ohno R, Sawai T. Extension of the substrate spectrum by an amino acid substitution at residue 219 in the *Citrobacter freundii* cephalosporinase. J Bacteriol 1990;172(8):4348–51.
72. Crémet L, Caroff N, Giraudeau C, et al. Detection of clonally related *Escherichia coli* isolates producing different CMY β-lactamases from a cystic fibrosis patient. J Antimicrob Chemother 2013;68(5):1032–5.
73. Matsumura N, Minami S, Mitsuhashi S. Sequences of homologous β-lactamases from clinical isolates of *Serratia marcescens* with different substrate specificities. Antimicrob Agents Chemother 1998;42(1):176–9.
74. Bour M, Fournier D, Jové T, et al. Acquisition of class C β-lactamase PAC-1 by ST664 strains of *Pseudomonas aeruginosa*. Antimicrob Agents Chemother 2019. https://doi.org/10.1128/AAC.01375-19.
75. Poirel L, Ortiz De La Rosa J-M, Kieffer N, et al. Acquisition of Extended-Spectrum β-Lactamase GES-6 Leading to Resistance to Ceftolozane-Tazobactam Combination in *Pseudomonas aeruginosa*. Antimicrob Agents Chemother 2019;63(1). https://doi.org/10.1128/AAC.01809-18.
76. Sid Ahmed MA, Abdel Hadi H, Hassan AAI, et al. Evaluation of *in vitro* activity of ceftazidime/avibactam and ceftolozane/tazobactam against MDR *Pseudomonas aeruginosa* isolates from Qatar. J Antimicrob Chemother 2019;74(12): 3497–504.
77. Khan A, Tran TT, Rios R, et al. Extensively Drug-Resistant *Pseudomonas aeruginosa* ST309 harboring tandem guiana extended spectrum β-lactamase enzymes: a newly emerging threat in the United States. Open Forum Infect Dis 2019;6(7):ofz273. https://doi.org/10.1093/ofid/ofz273.
78. Fraile-Ribot PA, Mulet X, Cabot G, et al. In vivo emergence of resistance to novel cephalosporin-β-lactamase inhibitor combinations through the duplication of amino acid D149 from OXA-2 β-Lactamase (OXA-539) in Sequence Type 235 *Pseudomonas aeruginosa*. Antimicrob Agents Chemother 2017;61(9). https://doi.org/10.1128/AAC.01117-17.
79. Arca-Suárez J, Fraile-Ribot P, Vázquez-Ucha JC, et al. Challenging antimicrobial susceptibility and evolution of resistance (OXA-681) during treatment of a long-term nosocomial infection caused by a *Pseudomonas aeruginosa* ST175 Clone. Antimicrob Agents Chemother 2019;63(10). https://doi.org/10.1128/AAC.01110-19.
80. Juan C, Zamorano L, Pérez JL, et al. Activity of a new antipseudomonal cephalosporin, CXA-101 (FR264205), against carbapenem-resistant and multidrug-resistant *Pseudomonas aeruginosa* clinical strains. Antimicrob Agents Chemother 2010;54(2):846–51.
81. Clinical and Laboratory Standards Institute (CLSI). M100: Performance Standards for Antimicrobial Susceptibility Testing. 30th edition. 2020.
82. Allergan USA, Inc. AVYCAZ (Ceftazidime and Avibactam) for Injection, for Intravenous Use. Madison (NJ): 2019.
83. Castanheira M, Farrell SE, Krause KM, et al. Contemporary diversity of β-lactamases among Enterobacteriaceae in the nine U.S. census regions and ceftazidime-avibactam activity tested against isolates producing the most prevalent β-lactamase groups. Antimicrob Agents Chemother 2014;58(2):833–8.
84. de Jonge BLM, Karlowsky JA, Kazmierczak KM, et al. In vitro susceptibility to ceftazidime-avibactam of carbapenem-nonsusceptible enterobacteriaceae isolates collected during the INFORM Global Surveillance Study (2012 to 2014). Antimicrob Agents Chemother 2016;60(5):3163–9.

85. Ehmann DE, Jahic H, Ross PL, et al. Kinetics of avibactam inhibition against Class A, C, and D β-lactamases. J Biol Chem 2013;288(39):27960–71.
86. Stone GG, Bradford PA, Yates K, et al. *In vitro* activity of ceftazidime/avibactam against urinary isolates from patients in a Phase 3 clinical trial programme for the treatment of complicated urinary tract infections. J Antimicrob Chemother 2017;72(5):1396–9.
87. Mazuski JE, Gasink LB, Armstrong J, et al. Efficacy and safety of ceftazidime-avibactam plus metronidazole versus meropenem in the treatment of complicated intra-abdominal infection: results from a randomized, controlled, double-blind, phase 3 program. Clin Infect Dis 2016;62(11):1380–9.
88. Carmeli Y, Armstrong J, Laud PJ, et al. Ceftazidime-avibactam or best available therapy in patients with ceftazidime-resistant Enterobacteriaceae and Pseudomonas aeruginosa complicated urinary tract infections or complicated intra-abdominal infections (REPRISE): a randomised, pathogen-directed, phase 3 study. Lancet Infect Dis 2016;16(6):661–73.
89. Bradley JS, Broadhurst H, Cheng K, et al. Safety and efficacy of ceftazidime-avibactam plus metronidazole in the treatment of children ≥3 months to <18 years with complicated intra-abdominal infection: results from a phase 2, randomized, controlled trial. Pediatr Infect Dis J 2019;38(8):816–24.
90. Wagenlehner FM, Sobel JD, Newell P, et al. Ceftazidime-avibactam versus doripenem for the treatment of complicated urinary tract infections, including acute pyelonephritis: RECAPTURE, a phase 3 randomized trial program. Clin Infect Dis 2016;63(6):754–62.
91. Torres A, Zhong N, Pachl J, et al. Ceftazidime-avibactam versus meropenem in nosocomial pneumonia, including ventilator-associated pneumonia (REPROVE): a randomised, double-blind, phase 3 non-inferiority trial. Lancet Infect Dis 2018; 18(3):285–95.
92. Bradley JS, Roilides E, Broadhurst H, et al. Safety and efficacy of ceftazidime-avibactam in the treatment of children ≥3 months to <18 years with complicated urinary tract infection: results from a phase 2 randomized, controlled trial. Pediatr Infect Dis J 2019;38(9):920–8.
93. O'Callaghan CH, Acred P, Harper PB, et al. GR 20263, a new broad-spectrum cephalosporin with anti-pseudomonal activity. Antimicrob Agents Chemother 1980;17(5):876–83.
94. Verbist L, Verhaegen J. GR-20263: a new aminothiazolyl cephalosporin with high activity against *Pseudomonas* and Enterobacteriaceae. Antimicrob Agents Chemother 1980;17(5):807–12.
95. Mushtaq S, Warner M, Livermore DM. *In vitro* activity of ceftazidime+NXL104 against *Pseudomonas aeruginosa* and other non-fermenters. J Antimicrob Chemother 2010;65(11):2376–81.
96. Endimiani A, Perez F, Bonomo RA. Cefepime: a reappraisal in an era of increasing antimicrobial resistance. Expert Rev Anti Infect Ther 2008;6(6): 805–24.
97. Lahiri SD, Mangani S, Durand-Reville T, et al. Structural Insight into Potent Broad-Spectrum Inhibition with Reversible Recyclization Mechanism: Avibactam in Complex with CTX-M-15 and *Pseudomonas aeruginosa* AmpC β-Lactamases. Antimicrob Agents Chemother 2013;57(6):2496–505.
98. Lahiri SD, Johnstone MR, Ross PL, et al. Avibactam and class C β-lactamases: mechanism of inhibition, conservation of the binding pocket, and implications for resistance. Antimicrob Agents Chemother 2014;58(10):5704–13.

99. Lohans CT, Brem J, Schofield CJ. New Delhi metallo-β-lactamase 1 catalyzes avibactam and aztreonam hydrolysis. Antimicrob Agents Chemother 2017; 61(12). https://doi.org/10.1128/AAC.01224-17.
100. Humphries RM, Yang S, Hemarajata P, et al. First report of ceftazidime-avibactam resistance in a KPC-3-expressing *Klebsiella pneumoniae* Isolate. Antimicrob Agents Chemother 2015;59(10):6605–7.
101. Spellberg B, Bonomo RA. Editorial commentary: ceftazidime-avibactam and carbapenem-resistant enterobacteriaceae: "we're gonna need a bigger boat." Clin Infect Dis 2016;63(12):1619–21.
102. Winkler ML, Papp-Wallace KM, Bonomo RA. Activity of ceftazidime/avibactam against isogenic strains of *Escherichia coli* containing KPC and SHV β-lactamases with single amino acid substitutions in the Ω-loop. J Antimicrob Chemother 2015;70(8):2279–86.
103. Livermore DM, Warner M, Jamrozy D, et al. *In vitro* selection of ceftazidime-avibactam resistance in Enterobacteriaceae with KPC-3 carbapenemase. Antimicrob Agents Chemother 2015;59(9):5324–30.
104. Shields RK, Chen L, Cheng S, et al. Emergence of ceftazidime-avibactam resistance due to plasmid-borne $bla_{\text{kpc-3}}$ mutations during treatment of carbapenem-resistant *Klebsiella pneumoniae* infections. Antimicrob Agents Chemother 2017; 61(3). https://doi.org/10.1128/AAC.02097-16.
105. Shields RK, Potoski BA, Haidar G, et al. Clinical outcomes, drug toxicity, and emergence of ceftazidime-avibactam resistance among patients treated for carbapenem-resistant enterobacteriaceae infections. Clin Infect Dis 2016; 63(12):1615–8.
106. Compain F, Arthur M. Impaired inhibition by avibactam and resistance to the ceftazidime-avibactam combination due to the D179Y substitution in the KPC-2 β-lactamase. Antimicrob Agents Chemother 2017;61(7). https://doi.org/10.1128/AAC.00451-17.
107. Shields RK, Nguyen MH, Press EG, et al. In vitro selection of meropenem resistance among ceftazidime-avibactam-resistant, meropenem-susceptible *Klebsiella pneumoniae* isolates with variant KPC-3 carbapenemases. Antimicrob Agents Chemother 2017;61(5). https://doi.org/10.1128/AAC.00079-17.
108. Giddins MJ, Macesic N, Annavajhala MK, et al. Successive emergence of ceftazidime-avibactam resistance through distinct genomic adaptations in bla_{KPC-2}-Harboring *Klebsiella pneumoniae* sequence type 307 isolates. Antimicrob Agents Chemother 2018;62(3). https://doi.org/10.1128/AAC.02101-17.
109. Göttig S, Frank D, Mungo E, et al. Emergence of ceftazidime/avibactam resistance in KPC-3-producing *Klebsiella pneumoniae in vivo*. J Antimicrob Chemother 2019;74(11):3211–6.
110. Castanheira M, Arends SJR, Davis AP, et al. Analyses of a ceftazidime-avibactam-resistant *Citrobacter freundii* Isolate Carrying $bla_{\text{KPC-2}}$ Reveals a Heterogenous Population and Reversible Genotype. mSphere 2018;3(5). https://doi.org/10.1128/mSphere.00408-18.
111. Shields RK, Nguyen MH, Hao B, et al. Colistin does not potentiate ceftazidime-avibactam killing of carbapenem-resistant enterobacteriaceae *in vitro* or suppress emergence of ceftazidime-avibactam resistance. Antimicrob Agents Chemother 2018;62(8). https://doi.org/10.1128/AAC.01018-18.
112. Gaibani P, Campoli C, Lewis RE, et al. *In vivo* evolution of resistant subpopulations of KPC-producing *Klebsiella pneumoniae* during ceftazidime/avibactam treatment. J Antimicrob Chemother 2018;73(6):1525–9.

113. Shields RK, Nguyen MH, Press EG, et al. Emergence of ceftazidime-avibactam resistance and restoration of carbapenem susceptibility in *klebsiella pneumoniae* carbapenemase-producing *K pneumoniae*: a case report and review of literature. Open Forum Infect Dis 2017;4(3):ofx101.
114. Shields RK, Nguyen MH, Chen L, et al. Pneumonia and renal replacement therapy are risk factors for ceftazidime-avibactam treatment failures and resistance among patients with carbapenem-resistant enterobacteriaceae infections. Antimicrob Agents Chemother 2018;62(5). https://doi.org/10.1128/AAC.02497-17.
115. Bidell MR, Lodise TP. Suboptimal clinical response rates with newer antibiotics among patients with moderate renal impairment: review of the literature and potential pharmacokinetic and pharmacodynamic considerations for observed findings. Pharmacotherapy 2018;38(12):1205–15.
116. Yasmin M, Fouts DE, Jacobs MR, et al. Monitoring Ceftazidime-Avibactam (CAZ-AVI) and Aztreonam (ATM) Concentrations in the Treatment of a Bloodstream Infection Caused by a Multidrug-Resistant *Enterobacter* sp. Carrying both KPC-4 and NDM-1 carbapenemases. Clin Infect Dis 2019. https://doi.org/10.1093/cid/ciz1155.
117. Wilson WR, Kline EG, Jones CE, et al. Effects of KPC Variant and Porin Genotype on the *In Vitro* activity of meropenem-vaborbactam against carbapenem-resistant enterobacteriaceae. Antimicrob Agents Chemother 2019;63(3). https://doi.org/10.1128/AAC.02048-18.
118. Galani I, Antoniadou A, Karaiskos I, et al. Genomic characterization of a KPC-23-producing *Klebsiella pneumoniae* ST258 clinical isolate resistant to ceftazidime-avibactam. Clin Microbiol Infect 2019;25(6):763.e5-e8.
119. Zhang P, Shi Q, Hu H, et al. Emergence of ceftazidime/avibactam resistance in carbapenem-resistant *Klebsiella pneumoniae* in China. Clin Microbiol Infect 2019. https://doi.org/10.1016/j.cmi.2019.08.020.
120. Athans V, Neuner EA, Hassouna H, et al. Meropenem-vaborbactam as salvage therapy for ceftazidime-avibactam-resistant *Klebsiella pneumoniae* bacteremia and abscess in a liver transplant recipient. Antimicrob Agents Chemother 2019;63(1). https://doi.org/10.1128/AAC.01551-18.
121. Venditti C, Nisii C, D'Arezzo S, et al. Molecular and phenotypical characterization of two cases of antibiotic-driven ceftazidime-avibactam resistance in bla_{KPC-3}-harboring *Klebsiella pneumoniae*. Infect Drug Resist 2019;12:1935–40.
122. Cano Á, Guzmán-Puche J, García-Gutiérrez M, et al. Use of carbapenems in the combined treatment of emerging ceftazidime/avibactam-resistant and carbapenem-susceptible KPC-producing *Klebsiella pneumoniae* infections: report of a case and review of the literature. J Glob Antimicrob Resist 2019. https://doi.org/10.1016/j.jgar.2019.11.007.
123. Gaibani P, Carla Re M, Campoli C, et al. Bloodstream infection caused by KPC-producing *Klebsiella pneumoniae* resistant to ceftazidime/avibactam: Epidemiology and genomic characterization. Clin Microbiol Infect 2019. https://doi.org/10.1016/j.cmi.2019.11.011.
124. Wozniak A, Paillavil B, Legarraga P, et al. Evaluation of a rapid immunochromatographic test for detection of KPC in clinical isolates of Enterobacteriaceae and *Pseudomonas* species. Diagn Microbiol Infect Dis 2019;95(2):131–3.
125. Hemarajata P, Humphries RM. Ceftazidime/avibactam resistance associated with L169P mutation in the omega loop of KPC-2. J Antimicrob Chemother 2019;74(5):1241–3.

126. Oueslati S, Iorga BI, Tlili L, et al. Unravelling ceftazidime/avibactam resistance of KPC-28, a KPC-2 variant lacking carbapenemase activity. J Antimicrob Chemother 2019;74(8):2239–46.
127. Räisänen K, Koivula I, Ilmavirta H, et al. Emergence of ceftazidime-avibactam-resistant Klebsiella pneumoniae during treatment, Finland, 2018. Euro Surveill 2019;24(19). https://doi.org/10.2807/1560-7917.ES.2019.24.19.1900256.
128. Mueller L, Masseron A, Prod'Hom G, et al. Phenotypic, biochemical and genetic analysis of KPC-41, a KPC-3 variant conferring resistance to ceftazidime-avibactam and exhibiting reduced carbapenemase activity. Antimicrob Agents Chemother 2019. https://doi.org/10.1128/AAC.01111-19.
129. Barnes MD, Winkler ML, Taracila MA, et al. *Klebsiella* pneumoniae carbapenemase-2 (KPC-2), substitutions at ambler position asp179, and resistance to ceftazidime-avibactam: unique antibiotic-resistant phenotypes emerge from β-lactamase protein engineering. mBio 2017;8(5). https://doi.org/10.1128/mBio.00528-17.
130. Papp-Wallace KM, Winkler ML, Taracila MA, et al. Variants of β-lactamase KPC-2 that are resistant to inhibition by avibactam. Antimicrob Agents Chemother 2015;59(7):3710–7.
131. Ourghanlian C, Soroka D, Arthur M. Inhibition by Avibactam and Clavulanate of the β-Lactamases KPC-2 and CTX-M-15 Harboring the Substitution N132G in the Conserved SDN Motif. Antimicrob Agents Chemother 2017;61(3). https://doi.org/10.1128/AAC.02510-16.
132. Both A, Büttner H, Huang J, et al. Emergence of ceftazidime/avibactam non-susceptibility in an MDR *Klebsiella pneumoniae* isolate. J Antimicrob Chemother 2017;72(9):2483–8.
133. Compain F, Dorchène D, Arthur M. Combination of amino acid substitutions leading to CTX-M-15-mediated resistance to the ceftazidime-avibactam combination. Antimicrob Agents Chemother 2018;62(9). https://doi.org/10.1128/AAC.00357-18.
134. Karlowsky JA, Biedenbach DJ, Kazmierczak KM, et al. Activity of Ceftazidime-Avibactam against Extended-Spectrum- and AmpC β-Lactamase-Producing Enterobacteriaceae Collected in the INFORM Global Surveillance Study from 2012 to 2014. Antimicrob Agents Chemother 2016;60(5):2849–57.
135. Karlowsky JA, Kazmierczak KM, Bouchillon SK, et al. In Vitro Activity of Ceftazidime-Avibactam against Clinical Isolates of Enterobacteriaceae and *Pseudomonas aeruginosa* Collected in Latin American Countries: Results from the INFORM Global Surveillance Program, 2012 to 2015. Antimicrob Agents Chemother 2019;63(4). https://doi.org/10.1128/AAC.01814-18.
136. Castanheira M, Doyle TB, Smith CJ, et al. Combination of MexAB-OprM overexpression and mutations in efflux regulators, PBPs and chaperone proteins is responsible for ceftazidime/avibactam resistance in *Pseudomonas aeruginosa* clinical isolates from US hospitals. J Antimicrob Chemother 2019;74(9):2588–95.
137. Stone GG, Smayevsky J, Kazmierczak K. Longitudinal analysis of the *in vitro* activity of ceftazidime-avibactam vs. *Pseudomonas aeruginosa*, 2012-2016. Diagn Microbiol Infect Dis 2020;96(1):114835.
138. Voulgari E, Kotsakis SD, Giannopoulou P, et al. Detection in two hospitals of transferable ceftazidime-avibactam resistance in *Klebsiella pneumoniae* due to a novel VEB β-lactamase variant with a Lys234Arg substitution, Greece, 2019. Euro Surveill 2020;25(2). https://doi.org/10.2807/1560-7917.ES.2020.25.2.1900766.

139. Livermore DM, Mushtaq S, Doumith M, et al. Selection of mutants with resistance or diminished susceptibility to ceftazidime/avibactam from ESBL- and AmpC-producing Enterobacteriaceae. J Antimicrob Chemother 2018;73(12):3336–45.
140. Lahiri SD, Giacobbe RA, Johnstone MR, et al. Activity of avibactam against *Enterobacter cloacae* producing an extended-spectrum class C β-lactamase enzyme. J Antimicrob Chemother 2014;69(11):2942–6.
141. Lahiri SD, Walkup GK, Whiteaker JD, et al. Selection and molecular characterization of ceftazidime/avibactam-resistant mutants in *Pseudomonas aeruginosa* strains containing derepressed AmpC. J Antimicrob Chemother 2015;70(6):1650–8.
142. Khil PP, Dulanto Chiang A, Ho J, et al. Dynamic emergence of mismatch repair deficiency facilitates rapid evolution of ceftazidime-avibactam resistance in *Pseudomonas aeruginosa* Acute infection. mBio 2019;10(5). https://doi.org/10.1128/mBio.01822-19.
143. Shields RK, Clancy CJ, Hao B, et al. Effects of *Klebsiella pneumoniae* carbapenemase subtypes, extended-spectrum β-lactamases, and porin mutations on the *in vitro* activity of ceftazidime-avibactam against carbapenem-resistant *K. pneumoniae*. Antimicrob Agents Chemother 2015;59(9):5793–7.
144. López-Hernández I, Alonso N, Fernández-Martínez M, et al. Activity of ceftazidime-avibactam against multidrug-resistance Enterobacteriaceae expressing combined mechanisms of resistance. Enferm Infecc Microbiol Clin 2017;35(8):499–504.
145. Humphries RM, Hemarajata P. Resistance to ceftazidime-avibactam in *Klebsiella pneumoniae* due to porin mutations and the increased expression of KPC-3. Antimicrob Agents Chemother 2017;61(6). https://doi.org/10.1128/AAC.00537-17.
146. Nelson K, Hemarajata P, Sun D, et al. Resistance to ceftazidime-avibactam is due to transposition of KPC in a porin-deficient strain of *Klebsiella pneumoniae* with increased efflux activity. Antimicrob Agents Chemother 2017;61(10). https://doi.org/10.1128/AAC.00989-17.
147. Giani T, Antonelli A, Sennati S, et al. Results of the Italian infection-Carbapenem Resistance Evaluation Surveillance Trial (iCREST-IT): activity of ceftazidime/avibactam against Enterobacterales isolated from urine. J Antimicrob Chemother 2020. https://doi.org/10.1093/jac/dkz547.
148. Coppi M, Di Pilato V, Monaco F, et al. Ceftazidime-avibactam resistance associated with increased bla_{KPC-3} gene copy number mediated by pKpQIL plasmid derivatives in ST258 *Klebsiella pneumoniae*. Antimicrob Agents Chemother 2020. https://doi.org/10.1128/AAC.01816-19.
149. Viala B, Zaidi FZ, Bastide M, et al. Assessment of the *In Vitro* activities of ceftolozane/tazobactam and ceftazidime/avibactam in a collection of beta-lactam-resistant enterobacteriaceae and *Pseudomonas aeruginosa* Clinical Isolates at Montpellier University Hospital, France. Microb Drug Resist 2019;25(9):1325–9.
150. Hackel M, Kazmierczak KM, Hoban DJ, et al. Assessment of the *In Vitro* Activity of Ceftazidime-Avibactam against Multidrug-Resistant Klebsiella spp. Collected in the INFORM Global Surveillance Study, 2012 to 2014. Antimicrob Agents Chemother 2016;60(8):4677–83.
151. Sader HS, Castanheira M, Flamm RK. Antimicrobial activity of ceftazidime-avibactam against gram-negative bacteria isolated from patients hospitalized

with pneumonia in U.S. Medical Centers, 2011 to 2015. Antimicrob Agents Chemother 2017;61(4). https://doi.org/10.1128/AAC.02083-16.

152. Sader HS, Castanheira M, Shortridge D, et al. Antimicrobial activity of ceftazidime-avibactam tested against multidrug-resistant enterobacteriaceae and *Pseudomonas aeruginosa* Isolates from U.S. Medical Centers, 2013 to 2016. Antimicrob Agents Chemother 2017;61(11). https://doi.org/10.1128/AAC.01045-17.
153. Zhang Y, Kashikar A, Brown CA, et al. Unusual *Escherichia coli* PBP 3 Insertion Sequence Identified from a Collection of Carbapenem-Resistant Enterobacteriaceae Tested *In Vitro* with a Combination of Ceftazidime-, Ceftaroline-, or Aztreonam-Avibactam. Antimicrob Agents Chemother 2017;61(8). https://doi.org/10.1128/AAC.00389-17.
154. Alm RA, Johnstone MR, Lahiri SD. Characterization of *Escherichia coli* NDM isolates with decreased susceptibility to aztreonam/avibactam: role of a novel insertion in PBP3. J Antimicrob Chemother 2015;70(5):1420–8.
155. Nichols WW, de Jonge BLM, Kazmierczak KM, et al. In V*itro* Susceptibility of Global Surveillance Isolates of *Pseudomonas aeruginosa* to Ceftazidime-Avibactam (INFORM 2012 to 2014). Antimicrob Agents Chemother 2016; 60(8):4743–9.
156. Torrens G, Cabot G, Ocampo-Sosa AA, et al. Activity of Ceftazidime-Avibactam against Clinical and Isogenic Laboratory </i>Pseudomonas aeruginosa</i> Isolates Expressing Combinations of Most Relevant β-Lactam Resistance Mechanisms. Antimicrob Agents Chemother 2016;60(10):6407–10.
157. Winkler ML, Papp-Wallace KM, Hujer AM, et al. Unexpected challenges in treating multidrug-resistant gram-negative bacteria: resistance to ceftazidime-avibactam in archived isolates of *Pseudomonas aeruginosa.* Antimicrob Agents Chemother 2015;59(2):1020–9.
158. Chalhoub H, Sáenz Y, Nichols WW, et al. Loss of activity of ceftazidime-avibactam due to MexAB-OprM efflux and overproduction of AmpC cephalosporinase in *Pseudomonas aeruginosa* isolated from patients suffering from cystic fibrosis. Int J Antimicrob Agents 2018;52(5):697–701.
159. Atkin SD, Abid S, Foster M, et al. Multidrug-resistant *Pseudomonas aeruginosa* from sputum of patients with cystic fibrosis demonstrates a high rate of susceptibility to ceftazidime-avibactam. Infect Drug Resist 2018;11:1499–510.
160. Sanz-García F, Hernando-Amado S, Martínez JL. Mutation-driven evolution of *Pseudomonas aeruginosa* in the presence of either ceftazidime or ceftazidime-avibactam. Antimicrob Agents Chemother 2018;62(10). https://doi.org/10.1128/AAC.01379-18.
161. Kazmierczak KM, Bradford PA, Stone GG, et al. In vitro activity of ceftazidime-avibactam and aztreonam-avibactam against OXA-48-Carrying Enterobacteriaceae Isolated as Part of the International Network for Optimal Resistance Monitoring (INFORM) Global Surveillance Program from 2012 to 2015. Antimicrob Agents Chemother 2018;62(12). https://doi.org/10.1128/AAC.00592-18.
162. Fröhlich C, Sørum V, Thomassen AM, et al. OXA-48-mediated ceftazidime-avibactam resistance is associated with evolutionary trade-offs. mSphere 2019;4(2). e00024-19.
163. Marshall S, Hujer AM, Rojas LJ, et al. Can ceftazidime-avibactam and aztreonam overcome β-lactam resistance conferred by metallo-β-lactamases in enterobacteriaceae? Antimicrob Agents Chemother 2017;61(4). https://doi.org/10.1128/AAC.02243-16.

164. Davido B, Fellous L, Lawrence C, et al. Ceftazidime-avibactam and aztreonam, an interesting strategy to overcome β-lactam resistance conferred by metallo-β-lactamases in enterobacteriaceae and *Pseudomonas aeruginosa*. Antimicrob Agents Chemother 2017;61(9). https://doi.org/10.1128/AAC.01008-17.
165. Biagi M, Wu T, Lee M, et al. Searching for the optimal treatment for metallo- and serine-β-lactamase producing enterobacteriaceae: aztreonam in combination with ceftazidime-avibactam or meropenem-vaborbactam. Antimicrob Agents Chemother 2019. https://doi.org/10.1128/AAC.01426-19.
166. Castanheira M, Mendes RE, Sader HS. Low Frequency of Ceftazidime-Avibactam Resistance among Enterobacteriaceae Isolates Carrying bla_{KPC} Collected in U.S. Hospitals from 2012 to 2015. Antimicrob Agents Chemother 2017;61(3). https://doi.org/10.1128/AAC.02369-16.
167. Melinta Therapeutics, Inc. VABOMERE (Meropenem and Vaborbactam) for Injection, for Intravenous Use. Lincolnshire (IL): 2019.
168. Kaye KS, Bhowmick T, Metallidis S, et al. Effect of meropenem-vaborbactam vs piperacillin-tazobactam on clinical cure or improvement and microbial eradication in complicated urinary tract infection: the TANGO I randomized clinical trial. JAMA 2018;319(8):788–99. https://doi.org/10.1001/jama.2018.0438.
169. Edwards JR, Turner PJ, Wannop C, et al. *In vitro* antibacterial activity of SM-7338, a carbapenem antibiotic with stability to dehydropeptidase I. Antimicrob Agents Chemother 1989;33(2):215–22. https://doi.org/10.1128/aac.33.2.215.
170. Papp-Wallace KM, Endimiani A, Taracila MA, et al. Carbapenems: past, present, and future. Antimicrob Agents Chemother 2011;55(11):4943–60. https://doi.org/10.1128/AAC.00296-11.
171. Hecker SJ, Reddy KR, Totrov M, et al. Discovery of a Cyclic Boronic Acid β-Lactamase Inhibitor (RPX7009) with Utility vs Class A Serine Carbapenemases. J Med Chem 2015;58(9):3682–92. https://doi.org/10.1021/acs.jmedchem.5b00127.
172. Lomovskaya O, Sun D, Rubio-Aparicio D, et al. Vaborbactam: Spectrum of Beta-Lactamase Inhibition and Impact of Resistance Mechanisms on Activity in Enterobacteriaceae. Antimicrob Agents Chemother 2017;61(11). https://doi.org/10.1128/AAC.01443-17.
173. Sun D, Rubio-Aparicio D, Nelson K, et al. Meropenem-Vaborbactam Resistance Selection, Resistance Prevention, and Molecular Mechanisms in Mutants of KPC-Producing *Klebsiella pneumoniae*. Antimicrob Agents Chemother 2017; 61(12). https://doi.org/10.1128/AAC.01694-17.
174. Pfaller MA, Huband MD, Mendes RE, et al. *In vitro* activity of meropenem/vaborbactam and characterisation of carbapenem resistance mechanisms among carbapenem-resistant Enterobacteriaceae from the 2015 meropenem/vaborbactam surveillance programme. Int J Antimicrob Agents 2018;52(2):144–50. https://doi.org/10.1016/j.ijantimicag.2018.02.021.
175. Lapuebla A, Abdallah M, Olafisoye O, et al. Activity of Meropenem Combined with RPX7009, a Novel β-Lactamase Inhibitor, against Gram-Negative Clinical Isolates in New York City. Antimicrob Agents Chemother 2015;59(8):4856–60. https://doi.org/10.1128/AAC.00843-15.
176. Zhou M, Yang Q, Lomovskaya O, et al. *In vitro* activity of meropenem combined with vaborbactam against KPC-producing Enterobacteriaceae in China. J Antimicrob Chemother 2018;73(10):2789–96. https://doi.org/10.1093/jac/dky251.
177. Castanheira M, Rhomberg PR, Flamm RK, et al. Effect of the β-Lactamase Inhibitor Vaborbactam Combined with Meropenem against Serine Carbapenemase-

Producing Enterobacteriaceae. Antimicrob Agents Chemother 2016;60(9): 5454–8. https://doi.org/10.1128/AAC.00711-16.

178. Griffith DC, Sabet M, Tarazi Z, et al. Pharmacokinetics/Pharmacodynamics of Vaborbactam, a Novel Beta-Lactamase Inhibitor, in Combination with Meropenem. Antimicrob Agents Chemother 2019;63(1). https://doi.org/10.1128/AAC.01659-18.
179. Shields RK, McCreary EK, Marini RV, et al. Early experience with meropenem-vaborbactam for treatment of carbapenem-resistant Enterobacteriaceae infections. Clin Infect Dis 2019. https://doi.org/10.1093/cid/ciz1131.
180. Merck & Co., Inc. RECARBRIO (imipenem, cilastatin, and relebactam) for injection, for intravenous Use. Whitehouse Station (NJ); 2019.
181. Livermore DM, Warner M, Mushtaq S. Activity of MK-7655 combined with imipenem against Enterobacteriaceae and *Pseudomonas aeruginosa*. J Antimicrob Chemother 2013;68(10):2286–90. https://doi.org/10.1093/jac/dkt178.
182. Motsch J, Murta de Oliveira C, Stus V, et al. RESTORE-IMI 1: A Multicenter, Randomized, Double-blind Trial Comparing Efficacy and Safety of Imipenem/Relebactam vs Colistin Plus Imipenem in Patients With Imipenem-nonsusceptible Bacterial Infections. Clin Infect Dis 2019. https://doi.org/10.1093/cid/ciz530.
183. Blizzard TA, Chen H, Kim S, et al. Discovery of MK-7655, a β-lactamase inhibitor for combination with Primaxin®. Bioorg Med Chem Lett 2014;24(3):780–5. https://doi.org/10.1016/j.bmcl.2013.12.101.
184. Lapuebla A, Abdallah M, Olafisoye O, et al. Activity of Imipenem with Relebactam against Gram-Negative Pathogens from New York City. Antimicrob Agents Chemother 2015;59(8):5029–31. https://doi.org/10.1128/AAC.00830-15.
185. Haidar G, Clancy CJ, Chen L, et al. Identifying Spectra of Activity and Therapeutic Niches for Ceftazidime-Avibactam and Imipenem-Relebactam against Carbapenem-Resistant Enterobacteriaceae. Antimicrob Agents Chemother 2017;61(9). https://doi.org/10.1128/AAC.00642-17.
186. Balabanian G, Rose M, Manning N, et al. Effect of porins and bla_{kpc} expression on activity of imipenem with Relebactam in *Klebsiella pneumoniae*: can antibiotic combinations overcome resistance? Microb Drug Resist 2018;24(7): 877–81.
187. Gomez-Simmonds A, Stump S, Giddins MJ, et al. Clonal Background, Resistance Gene Profile, and Porin Gene Mutations Modulate *In Vitro* Susceptibility to Imipenem-Relebactam in Diverse Enterobacteriaceae. Antimicrob Agents Chemother 2018;62(8). https://doi.org/10.1128/AAC.00573-18.
188. Galani I, Souli M, Nafplioti K, et al. *In vitro* activity of imipenem-relebactam against non-MBL carbapenemase-producing *Klebsiella pneumoniae* isolated in Greek hospitals in 2015-2016. Eur J Clin Microbiol Infect Dis 2019;38(6): 1143–50.
189. Lob SH, Hackel MA, Kazmierczak KM, et al. In Vitro Activity of imipenem-relebactam against gram-negative ESKAPE pathogens isolated by clinical laboratories in the united states in 2015 (results from the SMART global surveillance program). Antimicrob Agents Chemother 2017;61(6). https://doi.org/10.1128/AAC.02209-16.
190. Carpenter J, Neidig N, Campbell A, et al. Activity of imipenem/relebactam against carbapenemase-producing Enterobacteriaceae with high colistin resistance. J Antimicrob Chemother 2019;74(11):3260–3.
191. Hirsch EB, Ledesma KR, Chang K-T, et al. *In vitro* activity of MK-7655, a novel β-lactamase inhibitor, in combination with imipenem against carbapenem-

resistant Gram-negative bacteria. Antimicrob Agents Chemother 2012;56(7): 3753–7.

192. Horner C, Mushtaq S, Livermore DM. BSAC Resistance Surveillance Standing Committee. Potentiation of imipenem by relebactam for *Pseudomonas aeruginosa* from bacteraemia and respiratory infections. J Antimicrob Chemother 2019;74(7):1940–4.
193. Livermore DM. Interplay of impermeability and chromosomal β-lactamase activity in imipenem-resistant *Pseudomonas aeruginosa*. Antimicrob Agents Chemother 1992;36(9):2046–8.
194. Barnes MD, Bethel CR, Alsop J, et al. Inactivation of the *Pseudomonas*-Derived Cephalosporinase-3 (PDC-3) by Relebactam. Antimicrob Agents Chemother 2018;62(5). https://doi.org/10.1128/AAC.02406-17.
195. Young K, Painter RE, Raghoobar SL, et al. *In vitro* studies evaluating the activity of imipenem in combination with relebactam against *Pseudomonas aeruginosa*. BMC Microbiol 2019;19(1):150.
196. Lob SH, Hackel MA, Kazmierczak KM, et al. *In vitro* activity of imipenem-relebactam against gram-negative bacilli isolated from patients with lower respiratory tract infections in the United States in 2015 - Results from the SMART global surveillance program. Diagn Microbiol Infect Dis 2017;88(2):171–6.
197. Karlowsky JA, Lob SH, Kazmierczak KM, et al. *In vitro* activity of imipenem/relebactam against Gram-negative ESKAPE pathogens isolated in 17 European countries: 2015 SMART surveillance programme. J Antimicrob Chemother 2018;73(7):1872–9.
198. Karlowsky JA, Lob SH, Kazmierczak KM, et al. *In vitro* activity of imipenem-relebactam against Enterobacteriaceae and *Pseudomonas aeruginosa* isolated from intraabdominal and urinary tract infection samples - SMART Surveillance United States 2015-2017. J Glob Antimicrob Resist 2019. https://doi.org/10.1016/j.jgar.2019.10.028.

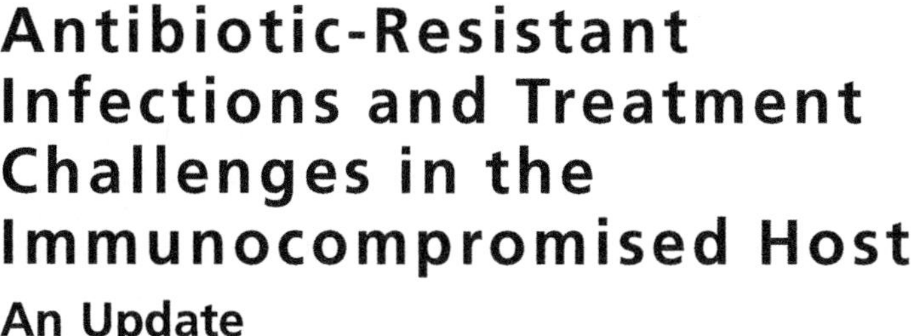

Antibiotic-Resistant Infections and Treatment Challenges in the Immunocompromised Host

An Update

Donald Dumford 3rd, MD, MPH[a,b,*], Marion J. Skalweit, MD, PhD[c,d]

KEYWORDS

• MDRO • Immunocompromise • Organ transplant recipient • HIV/AIDS
• Neutropenic host • Infection

KEY POINTS

- Rates of infection with multidrug-resistant organisms (MDRO) are increasing among immunocompromised persons, as greater numbers of MDRO are observed throughout the population.
- Inappropriate empirical antibiotic selection related to prevalence of MDRO in immunocompromised persons is common.
- Antibiotic prophylaxis and empirical antibiotic therapy influence the selection of these MDRO; susceptibility patterns vary among regions and even within hospitals.
- MDRO can be associated with worse outcomes among immunocompromised persons, and empirical antibiotic choices must be selected with the local antibiogram in mind.
- Studies are needed among immunocompromised persons to evaluate these novel approaches to improve outcomes.

INTRODUCTION

This article reviews antibiotic resistance, chemoprophylaxis and its effect on the human microbiome and infection, and treatment of bacterial infections in the growing number of patients with solid organ transplant (SOT) and in the neutropenic host. In addition, the role of antimicrobial stewardship in reducing exposure to unnecessary

[a] Department of Medicine, Northeast Ohio Medical University, 4209 St. Rt. 44, PO Box 95, Rootstown, OH 44272, USA; [b] Division of Infectious Diseases, Cleveland Clinic Akron General, 224 West Exchange Street, Suite 290, Akron, OH 44302, USA; [c] Case Western Reserve University School of Medicine, 2109 Adelbert Road, Cleveland, OH 44106, USA; [d] Louis Stokes Cleveland Department of Veterans Affairs, 10701 East Boulevard 111 (W), Cleveland, OH 44106, USA
* Corresponding author. Division of Infectious Diseases, Cleveland Clinic Akron General, 224 West Exchange Street, Suite 290, Akron, OH 44302.
E-mail address: Dumford@ccf.org

Infect Dis Clin N Am 34 (2020) 821–847
https://doi.org/10.1016/j.idc.2020.08.005

antibiotic exposure is also examined in the setting of neutropenic fever treatment. The antibiotic-resistant infections in persons with human immunodeficiency virus (HIV) and AIDS have been reviewed previously by the authors.[1] Most of the recent literature focuses on resistance in *Mycobacterium tuberculosis*, which shall be addressed in a subsequent chapter. Similarly, a literature review of the role of antibiotic resistance in infections in patients with primary and secondary immunodeficiencies, and associated infections, as well as fungal and viral resistance is beyond the scope of this article and will not be included. Specific mechanisms of resistance in both gram-negative and gram-positive bacteria, as well as newer treatment options will be addressed in other sections of this monograph and will only be briefly discussed in the context of the immunocompromised host.

THE IMMUNE SYSTEM AND HOST SUSCEPTIBILITY TO BACTERIAL PATHOGENS

As a brief introduction,[2,3] the immune system is divided into components that represent innate and adaptive immunity to bacterial pathogens. Innate immunity includes mucosal barriers and the skin, the complement system as well as cellular components such as dendritic cells and neutrophils and phagocytic cells in circulation and in tissues (eg, Langerhans cells, Kupffer cells, alveolar macrophages). Defects in innate immunity can be primary (congenital) or secondary (eg, related to other diseases or as adverse reactions to medications) and lead to specific susceptibility to bacterial pathogens. The adaptive immune response (B and T lymphocytes) includes both humoral and cell-mediated immune mechanisms. Some immunodeficiency states involve a combination of both defects in innate and adaptive immunity, for example, cytotoxic chemotherapy and the neutropenic host, common variable immunodeficiency, or AIDS. In recent years, the human microbiome is considered as an additional immune defense[4] whose disruption can contribute to susceptibility to specific pathogens, for example, *Clostridium difficile* infection, requiring unique treatments such as fecal microbiota transplant.[5]

SOLID ORGAN TRANSPLANTS

SOTs have saved many lives since their inception. In an analysis of United Network for Organ Sharing (UNOS) data from 1987 to 2012, estimates project that 2,270,859 life-years were saved with a mean of 4.3 life-years per organ transplant.[6] SOTs are associated with significant morbidity and mortality after transplant with infections being a major cause of complications of SOT. In an analysis of 156 deceased SOT recipients who underwent autopsy, infections were found to be the most common cause of mortality accounting for 41% of deaths (64/156) and typically occurring within the first year of transplantation.[7] Mortality due to infection varied by organ transplant type. In the heart transplant group, 21% of deaths were attributable to infection compared with 59.4% in the liver transplant group, 58.6% in the kidney transplant group, and 63.1% in the lung transplant group.[7] Of the 64 cases of infection-related mortality, bacterial infections accounted for the majority with 43 (67.1%) being linked to a specific pathogen or pathogens.[7] A high mortality in the first year posttransplant is not necessarily surprising given high incidence of infection during this time period compared with later time periods posttransplant. For example, Al-Hasan and colleagues[8] showed a drastically higher incidence of gram-negative bloodstream infections (BSIs) in the first month posttransplant at 210/1000 patient-years compared with 2 to 12 months and greater than 1 year posttransplant with incidence of 25.7 and 8.2 per 1000 patient-years during those time periods, respectively. However, even in the late posttransplant period of greater than 1 year, the incidence of gram-negative bacteremia in the SOT population was still 10-fold greater than that of the general population.[8] Bert and colleagues[9] also showed higher incidence of BSIs in the early posttransplant period, with 39% of BSIs occurring within 10 days after liver transplant, 27.8% occurring between days 11 and 30, and 17% occurring between days 31 and 90. As with other patient populations, infections due to antibiotic-resistant pathogens are a concern, especially with those considered multidrug resistant (MDR). In this review, issues regarding SOT and antimicrobial resistance are addressed, with a focus on the epidemiology of MDR organisms in this population, including incidence of antibiotic-resistant pathogens, risk factors for antibiotic-resistant pathogens, and mortality associated with antibiotic-resistant pathogens.

Prevalence of Antibiotic-Resistant Pathogens in Solid Organ Transplant

In studies looking at SOT patients and drug resistance, much of the focus seems to be on gram-negative pathogens. In the studies that included methicillin-resistant*Staphylococcus aureus* (MRSA) infections among total number of infections, MRSA accounted for 6.9% (96/1389) of all infections[10]{Bonatti H, 2009 #59}{Camargo, 2015 #5}{Song, 2014 #7}{Gagliotti C, 2018 #36}{Kiros T, 2019 #37}{El-Badrawy MK, 2017 #39}{Riera, 2015 #6}{Bert F1, 2010 #54}{Moreno, 2007 #15}. These ranged from only 1.81% (5/276 in Bodro and colleagues[10] and 6/332 in Moreno and colleagues) of BSIs being due to MRSA in 2 separate studies from Spain.{Bonatti H, 2009 #59}The highest was seen in the study from El-Badrawy and colleagues where 25% (3 of 12) patients with early pneumonia following liver transplant had MRSA.{Rana, 2015 #2} In narrowing our view to look at just *Staphylococcus aureus* isolates and the prevalence of methicillin resistance it is shown that methicillin resistance is fairly common in SOT patients. Among the studies reviewed, the prevalence of methicillin resistance among *S aureus isolates* was 49.7% (221/445).[9–22] This ranged from as low as 16.2% (6/37) in the study by Moreno and colleagues[21] to as high as 86% (60/70) in the study by Malinis and colleagues.[14] Malinis and colleagues[14] additionally compared their SOT population with a non-SOT population and found that the non-SOT population had a much lower prevalence of MRSA among *S aureus* isolates (86.2% vs 52%).

Several studies were reviewed that looked at the prevalence of vancomycin-resistant enterococci (VRE) among SOT patients with infection. Looking at prevalence of VRE among all infection, Kiros and colleagues[16] found that 18.2% (2 of 11) kidney transplant patients with bacteriuria had VRE. Macesic and colleagues[23] found that VRE accounted for 8.2% (8 of the 97) infections in their SOT population. Gagliotti and colleagues[15] found that 5.3% (4/75) of infections among liver transplant patients were VRE, but that none of the 113 lung transplant patients with infection had VRE. Among just enterococcal isolates, prevalence of VRE was variable. Four of the studies reviewed had assessed this with 28.7% (33/115) of the enterococcal isolates being VRE. Kiros and colleagues[16] found that 100% (2/2) of their enterococcal isolates were due to VRE, 22.2% (4/18 including 2/8 bacteria, 1/1 surgical site infections, and 1/5 biliary tract infections) due to enterococcus were VRE in the study by Gagliotti and colleagues,[15] and 44.8% (26/58) of bacteremic episodes due to enterococcus were VRE in the study by Kim and colleagues.[24] In regard to colonization, one study found that 51.5% (66/128) were found to be colonized with VRE.[23]

Drug resistance in gram-negative pathogens is frequent in the SOT population with many of the infections isolated being MDR or extremely drug resistant (XDR). Two studies looked at increasing rates of MDR, with Oriol and colleagues[25] finding an increase from 4.8% in 2007 to 2008 to 38.8% in 2015 to 2016 and Origuen and colleagues[26] finding an increase from 43.9% in 2002 to 2004 to 67.8% in 2011 to 2013.

In reviewing the data available on Enterobacteriaceae, the authors have chosen to focus on studies looking at extended-spectrum beta-lactamase (ESBL) producing and carbapenem-resistant Enterobacteriaceae (CRE). In the studies reviewed where incidence among the entire transplant populations is available and ESBL production was assessed, it was found that ESBL Enterobacteriaceae occurred in 4.9% (331/6723) of the total SOT population.[9,15,25,27–30] Of the studies reviewed where incidence among the entire transplant population is available and carbapenem resistance was reported, 4.8% (235/4907) developed a CRE infection.[9,15,29,31–36]

In studies where prevalence of ESBL production among Enterobacteriaceae was reported, 34.4% (280/812) of isolates were ESBL producing.[9,15,17,18,25,29,37,38] Two other studies reported cephalosporin resistance but did not specify if these were ESBL or not. In one, cefepime resistance was seen in 62 (83%) and ceftazidime resistance in 60 (80%) of their 75 Enterobacteriaceae.[35] The other found a much lower prevalence of cephalosporin resistance among their Enterobacteriaceae, with only 16.7% (24/144) being cephalosporin resistant.[21] For CRE, it was reported that 21.2% (110/518) of Enterobacteriaceae were CRE.[9,15–17,29,35] Oriol and colleagues[25] looked at change in prevalence of ESBL over time and found there was a substantial increase over the time of their study (7.1% at the start of the study in 2007–2008, increasing steadily to 34.7% in 2015–2016). In a similar study, Origuen and colleagues[26] found that carbapenemase production increased from none in 2002 to 2004 to 5% in 2011 to 2013. In addition to this, they also saw an increase in fluoroquinolone resistance from 36.6% to 54.5%, trimethoprim-sulfamethoxazole resistance from 68.5% to 81.6%, piperacillin-tazobactam resistance from 2.7% to 17.5%, gentamicin resistance from 11.3% to 19.7%, and nitrofurantoin resistance from 9.7% to 17.9%.[26]

Of the studies reviewed, where MDR *Pseudomonas aeruginosa* incidence among the entire transplant population was able to be determined, 0.73% (42/5716) of all SOT recipients developed an MDR *P aeruginosa* infection.[8,18,25,30] One study reported XDR *P aeruginosa* among the entire transplant populations and found that 0.13% (2/1569) developed XDR *P aeruginosa*.[35] Three studies did not specify if isolates were MDR or XDR, but in these 1.5% (25/1656) of patients developed carbapenem-resistant *P aeruginosa*.[9,15,30] Looking at prevalence of MDR or XDR among just *P aeruginosa* isolates, across 5 studies 43.3% (169/390) were MDR or XDR.[18,25,35,39,40] Unlike with Enterobacteriaceae, Oriol and colleagues[25] did not find a trend of increasing MDR among *P aeruginosa*.

Among studies reporting carbapenem resistance among *P aeruginosa*, 30.6% (119/389) were carbapenem resistant.[8,9,12,30,36,41,42] In addition, production of metallo-β-lactamase (MBL) production in *P aeruginosa* was assessed in 2 studies with Mlynarczyk and colleagues[41] finding 10.5% (24/228) prevalence whereas Men and colleagues[30] finding a 77.8% (7/9) prevalence.

In the reviewed studies, the incidence of carbapenem-resistant *Acinetobacter baumannii* among SOT recipients was 2.4% (148/6204).[15,35,36,43–46] Among *A baumannii* isolates, the prevalence of carbapenem resistance was 58.7% (175/298).[10,15,35,36,43–48] Two studies defined MDR and XDR status in *A baumannii*, with Men and colleagues[30] showing that 100% (24/24) of isolates were XDR and Kitazano and colleagues[47] showing that MDR occurred in 21 (63.6%) and XDR occurred in 7 (21.2%) of their 33 isolates. In addition, in the one study where MBL production was assessed, it was seen that 91.7% (22/24) *A baumannii* isolates produced MBL.[30]

Risk Factors for Antibiotic-Resistant Pathogens in Solid Organ Transplant

Across the studies reviewed, several factors were found to increase the risk for MDRO pathogens. Notable studies showed that specific types of transplants were risk factors with liver transplant significant in one study,[38] lung transplant in another,[36] and kidney transplant in a third[37]; however, the other studies did not show significance for any specific type of transplant so there may be no association. Risk factors that were found to be significant in more than one study included prior transplant,[10,39,49] length of stay before infection,[36,50] increasing age,[36,49] hemodialysis,[37,46] prior antibiotic use,[10,30,46,47,50] and nosocomial acquisition of infection.[35,39,40] Higher acuity of illness was found to be associated with resistant pathogens in several studies, with septic shock at onset (odds ratio[OR] of 2.8),[10] intensive care unit (ICU) admission (odds ratio [OR] 3.23,[50] higher Child-Turcotte-Pugh score (median of 24 in carbapenemase-producing group vs 18 in non-carbapenemase producing group, odds ratio [OR] 1.23),[23] and higher MELD (hazard ratio [HR] of 1.03 per each 1 point increasee,[34] being associated in 4 separate studies. Two studies found that endotracheal intubation was a risk factor MDRO.[30,34]

Several studies looked at risks for particular pathogens. Length of posttransplant intubation was found to a risk for CRE (odds ratio [OR] 1.94).[33] Giannella and colleagues[34] found that CRE colonization, combined transplant, prolonged mechanical ventilation, reintervention, and rejection were found to be significant risk factors for CRE infection. Presence of ESBL was found to be a risk factor for recurrence of ESBL urinary tract infection (UTI) in kidney transplant patients.[28]

Inappropriate Empirical Antibiotics

Assessing MDRO association with antibiotic use in the SOT population is important, as it is known that inappropriate antibiotics are associated with increased mortality. For example, the study by Kumar and colleagues[52] found that inappropriate antibiotics were associated with a 5-fold increase in risk of death in a nontransplant population. In the studies where there were data on inappropriate empirical antibiotics in the SOT population, it was found that inappropriate empirical antibiotic regimens were frequently used in patients with MDR pathogens. This was highest in the retrospective case series of ESBL infections in SOT patients by Winters and colleagues[53] where they found that 85% of empirical regimens for first episode of ESBL infections were inappropriate. Median time to change to appropriate therapy was reported as 3.5 days. Other studies with proportion of empirical antibiotics being inappropriate included 21.6% in resistant ESKAPE pathogens in the study by Bodro and colleagues, 38% in the study looking at incidence of ESBL-producing organisms in patients with Enterobacteriaceae bacteremia by Aguair and colleagues, 42.3% in the study of MDR *A baumannii* infections by Kim and colleagues, 57.5% in Liu and colleagues, 26% in Luo and colleagues, and 31.7% in Oriol and colleagues.[25,40,42,43,45,54] An additional study compared the prevalence of inappropriate antibiotics in patients with XDR pseudomonas bacteremia versus those without and found that patients with bacteremia because of XDR *P aeruginosa* more often received inadequate empirical antibiotic therapy (58% vs 22%; $P<.001$).[40]

The study by Aguair and colleagues[54] showed that use of appropriate empirical antibiotics was associated with increased mortality (6/10 [60%] of deaths vs 7/29 [24%] of survivors, $P = .056$). The investigators concluded that this paradox was attributable to selection bias, as these patients typically were sicker with higher Charlson comorbidity index and Pitt bacteremia scores.

Other studies did not find this paradoxic relationship between appropriate antibiotic use and mortality, as they found that appropriate antibiotics were protective. In the study by Kim and colleagues,[43] those patients who died were far more likely to have inadequate empirical antibiotics versus those who survived with a hazard ratio [HR] of 4.19; however, this was a study in which 75.7% of isolates were XDR, so antibiotic selection was very limited. In the study by de Gouvea and colleagues,[46] appropriate antibiotics were found to be associated with a 96% reduction in mortality (OR = 0.04). In the study by Men and colleagues,[30] 75% of patients with inappropriate antibiotics perished compared with 32% of those on appropriate antibiotics. Kitazano and colleagues[47] found that 43% of patients with inappropriate antibiotics died versus 11% of those with appropriate antibiotics. And, lastly, Lupei and colleagues[50] found that 28-day mortality for those on inappropriate antibiotics at 24 hours was 14%, compared with 2% of those on appropriate antibiotics. This last study investigated the risks associated with inappropriate antibiotics and found that younger age, longer courses of intravenous antibiotics before transplant, and longer length of stay before transplant were associated.[50]

Morbidity and Mortality Associated with Multidrug-Resistant Organisms

Mortality rates tend to be high in SOT patients with MDRO pathogens compared with nonresistant organism. This was seen in several studies: Bodro and colleagues[10] with 35.3% of patients with ESKAPE pathogens dying compared with 14.4% of patients with non-ESKAPE pathogens. In another study, patients with CRE had mortality of 24% compared with 10% of those without CRE.[55] Two studies looked specifically, at carbapenem-resistant *Klebsiella pneumoniae* (CR-KP) with findings of morality of 41.7% and 71% in those with CR-KP versus 19% and 14% in overall population, respectively.[29,32] In their study on patients with carbapenem-resistant *A baumannii*, Kim and colleagues[43] found that there was 50% morality in those with CRAB bacteremia, 10% in nonbacteremic, and 20.5% in non-CRAB bacteremia.

The risk of mortality does not seem to be related to the immunosuppression due to antirejection meds and may in fact be protective. Camargo and colleagues[12] showed statistically similar rates of mortality between the SOT group (34.5%) and the nontransplant group (40.5%). Patients with stem cell transplant were also included in this analysis and demonstrated a statistically significant decrease in mortality (16.7%) but were much more likely to have gram-positive infections with higher proportion of coagulase-negative staphylococci (CNS).[12] In another study by Kalil and colleagues[51] comparing bacteremic sepsis in transplant and nontransplant patient found that SOT was associated with a decreased risk of death when controlling for other factors. Twenty-eight–day mortality in the SOT group was 78% lower (HR = 0.22, $P = .001$) and 57% lower at 90 days (HR = 0.43, $P = .25$).[51] The other variables found to be significant on multivariate regression analysis included presence of comorbidities (OR = 8.2 [95% CI, 1.48–45.44], P = .016), SOFA score (OR = 1.2 [95% CI, 1.07–1.32], P = .001), presence of nosocomial infection (OR = 36.3 [95% CI, 9.71–135.96], P < .0001), appropriate initial antibiotics (OR = 0.04 [95% CI, .006–.23], P < .0001), and white blood cell (WBC) count (OR = 0.93 [95% CI, .89–.97], P < .0001).

One study looking at XDR *Acinetobacter baumannii* assessed type of therapy and mortality.[56] In the study all patients on monotherapy died.[56] Ten of eleven receiving colistin plus a noncarbapenem antibiotic died, including 0 of 7 on tigecycline plus colistin.[56] Sixteen of the twenty-one patients on colistin plus a carbapenem survived although the isolates should have been resistant to the carbapenem.[56] This may further support combination therapy for XDR pathogens.

In looking at other mortality risks, the following factors were seen to be associated with increased risk of mortality. Mortality was more commonly associated with increased severity of illness, whether it was by a specific system (Charlson

Comorbidity Index,[54] Pitt bacteremia score,[54] SOFA score,[49] APACHE II[47]) or by other objective data, for example, respiratory failure,[10] mechanical ventilation,[21,46] heart failure on admission,[50]multiorgan system failure,[50] and septic shock.[13,21]

THE NEUTROPENIC HOST

Early on in the treatment of hematologic malignancies in children and young adults, it was recognized that empirical antibiotics directed at bacterial pathogens including *Pseudomonas aeruginosa* were important in the supportive care of the neutropenic patient.[57] Considerations include host risk stratification using scoring systems such as Multinational Association Of Supportive Care In Cancer (MASCC),[58] type of cytotoxic chemotherapy, projected duration of neutropenia and whether granulocyte colony-stimulating factors can be used, and the use of antibiotic prophylaxis (fluoroquinolones, trimethoprim-sulfamethoxazole eg,). Clinical infectious disease syndromes will also dictate which pathogens are of greatest concern: severe mucositis syndromes and oral *Streptococcus* spp.; pneumonia and *P aeruginosa*, *Klebsiella pneumoniae*, *Streptococcus pneumoniae*, MRSA; skin and skin structure infections, device-related bacteremias and MRSA, *K. pneumoniae*, *A baumannii*; typhlitis-enteric gram-negative rods (GNRs), *Enterococcus* spp. including VRE; UTI-enteric gram-negative bacilli, *P aeruginosa*, MRSA, *Enterococcus* spp..[59]

The changing epidemiology of bacterial infections in neutropenic hosts reflects all of the host risks, as well as the emergence of antibiotic resistant pathogens in the hospital and the community.[60–62] More care is being delivered to patients with malignancies in the outpatient setting and thus the epidemiology reflects that of the community as well as the hospital (eg, CTX-M producing *Escherichia coli*, fluoroquinolone-resistant *Enterobacteriaceae* and *P aeruginosa*, *A baumannii*; community-acquired MRSA; penicillin-resistant *S pneumoniae*). Empirical antibiotic therapies must take the changing microbial landscape into consideration. The role of newer agents with antipseudomonal spectrum in empirical treatment of neutropenic fever has not yet been defined: ceftazidime-avibactam[63,64]; ceftolozane-tazobactam[63,65]; imipenem-cilastatin-relebactam and meropenem-vaborbactam[66]; plazomicin[67]; and cefiderocol.[68] Alternative gram-positive therapies such as ceftaroline, daptomycin, dalbavancin, oritavancin, linezolid, and tedizolid also offer possible prospects for treatment of infections with MDRO gram-positive organisms.[69]

Prevalence of Multidrug-Resistant Organisms in Patients with Cancer with Neutropenic Fever

The organisms responsible for bacteremic neutropenic fever have been well characterized during the many decades of clinical observation, and a shift in the type of organisms and antibiotic susceptibility phenotypes is noted. One of the most comprehensive early studies in 1993 showed that among 1051 BSIs in 9 French and 1 Belgian hospital, a total of 1147 isolates were obtained, with 86 blood cultures showing polymicrobial infection.[70] The other pathogens isolated included *E coli* (10.7%), *Klebsiella-Enterobacter-Serratia* (6.1%), other Enterobacteriaceae (2.2%), *P aeruginosa* (4.8%), other nonfermenters (4.7%), CNS (40.8%), *S aureus* (9.9%), streptococci (5.4%), enterococci (2.2%), anaerobes (3.4%), yeasts (3.5%), and other bacteria (6.9%). Antibiotic prophylaxis was not being used in patients at the time, but in 34.6% of the cases, patients were receiving systemic antibiotics when blood cultures were obtained. The role of antimicrobial resistance in outcomes for these patients was not addressed. It was noted, however, that gram-positive organisms predominated in patients with cancer at this time, reflecting a shift in pathogens due to the adoption of empirical antipseudomonal coverage.[57]

In more contemporary surveys that overlapped some with this very early period, Mebis and colleagues[71] and Ortega and colleagues[72] looked at all bloodstream isolates from patients with neutropenic fever from 1994 to 2008, and 1991 to 2012. In both large series, gram-positive organisms (namely CNS) predominated, but a shift in susceptibility to oxacillin-resistant CNS was observed.[71] Among *S aureus* isolates, the majority remained methicillin susceptible with 214 methicillin-susceptible *S aureus* (5.9%) and 48 (1.3%) MRSA.[71] During this time, standard practice evolved to administer oral fluoroquinolones to patients who were neutropenic and in the Mebis study, to use cefepime/amikacin for empirical therapy for febrile neutropenic patients. An increase of gram-negative isolates, namely *E coli* was foreshadowed in the latter period (2006–2012).[72] High rates of fluoroquinolone resistance were noted (66% Gram negatives[71] and 73% *E coli* isolates[72]). A reduced susceptibility of *P aeruginosa* strains to meropenem and cefepime was also noted. Resistance to cefotaxime, presumably because of the production of extended spectrum β-lactamases and other cephalosporinases, was noted in 26% of the *E coli* isolates.[73] Similar findings were reported in Australia in the period 2001 to 2010.[74]

However, in a large retrospective study conducted in France between 2003 and 2010,[75] examining 723 bacterial blood stream isolates researchers began to notice a definite predominance of gram-negative bacteria. Among 723 isolates, they found the following: gram-negative bacilli (70.8%) and gram-positive cocci (18.7%). The rate of MRSA was 6.45% and CNS 61.2%. Resistance to glycopeptides was not detected. In *E coli*, as in the *Klebsiella-Enterobacter-Serratia* group, a 27% resistance to fluoroquinolones was observed. Concerning *P aeruginosa*, 23.4% were resistant to penicillin and 13.1% were resistant to ceftazidime. The impermeability rate of imipenem was 9.3%. Increasing rates of gram-negative bacteria from less than 20% in 1996 to 80% in 2009 with a parallel decrease in gram-positive cocci (~80% in 1996 and ~5% in 2009) were noted. *E coli* isolates increased 2-fold, *K pneumoniae* isolates 3-fold, and there was a 2.5-fold increase in nonfermenters with increases in fluoroquinolone resistance to 25% of *E coli*. Four percent of *E coli* were ESBL producers. There was a concomitant 50% decrease in MRSA observed but no VRE were isolated. Gudiol and colleagues[76] compared 272 episodes of BSIs in adult neutropenic patients with cancer prospectively collected from January 1991 to December 1996 (first period), when quinolone prophylaxis was used, with 283 episodes recorded from January 2006 to March 2010 (second period), when antibacterial prophylaxis was stopped. Patients in the second period were significantly older and were more likely to have graft-versus-host disease and a urinary catheter in place, whereas the presence of a central venous catheter, parenteral nutrition, corticosteroids, and antifungal and quinolone prophylaxis were more frequent in the first period. More patients in the first period suffered from mucositis and soft tissue infection as the origin of BSIs, but an endogenous source was more common during the second period. Gram-positive BSI was more frequent in the first period (64% vs 41%; $P<.001$), mainly due to CNS and viridans group streptococci. Increases in MRSA BSI from 17% to 28.6% and enterococcal BSI (6% to 23%) were noted. In the second period gram-negative BSI increased (28% vs 49%; $P<.001$), mostly due to an increase in *K pneumoniae* isolates (7% to 21%). Quinolone susceptibilities were recovered, but MDR gram-negative BSI increased (3% to 11% with $P = .04$), including ESBL and AmpC hyper producers, MDR *P aeruginosa* and *A baumannii*, and *Stenotrophomonas maltophilia*. Blennow and colleagues[77] also reported on the increase in Gram negatives during this period.

In the intervening period through 2015, many investigators worldwide reported on the shift to more resistant gram-negative bacteria and the possible role of prophylactic fluoroquinolones in the selection of fluoroquinolone resistant bacteria, and ESBL producers, especially among Enterobacteriaceae (reviewed by[61,78–92]). Because of this Zhang and colleagues[93] looked at the issue of whether empirical oral fluoroquinolone therapy is appropriate in low-risk neutropenic patients in China who presented with fever and BSI: 38 patients were studied and 74% had bloodstream isolates with *E coli*, with 46% resistance to fluoroquinolones. Other isolates included 2 *K pneumoniae* (1 resistant to fluoroquinolones). In a Swiss pediatric neutropenic fever cohort,[94] although gram-positive organisms predominated overall, it was noted that in centers that did not use fluoroquinolone prophylaxis, more *P aeruginosa* isolates were found; greater fluoroquinolone-resistant gram-negative bacteria were recovered from centers where fluoroquinolone prophylaxis was used frequently. In academic medical centers in Italy, high rates of *P aeruginosa* BSIs (20% of all BSI) were observed in febrile neutropenic patients, with 33% to 70% MDR PSDA isolates reported.[91,92,95,96] Other centers have reported increasing rates of MDR *A baumannii* and other ESKAPE pathogens[8,80,81,87,95] including carbapenem-resistant *K pneumoniae* (35%).[91] Garza-Ramos and colleagues[97] also described a high prevalence of ESBL and GES carbapenemases in carbapenem-resistant-*P aeruginosa* in their hospitals. In their study, they observed 124 imipenem-resistant *P aeruginosa* with 36.2% producing carbapenemases of IMP, VIM, and GES types. ESBL GES-19 and carbapenemase GES-20 β-lactamases were most prevalent (84%).

More recently, because fluoroquinolone use is widespread throughout the world, an increase in the global prevalence of carbapenem-resistant organisms has been noted in patients with neutropenic fever, mainly in *P aeruginosa, Klebsiella* spp., and *Acinetobacter* spp. associated with median mortality of 50% and a 4.89-fold increase in MDRO associated with mortality.[98] The prevalence of highly resistant nonfermenting gram-negative bacilli (*P aeruginosa, A baumannii*, and *Stenotrophomonas maltophila*) also increased in patients with pediatric cancer with 25.8% of isolates showing an MDR phenotype.[99] A large prospective trial examining gram-negative blood stream infections 6 months after hematopoietic stem cell transplantation, a period in which 75% of the subjects still experienced profound neutropenia, found high rates of resistance among Enterobacteriaceae and nonfermenting rods, with half showing fluoroquinolone and cephalosporin resistance, 18.5% carbapenem resistance, and 35.2% multidrug resistance.[100] This study and others[101,102] bring into question the role of fluoroquinolones in prophylaxis (reviewed later).

Carbapenem-sparing regimens for BSIs with Enterobacteriaceae do not seem to be a viable option either according to one large noninferiority clinical trial ("MERINO") of piperacillin-tazobactam versus meropenem.[103] Some limitations of the MERINO trial were that there were more immunocompromised patients in the piperacillin-tazobactam arm, although the time to receipt of antibiotics was shorter in those subjects. Overall, initial microbiologically appropriate therapy was given in both arms of the study (67%). A large retrospective single center study from China revealed increased prevalence of MDR and XDR *E coli*, with 10% resistant to carbapenems.[104] A study from Egypt reveals an even more dire prevalence of 50% to 60% carbapenem resistance among bloodstream Enterobacteriaceae isolates from febrile neutropenic adult patients.[105] Similar high rates of resistance among Enterobacteriaceae were also reported among pediatric febrile neutropenic patients due to the presence of OXA-48, *Klebsiella pneumoniae* carbapenemase (KPC), and New Delhi metallo-β-lactamase.[106] Amikacin and tigecycline suspectibilities remained high in this center, although others report increasing resistance to tigecycline among other Enterobacteriaceae (*K pneumoniae*) associated with overexpression of efflux pump–associated genes *acrB, oqxB*, and regulatory genes *ramA* and *rarA*.[107] Many of these *K pneumoniae* isolates were also carbapenem and fluoroquinolone resistant. Finally, in a study of 109 neutropenic patients presenting with septic shock, Jung and colleagues[108] found that 30.3% had infections with MDRGram-negative bacteria with ESBL-producing *E coli* predominating. Approximately 49% of MDR bacteria were nonsusceptible to cefepime but not to piperacillin-tazobactam or carbapenems.

Gram-positive infections continued to predominate in some settings such as pediatric cancer hospitals[94,109,110] and were reported from one adult cancer hospital in Sweden[111] in earlier studies. These BSIs in febrile neutropenic patients were predominantly caused by CNS and viridans Streptococci, with relatively low rates of *S aureus* including MRSA and Enterococci including vancomycin-resistant Enterococci VRE. A recent study demonstrates why growing concern regarding glycopeptide resistance among CNS isolated from febrile neutropenic patients is warranted: Yamada and colleagues[112] showed that 20% of *S epidermidis* bloodstream isolates were resistant to teicoplanin. In 55.7% of patients with CNS bacteremia, teicoplanin was used as first-line therapy. Some studies noted an increase in the number of *S pneumoniae* isolates, especially those resistant to ceftazidime, among febrile neutropenic patients, prompting an inquiry into the rates of pneumococcal vaccination.[113,114]

An observational study of *Streptococcus mitis* bacteremia in pediatric febrile neutropenia conducted on isolates from the period 2010 to 213 revealed 30% resistance to penicillin, with high rates of toxic shock syndrome and multiorgan failure.[115] A recent single-institution survey of viridans streptococcal bacteremia in neutropenic patients revealed 45% of these isolates were *S mitis*, with only 5.9% resistance to penicillin.[116] Eighty-eight percent of the patients were on ciprofloxacin for necrotizing fasciitis (NF) prophylaxis in this cohort. Ampicillin resistance among Enterococci has also been associated with bacteremia in febrile neutropenic patients with mucositis who had prior exposure to penicillins and carbapenems.[117] Gudiol and colleagues[114] reported an increase in the number of vancomycin susceptible *Enterococcus faecium* isolates with high-level resistance to ampicillin and fluoroquinolones, related to the use of antibiotic prophylaxis in these patients. These investigators expressed concerns that this was a harbinger of future VRE infection, as vancomycin use increases in such patients. A recent study showed a 30.6% rate of VRE infection among febrile neutropenic children with Enterococcal bacteremia, although this did not have an impact on mortality.[118]

Limiting use of vancomycin has been associated with decreased rates of incident VRE infections in febrile neutropenic pediatric patients.[119] An even more frightening development is in a new MDR enterococcal phenotype—daptomycin and linezolid nonsusceptible VRE—in patients with immunosuppression, neutropenia, and recent invasive procedures.[120] Eighty-one isolates (36 bloodstream) were detected over a 5-year period. Exposure to daptomycin seems to be a risk factor for acquisition of this phenotype. Meta-analysis of gram-positive therapy and mortality suggests that there is no benefit to empirical gram-positive coverage in neutropenic fever patients.[121]

Risks for Multidrug-Resistant Organisms Pathogens in the Febrile Neutropenic Patient

Several excellent reviews are available[62,122,123] regarding risk factors for development of MDRO infections in oncology patients including patients with neutropenic fever. Colonization, previous infection, previous exposure to broad spectrum antibiotics, and/or prophylaxis with fluoroquinolones were associated with these types of infections, as well as advanced disease with severe presentation, prolonged hospitalization as well as the presence medical devices and instrumentation.[124,125]

Several additional studies have found similar associations between MDRO infections and febrile neutropenia. In a retrospective study of 747 blood stream infections in a 4-year period in Barcelona, Spain,[126] antibiotic exposures before neutropenic fever increased the odds of an MDRO being isolated 3.57-fold (95% confidence interval [CI] 1.63 to 7.80)—presence of a urinary catheter OR 2.41 (95% CI 1.01–5.74). In this series, 13.7% of the gram-negative bacteria isolated were MDR. In a separate study, these investigators found that carbapenem use was associated with increased rates of ampicillin-resistant, vancomycin-susceptible *E faecium* bacteremias.[127] In a Melbourne pediatric oncology hospital, antibiotic-resistant gram-negative BSIs were associated with high-intensity chemotherapy (OR 3.7, 95% confidence interval: 1.2–11.4), hospital-acquired bacteremia (OR 4.3, 95% confidence interval: 2.0–9.6), and isolation of antibiotic-resistant gram-negative bacteria from any site within the preceding 12 months (OR 9.9, 95% confidence interval: 3.8–25.5).[83] Kim and colleagues[128] showed that a hospital stay of greater than 2 weeks during the 3 months preceding bacteremia (adjusted OR, 5.887; 95% CI, 1.572 to 22.041) and the use of broad-spectrum cephalosporins in the 4 weeks before bacteremia (adjusted OR, 6.186; 95% CI, 1.616–23.683) were significantly related to the acquisition of ESBL-producing *Enterobacteriaceae*. However, the 30-day mortality for ESBL bacteremia and non-ESBL bacteremia were not significantly different (15% vs 5%; $P = .199$). A matched case-control (1:2) study in New York City hospitals including both pediatric and adult oncology ICU patients between February 2007 and January 2010 found that immunocompromised state (OR, 1.55; $P = .047$) and exposure to amikacin (OR, 13.81; $P<.001$), levofloxacin (OR, 2.05; $P = .005$), or trimethoprim-sulfamethoxazole (OR, 3.42; $P = .009$) were factors associated with extensively drug-resistant gram-negative bacilli health care–associated infections.[129] A retrospective chart review of 192 adults with cancer in China who were diagnosed with *Enterobacter* bacteremia evaluated risk factors and treatment outcomes associated with extended-spectrum cephalosporin resistance. Recent use of a third-generation cephalosporins, older age, tumor progression at last evaluation, recent surgery, and nosocomial acquisition were all associated with extended-spectrum cephalosporin-resistant *Enterobacter* bacteremia.[130]

Investigators in Mexico City evaluated the impact of fecal colonization with extended-spectrum β-lactamase-producing *E coli* for BSI, clinical outcome, and costs in patients with hematologic malignancies and severe neutropenia.[81] Colonization with ESBL *E coli* increased the risk of BSI by the same strain (relative risk = 3.4, 95% CI 1.5 to 7.8, $P = .001$), shorter time to death (74 ± 62 vs 95 ± 83 days, $P<.001$), longer hospital stay (64 ± 39 vs 48 ± 32 days, $P = .01$), and higher infection-related costs ($6528 ± $4348 vs $4722 ± $3173, $P = .01$). A difference in overall mortality between both groups was not reported. They concluded that stool colonization by ESBL *E coli* was associated with increased risk of BSI by this strain, longer hospital stays, and higher related costs. A contemporary review through 2017 of *E coli* BSI in a large teaching hospital in Great Britain found that more than one-third of cases were related to a gastrointestinal source and febrile neutropenia.[131] Forty-seven percent of these *E coli* isolates were resistant to ciprofloxacin, 37% to third-generation cephalosporins, and 22% to aminoglycosides. In a retrospective cohort analysis, Trecarichi and colleagues[132] examined risk factors for ESBL *E coli* BSIs at an Italian teaching hospital between 2016 and 2017 and using Cox proportional hazards methods, identified recent endoscopic procedures, culture-positive surveillance rectal swabs for multidrug-resistant bacteria, antibiotic prophylaxis with fluoroquinolones, and prolonged neutropenia as independent risk factors for BSIs caused by a third-generation cephalosporin-resistant *E coli*. Not surprisingly, however, Nesher and colleagues[133] at MD Anderson USA found in a 2-year retrospective review of all patients who received allogeneic hematopoietic stem cell transplants that the incidence of fecal colonization with *P aeruginosa*, including MDR strains was low and that the rate of infections with these bacteria was also low. The incidence of MDR *P aeruginosa* in the entire cohort was only 2.2% (18 of 794): 12 had positive surveillance stool cultures and 7 of these patients later developed MDR *P aeruginosa* infections. Older patients and patients with acute myelogenous leukemia (AML) were more likely to be colonized and to develop subsequent infection. Infection-related deaths were observed predominately during the first 30 days after infection. In this study, the positive predictive value of the *P aeruginosa* positive surveillance stool culture was only 23% for infection. Notably, 83% of the patients were on fluoroquinolones in the 30 days following HCT. Patients who were not colonized had a low chance of developing *P aeruginosa* infection. Most patients who developed infection did not have fecal colonization, suggesting a different source of infection.

Piperacillin-tazobactam is often administered as empirical therapy for neutropenic fever. Marini and colleagues[134] looked specifically at risk factors associated with infection with piperacillin-tazobactam resistant (PTZ-R) organisms using a retrospective cohort and multivariate analysis. This study reported that a 14.6% resistance rate is present among isolates with higher rates of mortality (29% vs 11%, $P = 0.024$) in the PTZ-R group. Other risk factors associated with PTZ-R infections were ICU admission, receipt of antibiotics for more than 14 days within the past 90 days, and respiratory infections. The investigators suggested that risk stratification of patients with neutropenic fever using this model in their hospital could define which patients would most benefit from combination empirical antibiotic therapy. Carbapenems are also used empirically in neutropenic fever. Micozzi and colleagues[135] instituted a rectal screening procedure to look for carbapenem-resistant *K pneumonia* in neutropenic patients. Rectal colonization and AML were independent risk factors for CR-KP bacteremia (occurring in 58% of carriers). These cases were associated with a high mortality (71%) in patients with AML and receipt of inadequate antimicrobial therapy initially.

Inappropriate Empirical Antibiotics

Given the profound immunosuppression associated with neutropenia in patients with cancer, reliance on early diagnosis and appropriate antibiotic selection would seem to be even more critical in this subset of patients with infectious disease. In a recent review,[92] antimicrobial resistance and/or the inadequacy of empirical antibiotic treatment have been frequently linked to a worse outcome in patients with cancer with BSIs caused by gram-negative isolates.

In one study,[136] immunocompetent patients with BSIs caused by ESBL-producing organisms who received inappropriate antibiotics (defined as receipt of treatment with an active antibiotic more than 72 hours after collection of the first positive blood culture) had an overall mortality of 38.2% when followed for a 21-day period. In their multivariate analysis, these investigators found that inadequate initial antimicrobial therapy (OR = 6.28; 95% CI = 3.18–12.42; $P<.001$) and unidentified primary infection site (OR = 2.69; 95% CI = 1.38–5.27; $P = .004$) were factors associated with mortality. The patients who received inappropriate empirical antibiotics (89 of 186 [47.8%]) were 3 times more likely to die compared with the adequately treated group (59.5% vs 18.5%; OR = 2.38; 95% CI = 1.76–3.22; $P<.001$). In a large study looking at hospitalized patients with cancer, Bodro and colleagues[79] showed that in patients with bacteremia with ESKAPE organisms, inappropriate empirical antibiotics were given more frequently (55.6% vs 21.5%, *P*<.001), were associated with more persistence of bacteremia (25% vs 9.7% *P*<.05), septic metastases (8% vs 4% *P*<.05), and early case fatality (23% vs 11% *P*<.05). In a subgroup analysis of data from 54 patients with an absolute neutrophil count less than 500/mm^3 in a larger study of *P aeruginosa* BSI in 234 patients with cancer[137] (n = 54), the patients who had appropriate empirical or targeted combination therapy showed better outcomes than those who underwent monotherapy or inappropriate therapy (*P*<.05). In a smaller study looking at MDR *P aeruginosa* bacteremias in patients with neutropenic fever, 6/22 patients received inappropriate antibiotics or developed resistance during therapy and demonstrated an increased mortality of 83.3% versus 27% in those who received appropriate antibiotics.[95] A retrospective study looking at *K pneumoniae* BSI in southern Europe[138] demonstrated a high rate of resistance in the hospitals studied: of 217 BSIs, 92 (42%) involved KPC-positive *K pneumoniae*, 49 (23%) ESBL-positive, and 1 (0.5%) metallo-β-lactamase–positive isolates. Appropriate empirical antibiotics were administered in 74% of infections caused by non-ESBL non-KPC strains versus 33% of ESBL and 23% of KPC cases (*P*<.0001). In multivariate analysis accounting for disease severity, inappropriate antibiotic therapy demonstrated close to a 2-fold higher rate of death (adjusted HR 1.9, 95% CI 1.1–3.4; *P* = .02). Even in lower risk patients, Zhang and colleagues[93] showed that inappropriate antibiotics in 22/38 patients led to higher rates of clinical deterioration (29%) and further infection (29%) but did not affect mortality in these low-risk neutropenic patients. In a study looking at risk of carbapenem-resistant *K pneumoniae*, Micozzi and colleagues[135] found that 80% of fatal BSI occurred while on inadequate therapy. Initial adequate antibiotic therapy was the single independent variable able to protect against death (*P* = .02).

One study examined BSI-related mortality in 400 patients who received hematopoietic stem cell transplants, before and after engraftment and found a difference in the rates of inappropriate antibiotic administration between the pre- and postengraftment periods.[114] In the preengraftment period, 17% of patients had a more than 48-hour delay in receipt of appropriate antibiotics, versus 27% in the postengraftment group. This resulted in greater ICU admissions (7% vs 25%) and a higher case fatality rate (4 vs 25%).[114] However, overall mortality in the cohort was not increased, and these investigators did not find an association with inappropriate antibiotics when looking at overall mortality, and this may be related to the fact that 50% of the patients on inappropriate antibiotics had central line–associated BSIs and central venous catheter lines were removed.

These investigators also looked prospectively at the administration of inappropriate antibiotics to patients with cancer with enterococcal BSIs and found that patients with *E faecium* were more likely to receive inappropriate antibiotics than patients with *Enterobacter faecalis* (44 vs 24%) but found significant difference in overall mortality was not present (30% *E faecium*, 26% *E faecalis*).[127] A mortality benefit to empirical linezolid therapy in children with febrile neutropenia colonized with VRE was also not found.[139] Similarly, an increase in mortality seen in patients with daptomycin-linezolid-vancomycin–resistant *E faecium* was not evident.[120] Likewise, in settings where CNS accounts for most of the MDR organisms, mortality is not increased as a result.[81]

Morbidity and Mortality Associated with Multidrug-Resistant Organisms

As has already been noted, the presence of MDRO and the receipt of inappropriate antibiotic therapy early on in infections are linked to increased mortality in neutropenic and other patients with cancer but there is a relationship between the specific type of infection and mortality, with higher mortality for MDR Gram negatives in most studies.[74,92,95,136] BSI with an MDR organism (OR 3.61, 95% CI: 1.40–9.32, P = .008) was an independent predictor of mortality at 7 days after a positive blood culture.[74]

In a pediatric setting, overall mortality was not affected by the presence of antibiotic-resistant gram-negative bacteria[83]; however, these investigators did show that antibiotic-resistant gram-negative infections were associated with longer median hospital length of stay (23.5 days vs 14.0 days; P = .0007), longer median ICU length of stay (3.8 days vs 1.6 days; P = .02), and a higher rate of invasive ventilation (15% vs 5.2%; P = .03). In addition, mortality was not increased in association with drug resistance in the setting of gram-positive infections[109,127] or in low-risk neutropenic patients.[93]

Mortality Risks and Multidrug-Resistant Organisms

Antimicrobial resistance and/or the inadequacy of empirical antibiotic treatment have been frequently linked to unfavorable outcomes in patients with cancer with BSI caused by gram-negative isolates.[92] BSIs with a MDRO (OR 3.61, 95% CI: 1.40–9.32, P = .008) was an independent predictor of mortality at 7 days after a positive blood culture.[74] In a large study of the effect of antibiotic resistance on outcomes in ICU patients including immunocompromised and neutropenic patients, multiple factors in both case and control subjects significantly predicted increased mortality at different time intervals after hospital-acquired infection diagnosis.[129] At 7 days, liver disease (HR, 5.52), immunocompromised state (HR, 3.41), and BSI (HR, 2.55) predicted mortality; at 15 days, age (HR, 1.02 per year increase), liver disease (HR, 3.34), and immunocompromised state (HR, 2.03) predicted mortality. Mortality at 30 days was predicted by age (HR, 1.02 per 1-year increase), liver disease (HR, 3.34), immunocompromised state (HR, 2.03), and hospitalization in a medical ICU (HR, 1.85). Infections caused by XDR-Gram negatives were associated with potentially modifiable factors. Moghnieh and colleagues[86] conducted a retrospective study of 75 episodes of bacteremia occurring in febrile neutropenic patients admitted to a hematology-oncology unit (2009–2012). Increased mortality was associated with MDRO BSI (22.7% died with extended spectrum cephalosporin resistance vs susceptible 3.8%; MDR bacteremia resulted in death in 4/7 [57%] versus 3/68 4.4% in non-MDR bacteremia patients). Risks associated with MDRO included carbapenem or piperacillin-tazobactam exposure greater than 4 days before the bacteremia. Two studies did not show an association between MDRO and mortality; in these studies, mortality in patients with neutropenic fever with BSI were associated with a septic shock presentation and polymicrobial sepsis.[73,89] Factors associated with lower mortality were isolation of CNS (OR 0·38, 95%CI 0·20 to 0·73, P = 0·004) and empirical therapy with amikacin (OR 0·50, 95% CI 0·29–0·88, P = 0·016)[73]; appropriate combination therapy also increased survival in patients with febrile neutropenia.[137] Carbapenems have been associated with a trend toward increased survival[140] in patients with neutropenic fever and ESBL-producing *E coli* and *K pneumoniae* BSI. However, increasing rates of carbapenem resistance are associated with increased mortality, given inadequate empirical coverage.[98,135]

P aeruginosa and MDR *P aeruginosa*,[91,95,137] ESBL-producing *E coli*, especially CTX-M-producing and ST131[141]; *K pneumoniae*[91,138] and *Enterobacter aerogenes*[130]; KPC and metallo-β-lactamase–producing *K. pneumoniae*[138] and *A baumannii*[91] were all associated with increased overall mortality in patients with cancer with neutropenic fever, adjusting for other risks such as degree of neutropenia, advanced or relapsed disease, APACHE score, age, septic shock, etc. typically associated with worse outcomes in immunocompromised patients. Discontinuation of prophylaxis with fluoroquinolones in some settings did not affect the overall mortality, only shifted the cause from gram-positive bacteria to gram-negative bacteria.[76]

Prophylaxis and the Role of the Microbiome

Early studies suggested that antibiotic prophylaxis (typically fluoroquinolones) targeting *P aeruginosa* reduced the number of febrile neutropenic episodes and reduced hospitalization. Some centers report decreased readmission rates and no increase in the incidence of *C difficile*–associated diarrhea with levofloxacin prophylaxis.[142] However, overall mortality is not reduced in individual studies. A meta-analysis in 2012 (including studies spanning 1973–2010) was able to demonstrate a mortality benefit in an era when fluoroquinolone resistance was rare.[143] A more recent meta-analysis that included RCTs and observational studies from 2006 to 2014 could only demonstrate a reduction in bacteremia but not overall mortality.[144] An appreciation for how fluoroquinolones alter gut microbiota,[145] MDRO Enterobacteriaceae especially *E coli* and *K pneumoniae* harboring ESBLs and fluoroquinolone-resistant determinants are selected through use of fluoroquinolones,[145,146] and overall mortality benefit of fluoroquinolones cannot be demonstrated, has led to a rethinking of the use of prophylaxis.[144,147,148]

Studies looking at fluoroquinolone prophylaxis generally have shown that prophylaxis tends to be used in higher risk neutropenic patients, is associated more often with not finding an etiologic agent for fever, and is associated with selection of fluoroquinolone-resistant and MDRO Gram negatives and inadequate empirical therapy.[149] It may also be associated with longer courses of carbapenems.[150] Prophylaxis may also benefit specific groups of neutropenic patients differently, for example, in one study, patients with multiple myeloma undergoing autologous *hematopoietic stem cell transplantation* (HSCT) experienced a benefit of levofloxacin therapy, whereas patients with lymphoma[151] and AML receiving reinduction chemotherapy[152] did not. A prospective study of children with acute lymphoblastic leukemia, looking at the development of ceftazidime-resistant *E coli* and *K pneumoniae* in stool, showed a significant increase in resistant organisms after 3 weeks in the children who received 20 mg/kg of ciprofloxacin compared with placebo.[146] A retrospective study in a cancer center that does not routinely administer fluoroquinolone prophylaxis demonstrated lower rates of 30-day mortality following BSI, lower rates of MDROs, and lower rates of ciprofloxacin resistance among GNRs compared with recent reports in the literature.[153] Another approach for patients colonized with CR-KP about to undergo allogeneic BMT is the "Turin bundle" consisting of oral gentamicin therapy 20 days pretransplant, avoidance of FQs (fluoroquinolone) during neutropenia, and use of combination tigecycline-piperacillin/tazobactam during fever and sepsis.[154] In the 5 patients described, all were alive and 60% had eradicated stool carriage of CR-KP.

So what if any prophylaxis affords the greatest benefit and lowest risk to the neutropenic patient? This clearly needs further study and is truly a "moving target." However, some encouraging data do exist in the literature. In a small retrospective study of 151 patients undergoing HSCT spanning 2005 to 2016, levofloxacin was compared with ciprofloxacin and found to reduce neutropenic fever episodes from 56.5% to 25.6% in HSCT patients.[155] Episodes of bacteremia decreased from 33% to 9% and were due to gram-positive organisms. Another study compared an older prophylaxis regimen, cotrimoxazole/colistin, to ciprofloxacin in a retrospective study.[156] In 2008, this center switched to ciprofloxacin as their prophylaxis for patients receiving induction chemotherapy for AML. They found that the incidence of NF, the rate of bacteremia, the types of bacteria isolated, and the rates of resistance and incidence of

CDAD were unchanged in the 2 prophylaxis eras. They pointed out that the COT/COL prophylaxis is also effective against *Pneumocystis jiroveci* and allows for use of fluoroquinolones in treatment of febrile neutropenia, if needed. In patients who have intolerance to fluoroquinolones, one center has begun to use oral fosfomycin as prophylaxis and in a small retrospective look at their experience, found similar rates of fever and infections when compared with FQs.[157] Reassuringly, they have not noted an increase in BSI with nonfermenters as a result of using fosfomycin. Another center has looked at the use of oral third-generation cephalosporins compared with levofloxacin, and although overall outcomes are similar, they noted an increased number of *Enterobacter* spp. infections in patients receiving cephalosporins.[158] Also, given the colocalization of resistance determinants for ESBLs and FQ resistance genes, use of third-generation cephalosporins as prophylaxis would not seem to afford much benefit in reducing MDRO selection in patients who receive them. Efforts to screen for colonization with MDROs at many body sites may yield means to risk stratify neutropenic patients as far as which empirical therapies would afford greatest coverage for potential resistant pathogens.[135,159–162]

The Role of Antimicrobial Stewardship and New Antibiotic Therapies

In the last 10 years, 12 antibiotics have been approved by Food and Drug Administration. These include 10 with clear potential in the treatment of MDRO infections in neutropenic patients: ceftaroline, dalbavancin, tedizolid, oritavancin, ceftolozane–tazobactam, ceftazidime–avibactam, meropenem-vaborbactam, imipenem-cilastatin-relebactam, plazomicin, and cefiderocol. As antimicrobial resistance has increased, some of these new agents have found their way into the therapeutic arsenal for patients with NF, and there are some compelling data to support their use.[163] The precise role of each agent has yet to be defined in neutropenic fever, but given increasing resistance trends, these antibiotics are a welcome addition to our armamentarium. Stewardship efforts to define local antibiograms, to help improve guideline concordance in antibiotic selection and management of lower risk patients with NF in the outpatient setting, adequate empirical therapy, improve time to first dose of antibiotic; to guide use of new antimicrobials[164]; to examine antimicrobial deescalation practices, and to reduce overall antibiotic exposures in neutropenic patients will be important steps to improving outcomes for patients with NF.[165,166] Questions regarding the duration of antibiotic therapy in neutropenic patients will still need to be answered with well-designed clinical trials.[167]

SUMMARY

Rates of infection with MDROs continue to increase among immunocompromised persons, as greater numbers of MDRO, including carbapenem-resistant organisms, are observed throughout the population. Antibiotic prophylaxis and empirical antibiotic therapy influence the selection of these MDRO; susceptibility patterns vary among regions and even within hospitals. The astute clinician is aware of his or her regional unique antibiogram. MDRO, especially gram-negative pathogens, can be associated with worse outcomes among immunocompromised persons, and empirical antibiotic choices must be selected with the local antibiogram in mind if appropriate lifesaving antibiotics are to be administered in a timely fashion. Other investigators in this monograph address the role of rapid diagnostics and newer agents for MDRO; studies are needed among immunocompromised persons to evaluate these novel approaches to improve outcomes.

DISCLOSURE

None.

REFERENCES

1. Dumford DM 3rd, Skalweit M. Antibiotic-Resistant Infections and Treatment Challenges in the Immunocompromised Host. Infect Dis Clin North Am 2016; 30(2):465–89.
2. Paul WE. Fundamental immunology. 7th edition. Lippincott Williams & Wilkins (LWW); 2102.
3. Owen J. Kuby immunology. 7th edition. W. H. Freeman; 2013.
4. Thaiss CA, Zmora N, Levy M, et al. The microbiome and innate immunity. Nature 2016;535(7610):65–74.
5. Drekonja D, Reich J, Gezahegn S, et al. Fecal Microbiota Transplantation for Clostridium difficile Infection: A Systematic Review. Ann Intern Med 2015; 162(9):630–8.
6. Rana A, Gruessner A, Agopian VG, et al. Survival benefit of solid-organ transplant in the United States. JAMA Surg 2015;150:252–9.
7. Sanroman Budino B, Vazquez Martul E, Pertega Diaz S, et al. Autopsy-determined causes of death in solid organ transplant recipients. Transplant Proc 2004;36:787–9.
8. Al-Hasan MN, Razonable RR, Eckel-Passow JE, et al. Incidence rate and outcome of Gram-negative bloodstream infection in solid organ transplant recipients. Am J Transplant 2009;9:835–43.
9. Bert F, Larroque B, Paugam-Burtz C, Janny S, et al. Microbial epidemiology and outcome of bloodstream infections in liver transplant recipients: an analysis of 259 episodes. Liver Transpl 2010;16:393–401.
10. Bodro M, Sabe N, Tubau F, et al. Risk factors and outcomes of bacteremia caused by drug-resistant ESKAPE pathogens in solid-organ transplant recipients. Transplantation 2013;96:843–84.
11. Bonatti HPT, Brandacher G, Hagspiel KD, et al. Pneumonia in solid organ recipients: spectrum of pathogens in 217 episodes. Transplant Proc 2009;41:371–4.
12. Camargo LF, Marra AR, Pignatari AC, et al. Nosocomial bloodstream infections in a nationwide study: comparison between solid organ transplant patients and the general population. Transpl Infect Dis 2015;17:308–13.
13. Song SH, Li XX, Wan QQ, et al. Risk factors for mortality in liver transplant recipients with ESKAPE infection. Transplant Proc 2014;46:3560–3.
14. Malinis MF, Mawhorter SD, Jain A, et al. Staphylococcus aureus bacteremia in solid organ transplant recipients: evidence for improved survival when compared with nontransplant patients. Transplantation 2012;93:1045–50.
15. Gagliotti C, Morsillo F, Moro ML, et al. Infections in liver and lung transplant recipients: a national prospective cohort. Eur J Clin Microbiol Infect Dis 2018;37: 399–407.
16. Kiros TAD, Ayenew Z, Tsige E. Bacterial Urinary Tract infection among adult renal transplant recipients at St. Paul's hospital millennium medical collect, Addis Ababa, Ethiopia. BMC Nephrol 2019;20:289.
17. El-Badrawy MK, El-Metwaly Ali R, Yassen A, et al. Early-onset pneumonia after liver trasnplant: microbial causes, risk factors, and outcomes, mansoura university, egypt, experience. Exp Clin Transplant 2017;5:547–53.
18. Riera J, Caralt B, Lopez I, et al. Ventilator-associated respiratory infection following lung transplantation. Eur Respir J 2015;45:726–37.

19. Liu TZY, Wan Q. Methicillin-resistant Staphylococcus aureus bacteremia among liver transplant recipients: epidemiology and associated risk factors for morbidity and mortality. Infect Drug Resist 2018;11:647–58.
20. Shields RKCC, Minces LR, Kwak EJ, et al. Staphylococcus aureus infections in the early period after lung transplantation: epidemiology, risk factors, and outcomes. J Heart Lung Transplant 2012;31:1199–206.
21. Moreno A, Cervera C, Gavalda J, et al. Bloodstream infections among transplant recipients: results of a nationwide surveillance in Spain. Am J Transplant 2007;7: 2579–86.
22. Florescu DFMA, Qiu F, Langnas AN, et al. Staphylococcus aureus infections after liver transplantation. Infection 2012;40:263–9.
23. Macesic NG-SA, Sullivan SB, Giddins MJ, et al. Genomic surveillance reveals diversity of multidrug-resistant organism colonization and infection: a prospective cohort study in liver transplant recipients. Clin Infect Dis 2018;67:905–12.
24. Kim YJJY, Choi HJ, You YK, et al. Impact of Enterococcal Bacteremia in Liver Transplant Recipients. Transplant Proc 2019;51:2766–70.
25. Oriol ISN, Simonetti AF, Lladó L, et al. Changing trends in the aetiology, treatment and outcomes of bloodstream infection occurring in the first year after solid organ transplantation: a single-centre prospective cohort study. Transpl Int 2017;30:903–13.
26. Origüen JF-RM, López-Medrano F, Ruiz-Merlo T, et al. Progressive increase of resistance in enterobacteriaceae urinary isolates from kidney. Transpl Infect Dis 2016;18:575–84.
27. Pilmis BSA, Join-Lambert O, Mamzer MF, et al. ESBL-producing enterobacteriaceae-related urinary tract infections in kidney transplant recipients: incidence and risk factors for recurrence. Infect Dis (Lond) 2015;47:714–8.
28. Alevizakos MND, Mylonakis E. Urinary tract infections caused by ESBL-producing Enterobacteriaceae in renal transplant recipients: a systematic review and meta-analysis. Transplant Infect Dis 2017;19:e12759.
29. Kalpoe JS, Sonnenberg E, Factor SH, et al. Mortality associated with carbapenem-resistant klebsiella pneumoniae infections in liver transplant recipients. Liver Transpl 2012;18:468–74.
30. Men TY, Wang JN, Li H, et al. Prevalence of multidrug-resistant gram-negative bacilli producing extended-spectrum beta-lactamases (ESBLs) and ESBL genes in solid organ transplant recipients. Transplant Infect Dis 2013;15:14–21.
31. Varotti GDF, Terulla A, Santori G, et al. Impact of carbapenem-resistant Klebsiella pneumoniae (CR-KP) infections in kidney transplantation. Transplant Infect Dis 2017;19:e12757.
32. Bergamasco MDBBM, de Oliveira Garcia D, Cipullo R, et al. Infection with Klebsiella pneumoniae carbapenemase (KPC)-producing K. pneumoniae in solid organ transplantation. Transplant Infect Dis 2012;13:198–205.
33. Cinar GKİ, Azap A, Kirimker OE, et al. Carbapenemase-Producing Bacterial Infections in Patients With Liver Transplant. Transplant Proc 2019;51:2461–5.
34. Giannella M, Bartoletti M, Campoli C, et al. The impact of carbapenemase-producing Enterobacteriaceae colonization on infection risk after liver transplantation: a prospective observational cohort study. Clin Microbiol Infect 2019;25: 1525–31.
35. Yuan XLT, Wu D, Wan Q. 11:. Epidemiology, susceptibility, and risk factors for acquisition of MDR/XDR gram-negative bacteria among kidney transplant recipients with urinary tract infections. Infect Drug Resist 2018;11:707–15.

36. Lanini S, Costa AN, Puro V, et al, Donor-Recipient Infection Collaborative Study, Group. Incidence of carbapenem-resistant gram negatives in Italian transplant recipients: a nationwide surveillance study. PLoS One 2015;10:e0123706.
37. Linares L, Cervera C, Hoyo I, et al. Klebsiella pneumoniae infection in solid organ transplant recipients: epidemiology and antibiotic resistance. Transplant Proc 2010;42:2941–3.
38. Linares L, Garcia-Goez JF, Cervera C, et al. Early bacteremia after solid organ transplantation. Transplant Proc 2009;41:2262–4.
39. Johnson LEDAE, Paterson DL, Clarke L, et al. Pseudomonas aeruginosa bacteremia over a 10-year period: multidrug resistance and outcomes in transplant recipients. Transpl Infect Dis 2009;11:227–34.
40. Bodro M, Sabe N, Tubau F, et al. Extensively drug-resistant Pseudomonas aeruginosa bacteremia in solid organ transplant recipients. Transplantation 2015; 99:616–22.
41. Mlynarczyk G, Sawicka-Grzelak A, Szymanek K, et al. Resistance to carbapenems among Pseudomonas aeruginosa isolated from patients of transplant wards. Transplant Proc 2009;41:3258–60.
42. Luo AZZ, Wan Q, Ye Q. The Distribution and Resistance of Pathogens Among Solid Organ Transplant Recipients with Pseudomonas aeruginosa Infections. Med Sci Monit 2016;22:1124–30.
43. Kim YJ, Yoon JH, Kim SI, et al. High mortality associated with Acinetobacter species infection in liver transplant patients. Transplant Proc 2011;43:2397–9.
44. Kim YJSS, Lee YD, CHoi HJ, et al. Carbapenem-resistant Acinetobacter baumanii bacteremia in liver transplant recipients. Transplant Proc 2018;50:1132–5.
45. Liu H, Ye QWQ, Zhou J. Predictors of mortality in solid-organ transplant recipients with infections caused by Acinetobacter baumanii. PLoS One 2015;10: e0130701.
46. de Gouvea EF, Martins IS, Halpern M, et al. The influence of carbapenem resistance on mortality in solid organ transplant recipients with Acinetobacter baumanii infection. BMC Infect Dis 2012;12:351.
47. Kitazono HRD, Grim SA, Clark NM, et al. Acinetobacter baumannii infection in solid organ transplant recipients. Clin Transplant 2015;29:227–32.
48. Reddy P, Zembower TR, Ison MG, et al. Transpl Infect Dis. Carbapenem-resistant Acinetobacter baumannii infections after organ transplantation. Transpl Infect Dis 2010;12:87–93.
49. Freire MP, Abdala E, Moura ML, et al. Risk factors and outcome of infections with Klebsiella pneumoniae carbapenemase-producing K. pneumoniae in kidney transplant recipients. Infection 2015;2015:315–23.
50. Lupei MI, Mann HJ, Beilman GJ, et al. Inadequate antibiotic therapy in solid organ transplant recipients is associated with a higher mortality rate. Surg Infect (Larchmt) 2010;11:33–9.
51. Kalil AC, Syed A, Rupp ME, et al. Is bacteremic sepsis associated with higher mortality in transplant recipients than in nontransplant patients? A matched case-control propensity-adjusted study. Clin Infect Dis 2015;60:216–22.
52. Kumar A, Ellis P, Arabi Y, et al. Initiation of inappropriate antimicrobial therapy results in a fivefold reduction of survival in human septic shock. Chest 2009; 136(5):1237–48.
53. Winters HA, Parbhoo RK, Schafer JJ, et al. Extended-spectrum beta-lactamase-producing bacterial infections in adult solid organ transplant recipients. Ann Pharmacother 2011;45:309–16.

54. Aguiar EB, Maciel LC, Halpern M, et al. Outcome of bacteremia caused by extended-spectrum beta-lactamase-producing Enterobacteriaceae after. Transplant Proc 2014;46:1753–6.
55. Lee KHHS, Yong D, Paik HC, et al. Acquisition of carbapenemase-producing enterobacteriaceae in solid organ transplantation recipients. Transplant Proc 2018;50:3748–55.
56. Shields RK, Clancy CJ, Gillis LM, et al. Epidemiology, clinical characteristics and outcomes of extensively drug-resistant Acinetobacter baumanni. PLoS One 2012;7:e52349.
57. Pizzo PA, Hathorn JW, Hiemenz J, et al. A randomized trial comparing ceftazidime alone with combination antibiotic therapy in cancer patients with fever and neutropenia. N Engl J Med 1986;315(9):552–8.
58. Freifeld AG, Bow EJ, Sepkowitz KA, et al. Clinical practice guideline for the use of antimicrobial agents in neutropenic patients with cancer: 2010 update by the infectious diseases society of america. Clin Infect Dis 2011;52(4):e56–93.
59. Escrihuela-Vidal F, Laporte J, Albasanz-Puig A, et al. Update on the management of febrile neutropenia in hematologic patients. Rev Esp Quimioter 2019; 32(Suppl 2):55–8.
60. Giacobbe DR, Mikulska M, Viscoli C. Recent advances in the pharmacological management of infections due to multidrug-resistant Gram-negative bacteria. Expert Rev Clin Pharmacol 2018;11(12):1219–36.
61. Mikulska M, Viscoli C, Orasch C, et al. Aetiology and resistance in bacteraemias among adult and paediatric haematology and cancer patients. J Infect 2014; 68(4):321–31.
62. Gustinetti G, Mikulska M. Bloodstream infections in neutropenic cancer patients: A practical update. Virulence 2016;7(3):280–97.
63. van Duin D, Bonomo RA. Ceftazidime/Avibactam and Ceftolozane/Tazobactam: Second-generation beta-Lactam/beta-Lactamase Inhibitor Combinations. Clin Infect Dis 2016;63(2):234–41.
64. Zhanel GG, Lawson CD, Adam H, et al. Ceftazidime-avibactam: a novel cephalosporin/beta-lactamase inhibitor combination. Drugs 2013;73(2):159–77.
65. Zhanel GG, Chung P, Adam H, et al. Ceftolozane/tazobactam: a novel cephalosporin/beta-lactamase inhibitor combination with activity against multidrug-resistant gram-negative bacilli. Drugs 2014;74(1):31–51.
66. Zhanel GG, Lawrence CK, Adam H, et al. Imipenem-Relebactam and Meropenem-Vaborbactam: Two Novel Carbapenem-beta-Lactamase Inhibitor Combinations. Drugs 2018;78(1):65–98.
67. Abdul-Mutakabbir JC, Kebriaei R, Jorgensen SCJ, et al. Teaching an Old Class New Tricks: A Novel Semi-Synthetic Aminoglycoside. Plazomicin *Infect Dis Ther* 2019;8(2):155–70.
68. Zhanel GG, Golden AR, Zelenitsky S, et al. Cefiderocol: A Siderophore Cephalosporin with Activity Against Carbapenem-Resistant and Multidrug-Resistant Gram-Negative Bacilli. Drugs 2019;79(3):271–89.
69. Tsoulas C, Nathwani D. Review of meta-analyses of vancomycin compared with new treatments for Gram-positive skin and soft-tissue infections: Are we any clearer? Int J Antimicrob Agents 2015;46(1):1–7.
70. Coullioud D, Van der Auwera P, Viot M, et al. Prospective multicentric study of the etiology of 1051 bacteremic episodes in 782 cancer patients. CEMIC (French-Belgian Study Club of Infectious Diseases in Cancer). Support Care Cancer 1993;1(1):34–46.

71. Mebis J, Jansens H, Minalu G, et al. Long-term epidemiology of bacterial susceptibility profiles in adults suffering from febrile neutropenia with hematologic malignancy after antibiotic change. Infect Drug Resist 2010;3:53–61.
72. Ortega M, Marco F, Soriano A, et al. Epidemiology and outcome of bacteraemia in neutropenic patients in a single institution from 1991-2012. Epidemiol Infect 2015;143(4):734–40.
73. Ortega M, Almela M, Soriano A, et al. Bloodstream infections among human immunodeficiency virus-infected adult patients: epidemiology and risk factors for mortality. Eur J Clin Microbiol Infect Dis 2008;27(10):969–76.
74. Macesic N, Morrissey CO, Cheng AC, et al. Changing microbial epidemiology in hematopoietic stem cell transplant recipients: increasing resistance over a 9-year period. Transpl Infect Dis 2014;16(6):887–96.
75. Bousquet A, Malfuson JV, Sanmartin N, et al. An 8-year survey of strains identified in blood cultures in a clinical haematology unit. Clin Microbiol Infect 2014; 20(1):O7–12.
76. Gudiol C, Bodro M, Simonetti A, et al. Changing aetiology, clinical features, antimicrobial resistance, and outcomes of bloodstream infection in neutropenic cancer patients. Clin Microbiol Infect 2013;19(5):474–9.
77. Blennow O, Ljungman P, Sparrelid E, et al. Incidence, risk factors, and outcome of bloodstream infections during the pre-engraftment phase in 521 allogeneic hematopoietic stem cell transplantations. Transpl Infect Dis 2014;16(1):106–14.
78. Montassier E, Batard E, Gastinne T, et al. Recent changes in bacteremia in patients with cancer: a systematic review of epidemiology and antibiotic resistance. Eur J Clin Microbiol Infect Dis 2013;32(7):841–50.
79. Bodro M, Gudiol C, Garcia-Vidal C, et al. Epidemiology, antibiotic therapy and outcomes of bacteremia caused by drug-resistant ESKAPE pathogens in cancer patients. Support Care Cancer 2014;22(3):603–10.
80. Chong Y, Yakushiji H, Ito Y, et al. Cefepime-resistant Gram-negative bacteremia in febrile neutropenic patients with hematological malignancies. Int J Infect Dis 2010;14(Suppl 3):e171–5.
81. Cornejo-Juarez P, Suarez-Cuenca JA, Volkow-Fernandez P, et al. Fecal ESBL Escherichia coli carriage as a risk factor for bacteremia in patients with hematological malignancies. Support Care Cancer 2015;24(1):253–9.
82. De Rosa FG, Motta I, Audisio E, et al. Epidemiology of bloodstream infections in patients with acute myeloid leukemia undergoing levofloxacin prophylaxis. BMC Infect Dis 2013;13:563.
83. Haeusler GM, Mechinaud F, Daley AJ, et al. Antibiotic-resistant Gram-negative bacteremia in pediatric oncology patients–risk factors and outcomes. Pediatr Infect Dis J 2013;32(7):723–6.
84. Lim CJ, Cheng AC, Kong DC, et al. Community-onset bloodstream infection with multidrug-resistant organisms: a matched case-control study. BMC Infect Dis 2014;14:126.
85. Marin M, Gudiol C, Ardanuy C, et al. Bloodstream infections in neutropenic patients with cancer: differences between patients with haematological malignancies and solid tumours. J Infect 2014;69(5):417–23.
86. Moghnieh R, Estaitieh N, Mugharbil A, et al. Third generation cephalosporin resistant Enterobacteriaceae and multidrug resistant gram-negative bacteria causing bacteremia in febrile neutropenia adult cancer patients in Lebanon, broad spectrum antibiotics use as a major risk factor, and correlation with poor prognosis. Front Cell Infect Microbiol 2015;5:11.

87. Papagheorghe R. Bloodstream infections in immunocompromised hosts. Roum Arch Microbiol Immunol 2012;71(2):87–94.
88. Rangaraj G, Granwehr BP, Jiang Y, et al. Perils of quinolone exposure in cancer patients: breakthrough bacteremia with multidrug-resistant organisms. Cancer 2010;116(4):967–73.
89. Rosa RG, Goldani LZ. Aetiology of bacteraemia as a risk factor for septic shock at the onset of febrile neutropaenia in adult cancer patients. Biomed Res Int 2014;2014:561020.
90. Sanz J, Cano I, Gonzalez-Barbera EM, et al. Bloodstream infections in adult patients undergoing cord blood transplantation from unrelated donors after myeloablative conditioning regimen. Biol Blood Marrow Transplant 2015;21(4): 755–60.
91. Trecarichi EM, Pagano L, Candoni A, et al. Current epidemiology and antimicrobial resistance data for bacterial bloodstream infections in patients with hematologic malignancies: an Italian multicentre prospective survey. Clin Microbiol Infect 2015;21(4):337–43.
92. Trecarichi EM, Tumbarello M. Antimicrobial-resistant Gram-negative bacteria in febrile neutropenic patients with cancer: current epidemiology and clinical impact. Curr Opin Infect Dis 2014;27(2):200–10.
93. Zhang S, Wang Q, Ling Y, et al. Fluoroquinolone resistance in bacteremic and low risk febrile neutropenic patients with cancer. BMC cancer 2015;15:42.
94. Miedema KG, Winter RH, Ammann RA, et al. Bacteria causing bacteremia in pediatric cancer patients presenting with febrile neutropenia–species distribution and susceptibility patterns. Support Care Cancer 2013;21(9):2417–26.
95. Cattaneo C, Antoniazzi F, Casari S, et al. P. aeruginosa bloodstream infections among hematological patients: an old or new question? Ann Hematol 2012; 91(8):1299–304.
96. Cattaneo C, Antoniazzi F, Tumbarello M, et al. Relapsing bloodstream infections during treatment of acute leukemia. Ann Hematol 2014;93(5):785–90.
97. Garza-Ramos U, Barrios H, Reyna-Flores F, et al. Widespread of ESBL- and carbapenemase GES-type genes on carbapenem-resistant Pseudomonas aeruginosa clinical isolates: a multicenter study in Mexican hospitals. Diagn Microbiol Infect Dis 2015;81(2):135–7.
98. Righi E, Peri AM, Harris PN, et al. Global prevalence of carbapenem resistance in neutropenic patients and association with mortality and carbapenem use: systematic review and meta-analysis. J Antimicrob Chemother 2017;72(3): 668–77.
99. Averbuch D, Avaky C, Harit M, et al. Non-fermentative Gram-negative rods bacteremia in children with cancer: a 14-year single-center experience. Infection 2017;45(3):327–34.
100. Averbuch D, Tridello G, Hoek J, et al. Antimicrobial Resistance in Gram-Negative Rods Causing Bacteremia in Hematopoietic Stem Cell Transplant Recipients: Intercontinental Prospective Study of the Infectious Diseases Working Party of the European Bone Marrow Transplantation Group. Clin Infect Dis 2017; 65(11):1819–28.
101. Hauck CG, Chong PP, Miller MB, et al. Increasing Rates of Fluoroquinolone Resistance in Escherichia coli Isolated From the Blood and Urine of Patients with Hematologic Malignancies and Stem Cell Transplant Recipients. Pathog Immun 2016;1(2):234–42.
102. Lubwama M, Phipps W, Najjuka CF, et al. Bacteremia in febrile cancer patients in Uganda. BMC Res Notes 2019;12(1):464.

103. Harris PNA, Tambyah PA, Lye DC, et al. Effect of piperacillin-tazobactam vs meropenem on 30-day mortality for patients with E coli or Klebsiella pneumoniae bloodstream infection and ceftriaxone resistance: a randomized clinical trial. JAMA 2018;320(10):984–94.
104. Ma J, Li N, Liu Y, et al. Antimicrobial resistance patterns, clinical features, and risk factors for septic shock and death of nosocomial E coli bacteremia in adult patients with hematological disease: A monocenter retrospective study in China. Medicine (Baltimore) 2017;96(21):e6959.
105. Tohamy ST, Aboshanab KM, El-Mahallawy HA, et al. Prevalence of multidrug-resistant Gram-negative pathogens isolated from febrile neutropenic cancer patients with bloodstream infections in Egypt and new synergistic antibiotic combinations. Infect Drug Resist 2018;11:791–803.
106. Kamel NA, El-Tayeb WN, El-Ansary MR, et al. Phenotypic screening and molecular characterization of carbapenemase-producing Gram-negative bacilli recovered from febrile neutropenic pediatric cancer patients in Egypt. PLoS One 2018;13(8):e0202119.
107. Elgendy SG, Abdel Hameed MR, El-Mokhtar MA. Tigecycline resistance among Klebsiella pneumoniae isolated from febrile neutropenic patients. J Med Microbiol 2018;67(7):972–5.
108. Jung SM, Kim YJ, Ryoo SM, et al. Cancer patients with neutropenic septic shock: etiology and antimicrobial resistance. Korean J Intern Med 2020;35(4): 979–87.
109. Ammann RA, Laws HJ, Schrey D, et al. Bloodstream infection in paediatric cancer centres–leukaemia and relapsed malignancies are independent risk factors. Eur J Pediatr 2015;174(5):675–86.
110. Wattier RL, Dvorak CC, Auerbach AD, et al. Repeat blood cultures in children with persistent fever and neutropenia: Diagnostic and clinical implications. Pediatr Blood Cancer 2015;62(8):1421–6.
111. Aust C, Tolfvenstam T, Broliden K, et al. Bacteremia in Swedish hematological patients with febrile neutropenia: bacterial spectrum and antimicrobial resistance patterns. Scand J Infect Dis 2013;45(4):285–91.
112. Yamada K, Namikawa H, Fujimoto H, et al. Clinical Characteristics of Methicillin-resistant Coagulase-negative Staphylococcal Bacteremia in a Tertiary Hospital. Intern Med 2017;56(7):781–5.
113. Garcia-Vidal C, Ardanuy C, Gudiol C, et al. Clinical and microbiological epidemiology of Streptococcus pneumoniae bacteremia in cancer patients. J Infect 2012;65(6):521–7.
114. Gudiol C, Garcia-Vidal C, Arnan M, et al. Etiology, clinical features and outcomes of pre-engraftment and post-engraftment bloodstream infection in hematopoietic SCT recipients. Bone Marrow Transplant 2014;49(6):824–30.
115. Nielsen MJ, Claxton S, Pizer B, et al. Viridans group streptococcal infections in children after chemotherapy or stem cell transplantation: a 10-year review from a tertiary pediatric hospital. Medicine (Baltimore) 2016;95(9):e2952.
116. Radocha J, Paterova P, Zavrelova A, et al. Viridans group streptococci bloodstream infections in neutropenic adult patients with hematologic malignancy: Single center experience. Folia Microbiol (Praha) 2018;63(2):141–6.
117. Hamada Y, Magarifuchi H, Oho M, et al. Clinical features of enterococcal bacteremia due to ampicillin-susceptible and ampicillin-resistant enterococci: An eight-year retrospective comparison study. J Infect Chemother 2015;21(7): 527–30.

118. Bae KS, Shin JA, Kim SK, et al. Enterococcal bacteremia in febrile neutropenic children and adolescents with underlying malignancies, and clinical impact of vancomycin resistance. Infection 2019;47(3):417–24.
119. Karandikar MV, Milliren CE, Zaboulian R, et al. Limiting vancomycin exposure in pediatric oncology patients with febrile neutropenia may be associated with decreased vancomycin-resistant enterococcus incidence. J Pediatr Infect Dis Soc 2020;9(4):428–36.
120. Greene MH, Harris BD, Nesbitt WJ, et al. Risk Factors and Outcomes Associated With Acquisition of Daptomycin and Linezolid-Nonsusceptible Vancomycin-Resistant Enterococcus. Open Forum Infect Dis 2018;5(10):ofy185.
121. Beyar-Katz O, Dickstein Y, Borok S, et al. Empirical antibiotics targeting gram-positive bacteria for the treatment of febrile neutropenic patients with cancer. Cochrane Database Syst Rev 2017;(6):CD003914.
122. Bassetti M, Righi E. Multidrug-resistant bacteria: what is the threat? Hematol Am Soc Hematol Educ Program 2013;2013:428–32.
123. Levene I, Castagnola E, Haeusler GM. Antibiotic-resistant Gram-negative Blood Stream Infections in Children With Cancer: A Review of Epidemiology, Risk Factors, and Outcome. Pediatr Infect Dis J 2018;37(5):495–8.
124. Gudiol C, Calatayud L, Garcia-Vidal C, et al. Bacteraemia due to extended-spectrum beta-lactamase-producing Escherichia coli (ESBL-EC) in cancer patients: clinical features, risk factors, molecular epidemiology and outcome. J Antimicrob Chemother 2010;65(2):333–41.
125. Kang CI, Chung DR, Ko KS, et al. Risk factors for infection and treatment outcome of extended-spectrum beta-lactamase-producing Escherichia coli and Klebsiella pneumoniae bacteremia in patients with hematologic malignancy. Ann Hematol 2012;91(1):115–21.
126. Gudiol C, Tubau F, Calatayud L, et al. Bacteraemia due to multidrug-resistant Gram-negative bacilli in cancer patients: risk factors, antibiotic therapy and outcomes. J Antimicrob Chemother 2011;66(3):657–63.
127. Gudiol C, Ayats J, Camoez M, et al. Increase in bloodstream infection due to vancomycin-susceptible Enterococcus faecium in cancer patients: risk factors, molecular epidemiology and outcomes. PLoS One 2013;8(9):e74734.
128. Kim SH, Kwon JC, Choi SM, et al. Escherichia coli and Klebsiella pneumoniae bacteremia in patients with neutropenic fever: factors associated with extended-spectrum beta-lactamase production and its impact on outcome. Ann Hematol 2013;92(4):533–41.
129. Patel SJ, Oliveira AP, Zhou JJ, et al. Risk factors and outcomes of infections caused by extremely drug-resistant gram-negative bacilli in patients hospitalized in intensive care units. Am J Infect Control 2014;42(6):626–31.
130. Huh K, Kang CI, Kim J, et al. Risk factors and treatment outcomes of bloodstream infection caused by extended-spectrum cephalosporin-resistant Enterobacter species in adults with cancer. Diagn Microbiol Infect Dis 2014;78(2):172–7.
131. Otter JA, Galletly TJ, Davies F, et al. Planning to halve Gram-negative bloodstream infection: getting to grips with healthcare-associated Escherichia coli bloodstream infection sources. J Hosp Infect 2019;101(2):129–33.
132. Trecarichi EM, Giuliano G, Cattaneo C, et al. Bloodstream infections caused by Escherichia coli in onco-haematological patients: Risk factors and mortality in an Italian prospective survey. PLoS One 2019;14(10):e0224465.

133. Nesher L, Rolston KV, Shah DP, et al. Fecal colonization and infection with Pseudomonas aeruginosa in recipients of allogeneic hematopoietic stem cell transplantation. Transpl Infect Dis 2015;17(1):33–8.
134. Marini BL, Hough SM, Gregg KS, et al. Risk factors for piperacillin/tazobactam-resistant Gram-negative infection in hematology/oncology patients with febrile neutropenia. Support Care Cancer 2015;23(8):2287–95.
135. Micozzi A, Gentile G, Minotti C, et al. Carbapenem-resistant Klebsiella pneumoniae in high-risk haematological patients: factors favouring spread, risk factors and outcome of carbapenem-resistant Klebsiella pneumoniae bacteremias. BMC Infect Dis 2017;17(1):203.
136. Tumbarello M, Sanguinetti M, Montuori E, et al. Predictors of mortality in patients with bloodstream infections caused by extended-spectrum-beta-lactamase-producing Enterobacteriaceae: importance of inadequate initial antimicrobial treatment. Antimicrob Agents Chemother 2007;51(6):1987–94.
137. Kim YJ, Jun YH, Kim YR, et al. Risk factors for mortality in patients with Pseudomonas aeruginosa bacteremia; retrospective study of impact of combination antimicrobial therapy. BMC Infect Dis 2014;14:161.
138. Girometti N, Lewis RE, Giannella M, et al. Klebsiella pneumoniae bloodstream infection: epidemiology and impact of inappropriate empirical therapy. Medicine (Baltimore) 2014;93(17):298–309.
139. Lisboa LF, Miranda BG, Vieira MB, et al. Empiric use of linezolid in febrile hematology and hematopoietic stem cell transplantation patients colonized with vancomycin-resistant Enterococcus spp. Int J Infect Dis 2015;33:171–6.
140. Chopra T, Marchaim D, Veltman J, et al. Impact of cefepime therapy on mortality among patients with bloodstream infections caused by extended-spectrum-beta-lactamase-producing Klebsiella pneumoniae and Escherichia coli. Antimicrob Agents Chemother 2012;56(7):3936–42.
141. Ha YE, Kang CI, Cha MK, et al. Epidemiology and clinical outcomes of bloodstream infections caused by extended-spectrum beta-lactamase-producing Escherichia coli in patients with cancer. Int J Antimicrob Agents 2013;42(5):403–9.
142. Lee SSF, Fulford AE, Quinn MA, et al. Levofloxacin for febrile neutropenia prophylaxis in acute myeloid leukemia patients associated with reduction in hospital admissions. Support Care Cancer 2018;26(5):1499–504.
143. Gafter-Gvili A, Fraser A, Paul M, et al. Antibiotic prophylaxis for bacterial infections in afebrile neutropenic patients following chemotherapy. Cochrane Database Syst Rev 2012;(1):CD004386.
144. Mikulska M, Averbuch D, Tissot F, et al. Fluoroquinolone prophylaxis in haematological cancer patients with neutropenia: ECIL critical appraisal of previous guidelines. J Infect 2018;76(1):20–37.
145. Chong Y, Shimoda S, Miyake N, et al. Incomplete recovery of the fecal flora of hematological patients with neutropenia and repeated fluoroquinolone prophylaxis. Infect Drug Resist 2017;10:193–9.
146. Tunyapanit W, Chelae S, Laoprasopwattana K. Does ciprofloxacin prophylaxis during chemotherapy induce intestinal microflora resistance to ceftazidime in children with cancer? J Infect Chemother 2018;24(5):358–62.
147. Horton LE, Haste NM, Taplitz RA. Rethinking antimicrobial prophylaxis in the transplant patient in the world of emerging resistant organisms-where are we today? Curr Hematol Malig Rep 2018;13(1):59–67.
148. Calitri C, Ruberto E, Castagnola E. Antibiotic prophylaxis in neutropenic children with acute leukemia: Do the presently available data really support this practice? Eur J Haematol 2018;101(6):721–7.

149. Carena AA, Jorge L, Bonvehi P, et al. [Levofloxacin prophylaxis in neutropenic patients]. Medicina 2016;76(5):295–303.
150. Nguyen AD, Heil EL, Patel NK, et al. A single-center evaluation of the risk for colonization or bacteremia with piperacillin-tazobactam- and cefepime-resistant bacteria in patients with acute leukemia receiving fluoroquinolone prophylaxis. J Oncol Pharm Pract 2016;22(2):303–7.
151. Satlin MJ, Vardhana S, Soave R, et al. Impact of prophylactic levofloxacin on rates of bloodstream infection and fever in neutropenic patients with multiple myeloma undergoing autologous hematopoietic stem cell transplantation. Biol Blood Marrow Transplant 2015;21(10):1808–14.
152. Ganti BR, Marini BL, Nagel J, et al. Impact of antibacterial prophylaxis during reinduction chemotherapy for relapse/refractory acute myeloid leukemia. Support Care Cancer 2017;25(2):541–7.
153. Conn JR, Catchpoole EM, Runnegar N, et al. Low rates of antibiotic resistance and infectious mortality in a cohort of high-risk hematology patients: A single center, retrospective analysis of blood stream infection. PLoS One 2017;12(5): e0178059.
154. De Rosa FG, Corcione S, Raviolo S, et al. Management of carbapenem-resistant K. pneumoniae in allogenic stem cell transplant recipients: the Turin bundle. The new microbiologica 2017;40(2):143–5.
155. Rambaran KA, Seifert CF. Ciprofloxacin vs. levofloxacin for prophylaxis in recipients of hematopoietic stem cell transplantation. J Oncol Pharm Pract 2019; 25(4):884–90.
156. Mayer K, Hahn-Ast C, Muckter S, et al. Comparison of antibiotic prophylaxis with cotrimoxazole/colistin (COT/COL) versus ciprofloxacin (CIP) in patients with acute myeloid leukemia. Support Care Cancer 2015;23(5):1321–9.
157. Zapolskaya T, Perreault S, McManus D, et al. Utility of fosfomycin as antibacterial prophylaxis in patients with hematologic malignancies. Support Care Cancer 2018;26(6):1979–83.
158. Yemm KE, Barreto JN, Mara KC, et al. A comparison of levofloxacin and oral third-generation cephalosporins as antibacterial prophylaxis in acute leukaemia patients during chemotherapy-induced neutropenia. J Antimicrob Chemother 2018;73(1):204–11.
159. Forcina A, Lorentino F, Marasco V, et al. Clinical impact of pretransplant multidrug-resistant gram-negative colonization in autologous and allogeneic hematopoietic stem cell transplantation. Biol Blood Marrow Transplant 2018;24(7): 1476–82.
160. Heidenreich D, Kreil S, Nolte F, et al. Multidrug-resistant organisms in allogeneic hematopoietic cell transplantation. Eur J Haematol 2017;98(5):485–92.
161. Sadowska-Klasa A, Piekarska A, Prejzner W, et al. Colonization with multidrug-resistant bacteria increases the risk of complications and a fatal outcome after allogeneic hematopoietic cell transplantation. Ann Hematol 2018;97(3):509–17.
162. Spinardi JR, Berea R, Orioli PA, et al. Enterococcus spp. and S. aureus colonization in neutropenic febrile children with cancer. Germs 2017;7(2):61–72.
163. Goodlet KJ, Nicolau DP, Nailor MD. In Vitro Comparison of Ceftolozane-Tazobactam to Traditional Beta-Lactams and Ceftolozane-Tazobactam as an Alternative to Combination Antimicrobial Therapy for Pseudomonas aeruginosa. Antimicrob Agents Chemother 2017;61(12). e01350-17.
164. Jean SS, Gould IM, Lee WS, et al, International Society of Antimicrobial Chemotherapy (ISAC). New drugs for multidrug-resistant gram-negative organisms: time for stewardship. Drugs 2019;79(7):705–14.

165. De Silva N, Jackson J, Steer C. Infections, resistance patterns and antibiotic use in patients at a regional cancer centre. Intern Med J 2018;48(3):323–9.
166. Kleinhendler E, Cohen MJ, Moses AE, et al. Empiric antibiotic protocols for cancer patients with neutropenia: a single-center study of treatment efficacy and mortality in patients with bacteremia. Int J Antimicrob Agents 2018;51(1):71–6.
167. Stern A, Carrara E, Bitterman R, et al. Early discontinuation of antibiotics for febrile neutropenia versus continuation until neutropenia resolution in people with cancer. Cochrane Database Syst Rev 2019;(1):CD012184.

Bacteremia due to Methicillin-Resistant *Staphylococcus aureus*

An Update on New Therapeutic Approaches

Marisa Holubar, MD, MS[a,*], Lina Meng, PharmD[b], William Alegria, PharmD[b], Stan Deresinski, MD[a]

KEYWORDS

• Methicillin • *Staphylococcus aureus* • MRSA • Bacteremia • Vancomycin • Daptomycin • Ceftaroline • Endocarditis

KEY POINTS

- Vancomycin and daptomycin, optimally dosed, are options for the initial management of methicillin-resistant *Staphylococcus aureus* (MRSA) bacteremia.
- There is insufficient clinical data to fully assess the roles of other antibiotics, including ceftaroline.
- Treatment options for persistent MRSA bacteremia or bacteremia due to vancomycin-intermediate or vancomycin-resistant strains include daptomycin, ceftaroline, and combination therapies.

INTRODUCTION

The emergence of antibiotic resistance and the continued high failure rate, including unacceptable mortality, in patients receiving standard therapies for methicillin-resistant *Staphylococcus aureus* (MRSA) bacteremia demonstrate the need for new therapeutic agents and approaches to this disease.

GLYCOPEPTIDES AND SEMISYNTHETIC LIPOGLYCOPEPTIDES

Vancomycin

Optimization of vancomycin administration is a critical factor in improving outcomes of patients with MRSA infection. Although it has been generally accepted that the

Financial Support. None reported.
Potential conflicts of interest. None.

[a] Division of Infectious Diseases and Geographic Medicine, Stanford University School of Medicine, 300 Pasteur Drive, Room L-134, Stanford, CA 94305-5105, USA; [b] Department of Quality, Patient Safety and Effectiveness, Stanford Health Care, 300 Pasteur Drive Lane 134, Stanford, CA 94305, USA
* Corresponding author.
E-mail address: mholubar@stanford.edu

Infect Dis Clin N Am 34 (2020) 849–861
https://doi.org/10.1016/j.idc.2020.04.003
id.theclinics.com

efficacy of vancomycin in *S aureus* bacteremia requires achievement of an area-under-the-curve (AUC) over 24 hours value greater than or equal to 400 times the minimum inhibition concentration (MIC) by broth microdilution ($AUC/MIC_{BMD} \geq 400$) and that a trough (Cmin) concentration of 15 to 20 mg/L is an accurate surrogate for this PK/PD index, recent evidence suggests these assumptions may be incorrect. Modeling studies demonstrated that unadjusted extrapolation of AUC from serum trough concentrations underestimated AUC by up to 25% and that AUCs varied between patients with similar trough results by up to 30-fold.[1] Furthermore, one meta-analysis suggests a threshold for increased concentration-related nephrotoxicity of AUC greater than or equal to 650 $\pm$ 100 mg/L, which is potentially problematic in the treatment of serious infections involving isolates with an MIC of 2 μg/mL.[2] The optimal exposure targets remain controversial because the proposed AUC targets are largely based on retrospective studies. One prospective observational study found that day 2 AUC values greater than 515 resulted in more nephrotoxicity but was not associated with lower treatment failures.[3] The addition of Bayesian analysis may allow for more precise individualized dosing, lower vancomycin exposures, and less nephrotoxicity.[1]

Semisynthetic Lipoglycopeptides

Dalbavancin, oritavancin, and telavancin are active *in vitro* against VISA. Telavancin and oritavancin are also active against VRSA and daptomycin nonsusceptible *S aureus*.[4] There is limited clinical data investigating the use of these drugs for MRSA bacteremia, but their pharmacokinetic properties are attractive for outpatient use.

Oritavancin

In a phase 2 study, oritavancin therapy was associated with microbiological success in greater than 79% of 84 patients with uncomplicated *S aureus* bacteremia.[5] The proportion due to MRSA (if any) was, however, not stated and, further complicating the analysis, the drug was administered in doses ranging from 5 to 10 mg/kg daily (in contrast to the recommended single 1200 mg dose.)

Dalbavancin

Among patients with MRSA bacteremia in phase 2 and 3 trials, all 38 dalbavancin recipients and 19 of 20 treated with comparator agents had clearance of bacteremia.[6]

Telavancin

In a retrospective analysis of patients with concurrent *S aureus* bacteremia in phase 3 trials, 20 patients with MRSA bacteremia receiving telavancin had clinical cure rates similar to those who received vancomycin.[7] Separately, 39 patients with cancer treated with telavancin for gram-positive bacteremias, including 9 due to MRSA, showed an 89% (32/36) clinical response rate without increased nephrotoxicity compared with vancomycin.[8] In a phase 2 study, all 5 patients with uncomplicated MRSA bacteremia treated with telavancin were cured.[9] Fourteen patients, 11 of whom had endocarditis, received salvage therapy with telavancin after a median duration of persistent bacteremia of 13 days.[10] All 10 with follow-up cultures had clearance of MRSA bacteremia, a median of 1 day (range, 1–3 days) after the therapeutic switch, although only 8 patients survived.

DAPTOMYCIN

Although Food and Drug Administration approved a dose of 6 mg/kg/d for MRSA bacteremia, higher doses are now commonly used and recommended,[11] but these may not reliably prevent the emergence of daptomycin nonsusceptibility.[12] One national retrospective cohort study of 371 adult patients with presumed persistent MRSA bacteremia whose therapy was changed to daptomycin within 7 days of initiating vancomycin found a survival benefit at 30 days in those who received daptomycin of greater than or equal to 7 mg/kg/d compared with those who received 6 mg/kg/d dosing (hazard ratio [HR] 0.31, 95% confidence interval [CI] 0.10–0.94).[13]

Murray and colleagues reported 85 patients with MRSA bacteremia with vancomycin MICs greater than or equal to 1.5 mg/dL whose therapy was switched to daptomycin (median dose 8.4 mg/kg/d after median of 1.7 days of vancomycin) and compared their outcomes with 85 matched historical controls treated only with vancomycin (median trough 17.6 μg/mL.) Patients treated with daptomycin experienced less frequent clinical failure and had a lower 30-day mortality rate.[14] Separately, Claeys and colleagues[15] found that the receipt of daptomycin (51.9% received $\geq$ 8 mg/kg/d) was associated with reduced clinical failure and 30-day mortality compared with vancomycin, regardless of the vancomycin MIC (measured with broth microdilution). In another retrospective analysis, when compared with vancomycin continuation, an early switch to daptomycin (median dose 6 mg/kg/d) was not associated with a significant difference in composite failure rate, but continued glycopeptide therapy was associated with an increased risk of nephrotoxicity.[16]

FIFTH-GENERATION CEPHALOSPORINS: CEFTAROLINE

Ceftaroline is active in vitro against hVISA and VISA, as well as against at least one VRSA strain, and exhibits a "see-saw" effect, with an inverse correlation between the MICs of ceftaroline and vancomycin.[17]

There are no randomized trials that compare ceftarolinemonotherapy with vancomycin or other agents. In a phase 4 registry study of *S aureus* bacteremia secondary either to acute bacterial skin and soft tissue infections (SSTIs) or to community-acquired bacterial pneumonia, clinical success in those with MRSA infection was reported in 18 of 32.[18] For many patients (the proportion was not reported), however, ceftaroline was administered together with a second antibiotic.

Ceftaroline has been used, often with an additional agent, as "salvage" therapy for patients with perceived failure of treatment of MRSA bacteremia with another antibiotic, but the definition of failure has been variable and, some cases, difficult to discern. In one such study, ceftaroline therapy was reported to achieve clinical success in 101 of the 129 patients with *S aureus* (92.5% MRSA) bacteremia, 92.0% of whom had endocarditis.[19] An unstated proportion, however, received ceftaroline in combination with a second antibiotic.

The relative efficacy of continuing the initial therapy (most with vancomycin) or switching to ceftaroline in patients with ongoing MRSA bacteremia was evaluated in a small case-control study with similar rates of microbiological cure in both groups (14/16 controls, 16/16 cases).[20]

Ceftaroline was administered to 31 patients after initial therapy with vancomycin or daptomycin; in 10 it was given in combination with another antibiotic, most frequently daptomycin.[21] Overall, microbiological cure was achieved in 64.5% (not all patients had test of cure) and clinical success in 74.2%, and the median duration of bacteremia after the switch to ceftarolinemonotherapy was 4 days (range, 1–8 days). Finally, after a change to ceftaroline therapy, blood cultures became negative in 1 to 5 days in 5 patients with persistent MRSA bacteremia, 2 of whom had endocarditis.[22]

OXAZOLIDINONES

Published information regarding the use of tedizolid for the treatment of bacteremia is limited. Bacteremia was present at enrollment in the ESTABLISH-1 and -2 trials of patients with SSTI in a small proportion of subjects.[23] In the 11 bacteremic patients who received tedizolid, 4 infections were due to *S aureus* (2 MSSA and 2 MRSA), whereas in the 16 who received linezolid, 9 were caused by *S aureus* (3 MSSA and 6 MRSA). All 11 tedizolid recipients and 11 of the 16 who were given linezolid responded to their assigned therapy.

The experience with linezolid may prove instructive in predicting the potential role of tedizolid in the treatment of MRSA bacteremia. A pooled analysis of 5 randomized trials found that clinical cure was achieved in 14 (56%) of 25 linezolid recipients and in 13 (46%) of 28 of the subset with MRSA infection given vancomycin, a difference that was not statistically significant.[24,25] In a prospective open randomized trial, clinical success at test-of-cure was achieved in 19 of 24 (79.2%) linezolid recipients and 16 of 21 (76.2%) of those given vancomycin.[26] In patients with persistent ($\geq$7 days) MRSA bacteremia while receiving vancomycin for at least 5 days, a switch to linezolid therapy (half also received a carbapenem) led to similar outcomes as seen in those in whom vancomycin was continued.[27]

Oxazolidinones are attractive oral step-down agents due to their bioavailability. In one prospective cohort study of adults with uncomplicated *S aureus* bacteremia (minority MRSA), Willekens and colleagues[28] compared clinical outcomes in patients switched to linezolid at days 3 to 9 of therapy compared with those treated with standard parenteral therapy. They found no difference in 30-day mortality or 90-day recurrence in these groups, but patients treated with linezolid experienced shorter hospitalizations (median 8 days vs 19 days, respectively.)

NEW-GENERATION TETRACYCLINES

The use of tigecycline in bacteremia is controversial due to its low serum levels with standard dosing.[29] In a pooled, retrospective data analysis of phase 3 clinical trials, 91 patients being treated with tigecycline developed secondary bacteremia.[30] In a prospective, randomized trial of patients with serious MRSA infections, 20 had documented MRSA bacteremia, 14 of whom received tigecycline and 6 received vancomycin. Clinical cure and microbiological eradication was 64.3% and 50% in tigecycline- and vancomycin-treated patients, respectively.[31]

Eravacycline, a fluorocycline, and omadacycline, an aminomethylcycline, have a similar spectrum of activity relative to tigecycline but with improved pharmacokinetic properties.[32] Both agents have *in vitro* activity against MRSA with favorable MIC_{50} and MIC_{90}values,[33,34] but data regarding their use of MRSA bacteremia are absent.

COMBINATION THERAPY

Combinations with Vancomycin

Vancomycin plus β-lactams

In a pooled data analysis of 156 patients from 2 separate retrospective studies,[35,36] bacteremia persistence for more than or equal to 5 days occurred in 24/90 (26.7%) patients given combination therapy with a β-lactam (piperacillin-tazobactam in more than half) and in 9/66 (43.9%; $P = .027$) given vancomycin alone, and was an independent predictor of persistence on multivariable analysis.[37] However, acute kidney injury (AKI) occurred in 18.9% of those given combination therapy and 7.6% ($P = .062$) of those receiving monotherapy and was similar in those who received a penicillin (piperacillin-tazobactam in 60%) when compared with those who received a cephalosporin. Clinical outcome, which was evaluated in only 1 of the 2 trials, reported that combination therapy was associated with a lower adjusted odds ratio for a composite clinical failure endpoint (0.237, 95% CI 0.057–0.982; P = .047), but no significant difference in 30-day all-cause mortality.[36]

In a retrospective study of 110 adults at a single center, combination therapy was associated with fewer treatment failures, a composite of clinical failure and persistent bacteremia on multivariable analysis.[38] There was no significant difference in 30-day mortality, and the median duration of bacteremia was 3 days in each group. Although piperacillin-tazobactam accounted for most of the β-lactam use, the incidence of nephrotoxicity did not differ.

In a retrospective study of adults with MRSA bacteremia in an 8-hospital health care system, 129 patients received vancomycin alone, whereas 229 received it in combination with cefepime.[39] Persistence of bacteremia for more than or equal to 7 days occurred less frequently in those receiving combination therapy (18.8% vs 31.0%, P = .008); there was no difference in recurrent bacteremia. After adjustment, there was no significant difference in 30-day mortality.

Published data regarding combination treatment with ceftaroline and vancomycin are limited to a very small number of patients for whom it was used as salvage and no conclusions regarding efficacy can be made.[40,41]

In the first randomized trial assessing combination therapy (CAMERA), 60 adults received either vancomycin (1.5 g twice daily) alone or with flucloxacillin (2 g every 6 hours for 7 days).[42] In this pilot study, the mean duration of bacteremia was 3 days in the monotherapy group and 1.94 days in those given combination therapy. Bacteremia persisted for more than 3 days in 8/29 (28%) and 4/31 (13%; P = .19) in the 2 groups, respectively. The time for 90% of subjects to clear their bacteremia was 4 days in the monotherapy arm and 9 days in the combination therapy group. Despite this apparently better microbiological efficacy, there were no significant differences between treatment arms with regard to mortality, relapse of MRSA bacteremia, metastatic infections, or need for intensive care unit admission.

This study served as prelude to a larger international randomized trial (CAMERA 2) with similar design.[43] Patients with MRSA bacteremia (only 4% had endocarditis) received either vancomycin or daptomycin45 at the discretion of the treating physician (approximately 99% received vancomycin) and were randomized to continue this alone or to receive it in combination with an anti-staphylococcal β-lactam, with the latter administered for 7 days. When tested by microbroth dilution, 95% had a vancomycin MIC <1 mcg/ml. Most of the combination group received flucloxacillin or cloxacillin, rather than cefazolin. The protocol specified that vancomycin be initiated with a 25 mg/kg loading dose with subsequent maintenance of a 15 to 20 mg/dL trough serum concentration while daptomycin be dosed at 6-10 mg/kg. The trial was stopped by the data and safety monitoring board after enrollment of 343 of a planned 440 subjects because of apparent futility as evidenced by an absence of effect on the composite outcome of death or complications by day 90, together with an imbalance in adverse events (acute kidney injury). There was no significant difference in the primary endpoint, a composite of 90-day mortality, persistence of bacteremia at day 5, and microbiological failure or relapsed infection. The incidence of bacteremia at day 5 was significantly reduced with combination therapy, but 21% in this group died compared to 16% of the monotherapy patients. AKI occurred in 30% of combination therapy recipients but in only 9% receiving monotherapy, with 7 and 2 requiring renal replacement therapy, respectively. AKI in the combination group predominantly occurred in those who received an anti-staphylococcal penicillin, mostly flucloxacillin rather than those who received cefazolin: 35% vs. 7%, respectively.

Vancomycin plus various non-β-lactam antibiotics
Retrospective studies have examined the addition of a variety of antibiotics to vancomycin, including rifampin, trimethoprim-sulfamethoxazole, fusidic acid, gentamicin, and doxycycline—sometimes with more than one of these agents—as salvage therapy.[44,45] There was no clear evidence benefit with use of these combinations.

In the ARREST trial, 758 patients with bacteremia due to *S aureus* were randomized to receive "standard antibiotics" together with either placebo or rifampin.[46] Only 47 (6%) of infections were caused by MRSA and, in this small subset of patients, the addition of rifampin to vancomycin or teicoplanin was not associated with benefit as determined by the number of patients reaching the composite endpoint (microbiological failure, recurrence, and/or death within 12 weeks), which occurred in 3/21 (14.3%) placebo recipients and 9/26 (34.6%) given rifampin (HR: 2.74, 0.74–10.15).

Combinations with Daptomycin

Daptomycin plus β-lactams
Among patients with MRSA bacteremia enrolled in a daptomycin registry study, most of whom had received prior antibiotic therapy, clinical or microbiological success was observed in 18 of 22 (82%) who received daptomycin in combination with a β-lactam antibiotic and in 27 of 34 (79%) who received this lipopeptide antibiotic without a β-lactam, a difference that was not significant.[47] The use of daptomycin in combination with rifampin, gentamicin, or vancomycin was not associated with a significant difference in outcome when compared with monotherapy.

The efficacy of salvage therapy with daptomycin and ceftaroline in combination was examined in patients at 10 medical centers with persistent staphylococcal bacteremia.[48] Of the 26 infections (including 14 with endocarditis), 22 were due to MRSA, including 2 VISA; 4 isolates were daptomycin nonsusceptible. Daptomycin monotherapy had failed in 12. The median duration of bacteremia before initiation of daptomycin plus ceftaroline was 10 days (range, 3–23 days) and was 2 days (range, 1–6 days) after.

In another retrospective report of salvage therapy, 7 patients with persistent or relapsed MRSA bacteremia who had sequentially failed vancomycin and daptomycin monotherapies cleared their bloodstreams a median of 1 day (range, 1–2 days) after the addition of a semisynthetic penicillin to daptomycin.[49]

In addition to these retrospective studies of their use as salvage, the combination of daptomycin and a β-lactam antibiotic has also been evaluated as primary (or at least early) therapy. Jorgensen and colleagues[50] performed a retrospective comparative cohort study to evaluate the effect of the addition of a β-lactam (cefepime in 43.0% and cefazolin in 25.0%) to daptomycin. Clinical failure (60-day crude mortality and/or 60-day MRSA bacteremia recurrence) occurred in 43 (27.4%) of daptomycin monotherapy patients and 9 (12.5%; $P = .013$) of those who received daptomycin plus a β-lactam, and the adjusted odds ratio for clinical failure was 0.386 (95% CI, 0.175–0.853). The median time to negative blood cultures was 66 hours, without a significant difference between treatment groups, and there were also no significant differences in the proportions with blood cultures positive at more than or equal to 5 days of daptomycin administration (27.5%) or at more than or equal to 7 days (27.9%). AKI occurred in 3 (2.9%) monotherapy and 7 (10.8%; $P = .046$) combination therapy patients.

Geriak and colleagues[51] enrolled adults with MRSA bacteremia in a prospective unblinded trial at 3 centers with randomization to receive either standard monotherapy with vancomycin (dosed to trough concentration of 15–20 mg/L) or daptomycin

(6–8 mg/kg/d) or combination of daptomycin and ceftaroline (600 mg every 8 h). Seventeen patients were randomized to combination therapy and 23 to monotherapy, which, by clinician choice, was vancomycin in 21 and daptomycin in 2 cases. The median interval from onset of bacteremia to initiation of study drugs was 2 days. The prespecified primary outcome was the duration of bacteremia, but the study was terminated (in the absence of a data and safety monitoring board or predetermined stopping rules) after 40 of a planned 50 patients were enrolled because of a mortality imbalance, with in-hospital death in 6/23 (26%) patients randomized to monotherapy and 0/17 ($P = .029$) to combination therapy. All deaths occurred in patients with endovascular infection, 2 of whom had stage IV lung cancer and the median duration of bacteremia was 3 days and did not differ between treatment groups. The results of this study are provocative and its interpretation has been challenged, in large part because of the small sample size and premature discontinuation.[52] As Geriak and colleagues[51] state, the results should only be considered as hypothesis generating.

Daptomycin plus trimethoprim-sulfamethoxazole

The addition of trimethoprim-sulfamethoxazole to daptomycin in 20 patients still bacteremic after having received a median of 5 days of receipt of the lipopeptide was associated with bloodstream clearance after a median of 2.5 days, although it was 6.5 days in the 6 patients infected with a daptomycin nonsusceptible strain.[53] Hyperkalemia occurred frequently during combination therapy.

In patients with bacteremia persisting for a median of 7 to 8 days on primary or secondary therapy, regimen was changed to daptomycin plus either ceftaroline (N = 23) or trimethoprim-sulfamethoxazole (N = 16) with a subsequent bacteremia duration of 2 days in each group.[54]

Trimethoprim-sulfamethoxazole plus ceftaroline

Vancomycin-based therapy was changed to a ceftaroline-based regimen in 29 patients (in combination with trimethoprim-sulfamethoxazole in 23), in 7 because of disease progression despite bacteremia clearance, and in 22 with persistent bacteremia for a median of 9.5 days. In the latter group, the subsequent duration of bacteremia was 2 days and microbiologic success was achieved in 26 (90%), but only 9 (31%) were considered treatment successes, which was defined as absence of clinical or microbiological recurrence at 6 weeks.[55]

Combinations with Fosfomycin

In a study published only in abstract form to date (although completed in January, 2018), Pujol and colleagues[56] randomized 155 patients (of a planned 206) with MRSA bacteremia at 18 centers in Spain to receive daptomycin (10 mg/kg/d) alone or with fosfomycin (2 g intravenously every 6 hours). Success (survival and clearance of bacteremia at day 7) was achieved at posttreatment day 7 in 69/74 (93.2%) recipients of combination therapy and 62/81 (76.5%) given daptomycin alone (absolute difference, 16.7%; 95% CI, 5.4%–27.7%). At the 6-week test of cure visit, the treatment was found to be successful in 40/74 (54.1%) and 34/81 (42%) in the combination and monotherapy groups, respectively (absolute difference 12%; 95% CI, 0%–27%). Microbiologic failure at the test-of-cure visit was observed in none of the combination therapy recipients but occurred in 9 monotherapy patients ($P = .009$). Patients receiving daptomycin plus fosfomycin were numerically more likely to suffer an adverse event leading to discontinuation of the drug—6/74 (8.1%) versus 3/81 (3.7%); $P = .31$.

Fosfomycin plus imipenem

Sixteen patients with persistent (N = 14) or relapsed (N = 2) MRSA bacteremia who had received a median of 9.5 days of antibiotic therapy (mostly vancomycin, but daptomycin in 2 cases) were treated with the combination of imipenem and fosfomycin with bloodstream clearance within 72 hours in each case and with a clinical success rate of 69%.[57]

Investigators attempted to follow-up on this observation with a multicenter open-label randomized clinical trial, which, unfortunately, was aborted after "flawed enrollment" of only 15 of the planned 50 patients.[58] Eight of the 15 had endocarditis and the remaining 7 had complicated bacteremia. All 8 patients randomized to receive fosfomycin plus imipenem had negative blood cultures at day 3 as did 6/7 receiving vancomycin. Cure was achieved in 4 (50%) and 3 (43%), respectively.

NEW AGENTS

Delafloxacin

Delafloxacin is a non-zwitterionic fluoroquinolone with enhanced activity against MRSA strains resistant to earlier generation fluoroquinolones.[59]

Although clinical data in patients with MRSA bacteremia are nonexistent, in a pooled analysis from phase 3 trials of patients with acute bacterial SSTIs, microbiological response at follow-up in patients with MRSA was similar between delafloxacin- and vancomycin/aztreonam-treated patients (98.1% vs 98.0%, respectively).[60] In a subgroup of patients with concomitant *S aureus* bacteremia at baseline (n = 6), 83.3% were labeled clinical responders at 48 to 72 hours and at day 14 ± 1.[61] It should be noted, however, that delafloxacin nonsusceptibility has been reported.[62]

SUMMARY

The lack of high-level evidence precludes definitive conclusions regarding optimal therapy of MRSA bacteremia. However, based on the available data and experience the following can be proposed:

- Vancomycin and daptomycin, optimally dosed, are options for initial management.
- Ceftaroline may be a promising alternative, but its broad spectrum of activity is not desirable when used as a definitive therapy.
- Relative to vancomycin alone, the combination of vancomycin with a variety of β-lactam antibiotics is associated with a shortened duration of bacteremia, but without significant clinical benefit, whether used as primary or salvage therapy. In addition, the use of piperacillin-tazobactam or flucloxacillin is associated with an increased risk of AKI, whereras cefazolin seems safe. Studies in other contexts suggest that cefepime and meropenem are also safe in this regard.
- The use of rifampin in combination with vancomycin does not seem to improve the efficacy of vancomycin given alone.
- Daptomycin combinations with various β-lactams are associated with a shorter duration of bacteremia compared with daptomycin monotherapy, with some studies also suggesting a clinical benefit. Of note is that there are no comparative studies that have examined the relative efficacy of ceftaroline alone.
- Other combinations that may deserve clinical investigation include daptomycin or ceftaroline plus trimethoprim-sulfamethoxazole and fosfomycin with daptomycin or imipenem.

REFERENCES

1. Neely MN, Youn G, Jones B, et al. Are vancomycin trough concentrations adequate for optimal dosing? Antimicrob Agents Chemother 2014;58(1):309–16.
2. Aljefri DM, Avedissian SN, Rhodes NJ, et al. Vancomycinarea under the curve and acute kidney injury: a meta-analysis. Clin Infect Dis 2019;69(11):1881–7.
3. Lodise TP, Rosenkranz SL, Finnemeyer M, et al. The Emperor's new clothes: prospective observational evaluation of the association between initial vancomycin exposure and failure rates among adult hospitalized patients with MRSAbloodstream infections (PROVIDE). Clin Infect Dis 2020;70(8):1536–45.
4. Zhanel GG, Calic D, Schweizer F, et al. New lipoglycopeptides: a comparative review of dalbavancin, oritavancin and telavancin. Drugs 2010;70(7):859–86.
5. Karaoui LR, El-Lababidi R, Chahine EB. Oritavancin: an investigational lipoglycopeptide antibiotic. Am J Health SystPharm 2013;70(1):23–33.
6. Rappo U, Gonzalez P, Akinapelli K, et al. Outcomes in patients with Staphylococcus aureus bacteraemia treated with dalbavancin in clinical trials. Paper presented at: European Congress of Clinical Microbiology & Infectious Diseases. Vienna, Austria, April 22 - 25, 2017, 2017.
7. Wilson SE, Graham DR, Wang W, et al. Telavancin in the treatment of concurrent staphylococcus aureus bacteremia: a retrospective analysis of ATLAS and ATTAIN studies. Infect Dis Ther 2017;6(3):413–22.
8. Chaftari AM, Hachem R, Jordan M, et al. Case-control study of Telavancin as an alternative treatment for gram-positive bloodstream infections in patients with cancer. Antimicrob Agents Chemother 2016;60(1):239–44.
9. Stryjewski ME, Lentnek A, O'Riordan W, et al. A randomized Phase 2 trial of telavancin versus standard therapy in patients with uncomplicated Staphylococcus aureus bacteremia: the ASSURE study. BMC Infect Dis 2014;14:289.
10. Ruggero MA, Peaper DR, Topal JE. Telavancin for refractory methicillin-resistant Staphylococcus aureus bacteremia and infective endocarditis. Infect Dis 2015; 47(6):379–84.
11. Baddour LM, Wilson WR, Bayer AS, et al. Infective endocarditis in adults: diagnosis, antimicrobial therapy, and management of complications: a scientific statement for healthcare professionals from the American Heart Association. Circulation 2015;132(15):1435–86.
12. Gasch O, Camoez M, Dominguez MA, et al. Emergence of resistance to daptomycin in a cohort of patients with methicillin-resistant Staphylococcus aureus persistent bacteraemia treated with daptomycin. J AntimicrobChemother 2014; 69(2):568–71.
13. Timbrook TT, Caffrey AR, Luther MK, et al. Association of higher daptomycin dose (7 mg/kg or Greater) with improved survival in patients with methicillin-resistant staphylococcus aureus bacteremia. Pharmacotherapy 2018;38(2):189–96.
14. Smith JR, Claeys KC, Barber KE, et al. High-dose daptomycin therapy for staphylococcal endocarditis and when to apply it. Curr Infect Dis Rep 2014;16(10):429.
15. Claeys KC, Zasowski EJ, Casapao AM, et al. Daptomycinimproves outcomes regardless of Vancomycin MIC in a propensity-matched analysis of methicillin-resistant Staphylococcus aureusbloodstream infections. Antimicrob Agents Chemother 2016;60(10):5841–8.
16. Moise PA, Culshaw DL, Wong-Beringer A, et al. Comparative effectiveness of vancomycin versus daptomycin for MRSAbacteremia with vancomycinMIC >1 mg/L: a multicenter evaluation. ClinTher 2016;38(1):16–30.

17. Espedido BA, Jensen SO, van Hal SJ. Ceftarolinefosamil salvage therapy: an option for reduced-vancomycin-susceptible MRSAbacteraemia. J AntimicrobChemother 2015;70(3):797–801.
18. Vazquez JA, Maggiore CR, Cole P, et al. CeftarolineFosamil for the treatment of staphylococcus aureus bacteremia secondary to acute bacterial skin and skin structure infections or community-acquired bacterial pneumonia. Infect Dis ClinPract 2015;23(1):39–43.
19. Casapao AM, Davis SL, Barr VO, et al. Large retrospective evaluation of the effectiveness and safety of ceftarolinefosamil therapy. Antimicrob Agents Chemother 2014;58(5):2541–6.
20. Paladino JA, Jacobs DM, Shields RK, et al. Use of ceftaroline after glycopeptide failure to eradicate meticillin-resistant Staphylococcus aureusbacteraemia with elevated vancomycin minimum inhibitory concentrations. Int J Antimicrob Agents 2014;44(6):557–63.
21. Polenakovik HM, Pleiman CM. Ceftaroline for meticillin-resistant Staphylococcus aureusbacteraemia: case series and review of the literature. Int J Antimicrob Agents 2013;42(5):450–5.
22. Ho TT, Cadena J, Childs LM, et al. Methicillin-resistant Staphylococcus aureusbacteraemia and endocarditis treated with ceftaroline salvage therapy. J AntimicrobChemother 2012;67(5):1267–70.
23. Burdette SD, Trotman R. Tedizolid: the first once-daily oxazolidinone class antibiotic. Clin Infect Dis 2015;61(8):1315–21.
24. Shorr AF, Kunkel MJ, Kollef M. Linezolid versus vancomycin for Staphylococcus aureusbacteraemia: pooled analysis of randomized studies. J AntimicrobChemother 2005;56(5):923–9.
25. Shorr AF, Lodise TP, Corey GR, et al. Analysis of the phase 3 ESTABLISH trials of tedizolid versus linezolid in acute bacterial skin and skin structure infections. Antimicrob Agents Chemother 2015;59(2):864–71.
26. Wilcox MH, Tack KJ, Bouza E, et al. Complicated skin and skin-structure infections and catheter-related bloodstream infections: noninferiority of linezolid in a phase 3 study. Clin Infect Dis 2009;48(2):203–12.
27. Park HJ, Kim SH, Kim MJ, et al. Efficacy of linezolid-based salvage therapy compared with glycopeptide-based therapy in patients with persistent methicillin-resistant Staphylococcus aureus bacteremia. J Infect 2012;65(6):505–12.
28. Willekens R, Puig-Asensio M, Ruiz-Camps I, et al. Early oral switch to linezolid for low-risk patients with Staphylococcus aureus bloodstream infections: a propensity-matched cohort study. Clin Infect Dis 2019;69(3):381–7.
29. Stein GE, Babinchak T. Tigecycline: an update. DiagnMicrobiol Infect Dis 2013;75(4):331–6.
30. Gardiner D, Dukart G, Cooper A, et al. Safety and efficacy of intravenous tigecycline in subjects with secondary bacteremia: pooled results from 8 phase III clinical trials. Clin Infect Dis 2010;50(2):229–38.
31. Florescu I, Beuran M, Dimov R, et al. Efficacy and safety of tigecycline compared with vancomycin or linezolid for treatment of serious infections with methicillin-resistant Staphylococcus aureus or vancomycin-resistant enterococci: a Phase 3, multicentre, double-blind, randomized study. J AntimicrobChemother 2008;62(Suppl1):i17–28.
32. Rodvold KA, Burgos RM, Tan X, et al. Omadacycline: a review of the clinical pharmacokinetics and pharmacodynamics. ClinPharmacokinet 2020;59(4):409–25.

33. Huband MD, Pfaller MA, Shortridge D, et al. Surveillance of omadacycline activity tested against clinical isolates from the United States and Europe: Results from the SENTRY Antimicrobial Surveillance Programme, 2017. J Glob Antimicrob Resist 2019;19:56–63.
34. Sutcliffe JA, O'Brien W, Fyfe C, et al. Antibacterial activity of eravacycline (TP-434), a novel fluorocycline, against hospital and community pathogens. Antimicrob Agents Chemother 2013;57(11):5548–58.
35. Dilworth TJ, Ibrahim O, Hall P, et al. Beta-Lactams enhance vancomycin activity against methicillin-resistant Staphylococcus aureus bacteremia compared to vancomycin alone. Antimicrob Agents Chemother 2014;58(1):102–9.
36. Casapao AM, Jacobs DM, Bowers DR, et al. Early administration of adjuvant beta-lactam therapy in combination with vancomycin among patients with methicillin-resistant Staphylococcus aureusbloodstream infection: a retrospective, multicenter analysis. Pharmacotherapy 2017;37(11):1347–56.
37. Dilworth TJ, Casapao AM, Ibrahim OM, et al. Adjuvant beta-lactam therapy combined with vancomycin for methicillin-resistant staphylococcus aureus bacteremia: does beta-lactam class matter? Antimicrob Agents Chemother 2019; 63(3) [pii:e02211-18].
38. Truong J, Veillette JJ, Forland SC. Outcomes of Vancomycin plus a beta-Lactam versus Vancomycinonly for treatment of methicillin-resistant Staphylococcus aureusbacteremia. Antimicrob Agents Chemother 2018;62(2) [pii:e01554-17].
39. Zasowski EJ, Trinh TD, Atwan SM, et al. The impact of concomitant empiric Cefepime on patient outcomes of methicillin-resistant staphylococcus aureus bloodstream infections treated with vancomycin. Open Forum Infect Dis 2019;6(4): ofz079.
40. Hornak JP, Anjum S, Reynoso D. Adjunctive ceftaroline in combination with daptomycin or vancomycin for complicated methicillin-resistant Staphylococcus aureus bacteremia after monotherapy failure. TherAdv Infect Dis 2019;6. 2049936119886504.
41. Gritsenko D, Fedorenko M, Ruhe JJ, et al. Combination therapy with vancomycin and ceftaroline for refractory methicillin-resistant staphylococcus aureus bacteremia: a case series. ClinTher 2017;39(1):212–8.
42. Davis JS, Sud A, O'Sullivan MVN, et al. Combination of Vancomycin and beta-Lactam therapy for methicillin-resistant staphylococcus aureus bacteremia: a pilot multicenter randomized controlled trial. Clin Infect Dis 2016;62(2):173–80.
43. Davis JS, Lye D, Nelson J. Combination antibiotic therapy for methicillin-resistant Staphylococcus aureus bacteraemia: the CAMERA2 randomised controlled trial Paper presented at: 29th European Congress of Clinical Microbiology & Infectious Diseases. Netherlands, 2019.
44. Seah J, Lye DC, Ng TM, et al. Vancomycinmonotherapy vs. combination therapy for the treatment of persistent methicillin-resistant Staphylococcus aureus bacteremia. Virulence 2013;4(8):734–9.
45. Jang HC, Kim SH, Kim KH, et al. Salvage treatment for persistent methicillin-resistant Staphylococcus aureus bacteremia: efficacy of linezolid with or without carbapenem. Clin Infect Dis 2009;49(3):395–401.
46. Thwaites GE, Scarborough M, Szubert A, et al. Adjunctive rifampicin for Staphylococcus aureusbacteraemia (ARREST): a multicentre, randomised, double-blind, placebo-controlled trial. Lancet 2018;391(10121):668–78.
47. Moise PA, Amodio-Groton M, Rashid M, et al. Multicenter evaluation of the clinical outcomes of daptomycin with and without concomitant beta-lactams in patients

with Staphylococcus aureus bacteremia and mild to moderate renal impairment. Antimicrob Agents Chemother 2013;57(3):1192–200.
48. Sakoulas G, Brown J, Lamp KC, et al. Clinical outcomes of patients receiving daptomycin for the treatment of Staphylococcus aureus infections and assessment of clinical factors for daptomycin failure: a retrospective cohort study utilizing the Cubicin Outcomes Registry and Experience. ClinTher 2009;31(9): 1936–45.
49. Dhand A, Sakoulas G. Daptomycin in combination with other antibiotics for the treatment of complicated methicillin-resistant Staphylococcus aureus bacteremia. ClinTher 2014;36(10):1303–16.
50. Jorgensen SCJ, Zasowski EJ, Trinh TD, et al. Daptomycin plus beta-lactam combination therapy for methicillin-resistant Staphylococcus aureus bloodstream infections: a retrospective, comparative cohort study. Clin Infect Dis 2019. [Epub ahead of print].
51. Geriak M, Haddad F, Rizvi K, et al. Clinical data on daptomycin plus ceftaroline versus standard of care monotherapy in the treatment of methicillin-resistant staphylococcus aureus bacteremia. Antimicrob Agents Chemother 2019;63(5) [pii:e02483-18].
52. Kalil AC, Holubar M, Deresinski S, et al. Is daptomycin plus ceftaroline associated with better clinical outcomes than standard of care monotherapy for staphylococcus aureus bacteremia? Antimicrob Agents Chemother 2019;63(11) [pii: e00900-19].
53. Steed ME, Werth BJ, Ireland CE, et al. Evaluation of the novel combination of high-dose daptomycin plus trimethoprim-sulfamethoxazole against daptomycin-nonsusceptible methicillin-resistant Staphylococcus aureus using an in vitro pharmacokinetic/pharmacodynamic model of simulated endocardialvegetations. Antimicrob Agents Chemother 2012;56(11):5709–14.
54. ZasowskiEJ, Claeys KC, Roberts KD, et al. Retrospective Evaluation of Daptomycin (DAP) plus Ceftarolinefosamil (CPT) versus DAP plus Sulfamethoxazole/ Trimethoprim (SMX/TMP) for Methicillin-Resistant Staphylococcus aureus Bloodstream Infections (BSI). Paper presented at: 25th European Congress of Clinical Microbiology and Infectious Diseases. Cogenhagen, Denmark, 2015.
55. Fabre V, Ferrada M, Buckel WR, et al. Ceftaroline in combination with trimethoprim-sulfamethoxazole for salvage therapy of methicillin-resistant staphylococcus aureus bacteremia and endocarditis. Open Forum Infect Dis 2014; 1(2):ofu046.
56. Pujol M, Miro J-M, Shaw E, et al. LB3.Daptomycinplus fosfomycin vs. daptomycinmonotherapy for methicillin-resistant staphylococcus aureus bacteremia: a multicenter, randomized, clinical trial. Open Forum Infect Dis 2018;5(suppl_1): S760.
57. del Rio A, Gasch O, Moreno A, et al. Efficacy and safety of fosfomycin plus imipenem as rescue therapy for complicated bacteremia and endocarditis due to methicillin-resistant Staphylococcus aureus: a multicenter clinical trial. Clin Infect Dis 2014;59(8):1105–12.
58. Pericas JM, Moreno A, Almela M, et al. Efficacy and safety of fosfomycin plus imipenem versus vancomycin for complicated bacteraemia and endocarditis due to methicillin-resistant Staphylococcus aureus: a randomized clinical trial. ClinMicrobiol Infect 2018;24(6):673–6.
59. Kocsis B, Domokos J, Szabo D. Chemical structure and pharmacokinetics of novel quinolone agents represented by avarofloxacin, delafloxacin, finafloxacin, zabofloxacin and nemonoxacin. Ann ClinMicrobiolAntimicrob 2016;15(1):34.

60. Giordano PA, Pogue JM, Cammarata S. Analysis of pooled phase III efficacy data for delafloxacin in acute bacterial skin and skin structure infections. Clin Infect Dis 2019;68(Supplement_3):S223–32.
61. Baxdela [package insert]. Lincolnshire (IL): Melinta Therapeutics, Inc; 2019.
62. Iregui A, Khan Z, Malik S, et al. Emergence of Delafloxacin-Resistant Staphylococcus aureus in Brooklyn, NY. Clin Infect Dis 2020;70(8):1758–60.

Drug-Resistant Tuberculosis

A Glance at Progress and Global Challenges

Khalid M. Dousa, MD[a,1], Sebastian G. Kurz, MD, PhD[b,1], Charles M. Bark, MD[c], Robert A. Bonomo, MD[d,e,f,g,h,i,j], Jennifer J. Furin, MD, PhD[a,k,*]

KEYWORDS

• Mycobacterium tuberculosis • Drug resistance • Antibiotics

KEY POINTS

- Multidrug-resistant *Mycobacterium tuberculosis* is a major public health threat in many countries, and its management poses a significant economic burden, especially in resource-limited areas.
- Treatment requires a programmatic approach with access to laboratory services, an array of second-line medications, and adequate clinical resources.
- The landscape of multidrug-resistant *M tuberculosis* has undergone major changes within recent years.
- We have seen rapid developments in diagnostic techniques with whole genome sequencing–based drug susceptibility prediction now in reach, an array of new drugs that transform treatment regimens to purely oral formulations, and a steady stream of multinational trials that inform us about most efficient combinations.

Continued

[a] Division of Infectious Diseases & HIV Medicine, University Hospitals Cleveland Medical Center, Case Western Reserve University, 10900 Euclid Avenue, Cleveland, OH 44106, USA; [b] Mount Sinai National Jewish Health Respiratory Institute, 10 East 102nd Street, New York City, NY 10029, USA; [c] Division of Infectious Diseases, MetroHealth Medical Center, 2500 MetroHealth Drive, Cleveland, OH 44109, USA; [d] Department of Medicine, Case Western Reserve University School of Medicine, 10900 Euclid Avenue, Cleveland, OH 44106, USA; [e] Department of Pharmacology, Case Western Reserve University School of Medicine, 10900 Euclid Avenue, Cleveland, OH 44106, USA; [f] Department of Molecular Biology and Microbiology, Case Western Reserve University School of Medicine, 10900 Euclid Avenue, Cleveland, OH 44106, USA; [g] Department of Biochemistry, Case Western Reserve University School of Medicine, 10900 Euclid Avenue, Cleveland, OH 44106, USA; [h] Department of Proteomics and Bioinformatics, Case Western Reserve University School of Medicine, 10900 Euclid Avenue, Cleveland, OH 44106, USA; [i] Medical Service and GRECC, Louis Stokes Cleveland Department of Veterans Affairs Medical Center, Cleveland, OH, USA; [j] CWRU-Cleveland VAMC Center for Antimicrobial Resistance and Epidemiology (Case VA CARES), Cleveland, OH, USA; [k] Department of Global Health and Social Medicine, Harvard Medical School, 641 Huntington Avenue, Boston, MA 02115, USA
[1] These authors contributed equally to this article.
* Corresponding author. Department of Global Health and Social Medicine, Harvard Medical School, 641 Huntington Avenue, Boston, MA 02115.
E-mail address: jjf38@case.edu

Infect Dis Clin N Am 34 (2020) 863–886
https://doi.org/10.1016/j.idc.2020.06.001

Continued

- Our hope is that the current momentum continues to keep the ambitious goal to end tuberculosis in 2030 in reach.

BACKGROUND

Multidrug-resistant *Mycobacterium tuberculosis* (MDR TB) continues to be a major public health threat in many countries, and its management poses a significant economic burden especially in resource-limited areas. Treatment of MDR TB requires a programmatic approach with access to laboratory services, an array of second-line medications, and adequate clinical resources. More challenging are the vulnerable patient groups, including patients co-infected with human immunodeficiency virus, children, pregnant women, and migrants, who become infected owing to limitations in drug selection, high incidence of medication adverse events, and a lack of adherence strategies. It has become clear that most patients infected with MDR TB contract the disease by transmission of already resistant strain.[1] Acquired resistance to anti-TB drugs can develop owing to subtherapeutic levels, drug concentration in lung parenchyma, efflux pumps, and nonadherence to medication regimens.[2] MDR TB is defined as resistant to both rifampin and isoniazid, which serve as the basis for anti-TB therapy. Extensive drug-resistant *M tuberculosis* (XDR TB) is defined as strains resistant to isoniazid and rifampin, plus any fluoroquinolone and at least 1 of 3 injectable agent (ie, amikacin, kanamycin, or capreomycin).[3]

In 2000, the United Nations (UN) partnered with Stop TB to establish targets that include (i) to halt and reverse TB incidence and (ii) to decrease TB prevalence and mortality by 50% by 2015. The World Health Organization (WHO) proclaimed the accomplishment of these targets in October 2015. Assisted by regional, national, and global efforts, the new formidable aim of "Ending the TB epidemic by 2030" has been incorporated into the UN's Sustainable Development goals covering the period between 2016 and 2035. In 2017, the commitment to End TB epidemic was affirmed at the global ministerial conference of TB (Moscow in November 2017) and later reaffirmed at the first ever historic and unprecedented UN high-level meeting on TB (held at the UN headquarters in New York, September 2018).[4,5] Strategies and indicators to reduce TB incidence and TB-related mortality and avoiding catastrophic costs for TB-affected families was incorporated into WHO's thirteenth General Program of Work.[6] To reach these goals within the End TB Strategy, effective control and successful treatment of MDR and XDR TB will be paramount, because failure to do so will negatively impact all 3 indicators of this strategy.

According to the Centers for Disease Control and Prevention (CDC) analysis (October 2018), 9025 TB cases were reported in the United States, a 0.7% decrease from 2017. The national incidence rate was 2.8 cases per 100,000 persons, a 1.3% decrease from 2017. An estimated 70% of reported cases of TB in 2018 were among persons born outside the United States. The proportion of patients with drug-resistant TB has remained stable for the last 20 years. In 2018, 98 cases were reported, 30 fewer than in 2017.

The most common primary drug resistance phenotype is resistance to isoniazid. Isoniazid monoresistance was reported in 507 cases (9.4% of drug susceptible cases), and combined isoniazid and rifampicin resistance in 98 cases (MDR TB, 1.5% of cases). XDR TB is rare in United States, with only 1 case reported in 2018.

According to the WHO Global Tuberculosis Report 2019, one-half of a million new cases of rifampicin resistance TB were reported in 2018 (Global Tuberculosis Report 2019), 78% of which were MDR TB, with nearly one-half of these cases reported from India (27%), China (14%), and the Russian Federation (9%). They found that 3.4% of new TB cases and 18% of previously treated cases had multidrug-resistant TB or rifampicin-resistant TB (MDR/RR-TB), with the highest percentage (>50% in previously treated cases) in countries of the former Soviet Union.

DRUG SUSCEPTIBILITY TESTING

Drug susceptibility testing (DST) is a prerequisite for treating drug-resistant tuberculosis. Phenotypic testing, which is based on the detection of growth inhibition during the presence of a drug is still considered the gold standard. However, it requires considerable laboratory resources and has a long turnaround time, which may lead to patients being exposed to suboptimal empiric treatment regimens with the potential to develop further resistance. Worldwide, the proportion method is most commonly performed, which compared growth of a 100 times diluted inoculum on drug-free medium with inoculum growth on medium containing a predefined critical concentration of drug. This method has been adapted to semiautomated liquid systems (BACTEC MGIT, Becton, Dickinson and Company, Franklin Lakes, NJ), which are now the preferred method owing to standardized media and rapid turnaround time.[7]

In *M tuberculosis*, drug resistance is determined by chromosomal mutations and, for the majority of first-line drugs, resistance has been conferred to discrete and predictable base alterations. For example, resistance to rifampicin is caused by mutations within a confined region of the messenger RNA polymerase gene *rpoB* in 95% of cases, which is readily detectable by molecular probes. For other drugs, resistance mechanisms are more complex and can be caused by several gene mutations (**Table 1**). During the last decade, molecular assays were developed, which led to the rapid identification of cases and early detection of resistant strains. The GeneXpert (Cepheid, Sunnyvale, CA), which has been endorsed by the WHO, uses polymerase chain reaction technology in a single cartridge and offers identification of *M tuberculosis* and detection of rifampicin resistance at the same time, which is a surrogate marker for MDR TB. In 2017, a new version, the GeneXpert Mtb/Rif Ultra, was introduced with increased sensitivity to detect *M tuberculosis* in smear negative samples. Initial performance characteristics revealed an improved overall sensitivity of 87.5% compared with 81.0% in the GeneXpert, and for smear negative sputum samples an increased sensitivity of 78.9% versus 66.1%, with both

Table 1
First-line drugs, their target protein function, and resistance mechanisms

Drug	Target Protein	Function	Resistance Mechanism
Rifampicin	RNA polymerase subunit β	Transcription	Lack of binding
Isoniazid	KatG: catalase-peroxidase InhA: Enoyl-ACP reductase	Prodrug activation Fatty acid synthesis	Loss of function Promoter: overexpression Impaired binding (INH-NAD)
Pyrazinamide	PncA: pyrazinidase	Prodrug activation	Loss of function
Ethambutol	EmbB: arabinosyl transferase	Arabinogalactan synthesis	Impaired binding

tests having specificity of 98.7%. Rifampicin detection remained highly accurate (sensitivity of 94%, specificity of 98%) with improved ability to detect rifampicin resistance in mixed cultures.[8]

Other tests based on line-probe technology are designed to detect resistance mutations for a larger set of drugs. They offer high accuracy for an array of first- and second-line drugs and were endorsed by the WHO (GenoType MDRplus and MTBDR*sl*, Hain Lifescience, Germany; Nipro NTM+MDRTB, Nipro, Japan).[9,10] Compared with the automatized Cepheid system, they require additional laboratory capacity.

With the advent of quick, reliable and affordable sequencing technology, whole genome sequencing (WGS) has been established at least in high resource countries, which shows good correlation with phenotypic resistance testing. The first study that applied WGS to the 5 resistance mutations harboring genes *rpoB*, *katG*, *pncA*, *gyrA*, and *rrs* (16S), found a 100% concordance with phenotypic DST testing in a collection of 26 strains from South Africa, which contained 4 MDR, 7 XDR, and 5 susceptible strains.[11]

In 2013, a case of XDR TB was reported in which WGS from a culture isolate that had grown within 3 days correctly identified a complex resistance profile, which correlated with subsequent phenotypic testing.[12] These reports served as a proof of principle and established a foundation for large-scale studies that evaluated thousands of strains.

A large study used DST and WGS data of a training set of 2099 strains to develop an algorithm for resistance prediction, which was then applied on an independent validation set of 1552 strain genomes. The collections comprised strains from various regions of the world with an overall resistance rate of 7.2%. During the development of the algorithm, the researchers initially focused on 23 candidate genes known to be associated with resistance for specific drugs and then expanded to other regions in the genome. Overall, 112 mutations were classified as resistance determining and 772 as benign, and 101 remained unclassified. In the validation set, the mutations predicted DST phenotypes with a sensitivity of 92.3% and specificity of 98.4%.[13] A large follow-up study of 10,209 isolates from 16 countries across 6 continents revealed a high accuracy, with 97.9% correct prediction of fully susceptible strains (48% of the isolates).[14] The study met the WHO target profiles for new molecular assays of more than 90% sensitivity and 95% specificity for all first-line drugs except for specificity for ethambutol (93.6%). A prospective study of WGS and phenotypic DST demonstrated feasibility of genomic species diagnostic and susceptibility prediction beyond first-line drugs across a network of 8 laboratories in Europe and North America and demonstrated the high value of WGS for *M tuberculosis* management programs and public health.[15]

With the exponential number of available genomic data comes the need to systematically evaluate genomic mutations. A standardized approach for interpreting the association between mutations and phenotypic drug resistance using a grading system of confidence has been proposed.[16] Overall, the prospect of more widespread use of WGS to allow for rapid diagnosis of drug resistance and prompt implementation of a treatment plan is within reach. Hopefully, with the decrease in labor, laboratory materials, and space in high-containment facilities, this technology will be available to lower income countries that share the major burden of *M tuberculosis* in the world.

Is the entire DST phenotype determined by WGS? Not entirely, as shown by another large study: an in-depth analysis of drug-susceptible *M tuberculosis* strains that caused relapse revealed that higher minimum inhibitory concentration values for isoniazid and rifampicin, but still well below the resistance breakpoint correlated with risk of treatment relapse. WGS comparison of high and low resistance strain failed to identify mutations that would explain these subtle differences in drug susceptibility.[17]

TREATMENT OF DRUG-RESISTANT *M TUBERCULOSIS* INFECTIONS

The treatment paradigms used for rifampicin-resistant forms of *M tuberculosis* (RR-TB) infections has radically changed during the past 5 years.[18] The use of newer and repurposed drugs—including bedaquiline, delamanid, linezolid, and clofazimine—has led to marked improvements in treatment outcomes for people, even those with the most highly resistant strains.[19] Novel drug combinations have also resulted in shorter regimens (9–12 months) that are injectable-free that can achieve cure in a majority of individuals.[20]

Treatment recommendations from normative bodies—including the WHO,[21] the CDC, the European Respiratory Society, the American Thoracic Society, and the Infectious Diseases Society of America[22]—are grounded in a more robust evidence base from both observational cohorts and randomized controlled trials. Increasing recognition and attention is also being given to the individual support needs and human rights of all persons living with RR-TB, and how essential it is to address these needs to optimize treatment success, even in the setting of more effective and tolerable treatment regimens.[23] This section reviews data on individual second-line drugs, treatment approaches for RR-TB, recommendations in vulnerable populations, and optimal support for persons diagnosed with RR-TB. We also discuss updated recommendations for the treatment of isoniazid monoresistant TB and for the treatment of RR-TB infection (ie, preventive therapy for RR-TB).

Second-Line Drugs

For the first time in almost 50 years, there are now novel agents available to treat RR-TB (including bedaquiline and delamanid) as well as increasing use of repurposed drugs (including linezolid, clofazimine, and the carbapenems) that have resulted in more robust regimens.[23] Many of these agents were assessed in randomized controlled trials—the first ever done in the field of RR-TB.[24] Data from these trials were combined with an individual patient data (IPD) meta-analysis of nearly 13,000 patient records[25] to lead to updated WHO recommendations on the use of individual drugs for the treatment of RR-TB.[26]

In the IPD meta-analysis, 3 medications were associated with improved outcomes and decreased mortality among people treated for RR-TB: bedaquiline, linezolid, and the third-generation fluoroquinolones (levofloxacin or moxifloxacin). Two medications—clofazimine and cycloserine/terizidone—were associated with improved outcomes, but not with decreased mortality. The use of delamanid was associated with improved treatment outcomes, but very few patients in the IPD had received delamanid. Ethambutol and pyrazinamide were associated with improved outcomes, but only among people whose *M tuberculosis* strains demonstrated documented susceptibility to these drugs. Amikacin and streptomycin were associated with improved treatment outcomes among those whose strains had documented susceptibility to them, but the logistics of administration and the high rates of toxicity—most notably permanent hearing loss and renal failure—were significant drawbacks to their routine use.

The carbapenems—including imipenem and meropenem—when given with clavulanic acid (only available as amoxicillin/clavulanic acid combination) were associated with improved outcomes, but there were only a small number of persons who had received these medications and the logistics of long-term intravenous administration were factors that are seen as limiting their use. Ethionamide/prothioamide and para-aminosalicylic acid were both associated with worse treatment outcomes, even among people whose strains of TB were susceptible to them. The same was true of kanamycin. Capreomycin was actually found to be associated with both worse treatment outcomes and increased mortality.

These data and those from randomized controlled trials led to the WHO developing a new priority grouping for second-line drugs (**Table 2**). Of note, the drugs ethionamide/prothioamide and para-aminosalicylic acid are only recommended for people with limited treatment options, and the drugs kanamycin and capreomycin are not recommended for use in the treatment of RR-TB. The CDC recommendations in general align with the WHO recommendations (**Table 3**), although they only strongly recommend the use of bedaquiline and a fluoroquinolone (either levofloxacin or moxifloxacin), with the recommendation for linezolid being conditional (although the drug is still given priority when designing a treatment regimen).

Table 4 summarizes the data on each of the individual second-line drugs, including the mechanism of action, recommended doses, the types of data supporting their use, important adverse events, and other notable information regarding each of the second-line medications.

Treatment Approaches

In the past, the treatment of RR-TB was characterized by long (18–24 month), highly toxic regimens that achieved success in only about 50% of people who received therapy.[27] Of particular concern was the reliance on injectable medications—including kanamycin, capreomycin, and amikacin—as a core part of RR-TB treatment, even though there was limited evidence supporting their use and significant evidence showing they caused permanent hearing loss in as many as 60% of people who received them.[28] In 2018, the WHO recommended that 3 potential treatment options could be used for people who are diagnosed with RR-TB.[29]

1. An all-oral regimen of 4 to 5 drugs lasting 18 to 20 months that contained the medications bedaquiline, linezolid, and a fluoroquinolone as essential medications and did not use the injectable agents;
2. A shorter 9- to 12-month regimen containing 7 drugs—including the injectable agent—based on the "Bangladesh" regimen and assessed in the STREAM study[30]; or
3. An all-oral regimen of 4 to 5 drugs lasting 9 to 12 months that contained bedaquiline, linezolid, a third-generation fluoroquinolone, and clofazimine as core backbone agents, with the regimen administered under operational research conditions.

The data supporting these recommendations came from several sources. The first data were from the IPD meta-analysis, which suggested that the optimal treatment duration should be between 18 and 24 months and the optimal number of drugs in the regimen should be between 4 and 5 for the initial phase of treatment and 3 and 4 for the continuation phase of treatment. It was notable that most records included in this IPD did not receive bedaquiline, linezolid, or delamanid.

The second source of data was a randomized controlled trial done comparing a 9-month regimen with a 12-month regimen of 7 drugs known as the "STREAM" study.[31] In this study, people with RR-TB who did not have resistance to either a fluoroquinolone or an injectable agent were randomized to receive either a standard of care regimen (depending on local recommendations) or a 9- to 12-month regimen consisting of kanamycin (given for 4–6 months), high-dose isoniazid (given for 4–6 months), ethionamide (given for 4–6 months), high-dose moxifloxacin, clofazimine,

Table 2
WHO grouping of second-line TB medications

Group	Medications	Recommendation	Comments
A (include all 3 medicines)	Bedaquiline	Strong	Moderate certainty in estimates of effect
	Linezolid	Strong	Moderate certainty in estimates of effect
	Levofloxacin or moxifloxacin	Strong	Moderate certainty in estimates of effect
B (add 1 or both medicines)	Clofazimine	Conditional	Very low certainty in estimates of effect
	Cycloserine/ terizidone	Conditional	Very low certainty in estimates of effect
C (add medications as needed to complete the regimen; medications listed in the order in which they should be used)	Ethambutol	Conditional	Very low certainty in estimates of effect, should only be used in settings where there is no documented evidence of resistance
	Delamanid	Conditional	Moderate certainty in estimates of effect
	Pyrazinamide	Conditional	Very low certainty in estimates of effect
	Imipenem or meropenem plus clavulanic acid	Conditional	Very low certainty in estimates of effect
	Amikacin	Conditional	Very low certainty in estimates of effect, should only be used in settings of documented susceptibility and where formal hearing assessments can be routinely performed
	Ethionamide/ prothionamide	Conditional recommendation against its use	Very low certainty in estimates of effect, should only be used in persons without documented resistance and in whom there are limited treatment options
	Para-aminosalicyclic acid	Conditional recommendation against its use	Very low certainty in estimates of effect, should only be used in persons without documented resistance and in whom there are limited treatment options

From Organization WH. The use of molecular line probe assay for the detection of resistance to isoniazid and rifampicin: policy update. 2016; with permission.

Table 3
US CDC groupings of second-line drugs

Drug	Recommendation For	Recommendation Against	Certainty in the Evidence
Bedaquiline	Strong	—	Very low
Levofloxacin	Strong	—	Very low
Moxifloxacin	Strong	—	Very low
Linezolid	Conditional	—	Very low
Clofazimine	Conditional	—	Very low
Cycloserine	Conditional	—	Very low
Amikacin	Conditional	—	Very low
Ethambutol	Conditional	—	Very low
Pyrazinamide	Conditional	—	Very low
Carbapenems plus clavulanic acid	Conditional	—	Very low
Delamanid	Conditional	—	Very low
Ethionamide/ prothionamide	—	Conditional	Very low
Kanamycin	—	Conditional	Very low
Para-aminosalcylic acid	—	Conditional	Very low
Capreomycin	—	Conditional	Very low
Macrolides	—	Strong	Very low
Amoxicillin-clavulanic acid	—	Strong	Very low

From Zumla A, Petersen E. The historic and unprecedented United Nations General Assembly High Level Meeting on Tuberculosis (UNGA-HLM-TB)-'United to End TB: An Urgent Global Response to a Global Epidemic'. *Int J Infect Dis.* 2018;75:118-120; with permission.

pyrazinamide, and ethambutol given for the entire duration of the regimen. The study found that the shorter experimental regimen was noninferior compared with the longer regimen (favorable outcomes of 79.8% achieved in the longer regimen compared with 78.8% in the experimental shorter regimen; 95% confidence interval, −7.5 to 9.0; $P = .02$). However, although the rates of loss to follow-up were significantly lower in the shorter experimental regimen, rates of treatment failed, recurrent TB, and mortality were all higher in the shorter experimental regimen, and in the sensitivity analysis there was a trend toward higher mortality among people living with human immunodeficiency virus. Both groups had similar rates of adverse events. Notably, almost none of the participants in the longer regimen received bedaquiline, linezolid, or delamanid. Although the results of the study did demonstrate noninferiority in terms of the composite favorable outcome, the higher rates of poor bacteriologic outcomes in the shorter regimen led to some controversy around the recommendation for use of the shorter regimen,[30] and this regimen has not been recommended for use by the CDC. In addition to concerns about the efficacy of the shorter 9- to 12 month regimen, concerns were raised about the continued use of the injectable agent in the regimen and that the regimen did not contain drugs that were associated with improved outcomes and decreased mortality (ie, bedaquiline and linezolid) and did contain medications associated with worse treatment outcomes (ethionamide).[32] For this reason, the WHO also offered countries the third option of using all-oral shorter regimens

Table 4
Second-line drugs used for the treatment of RR-TB (in alphabetical order)

Medication	Mechanism of Action	Dosing Recommendations	Evidence to Support Use	Important Adverse Events	Drug–Drug Interactions	Comments
Amikacin	Aminoglycoside that interferes with mycobacterial ribosomal reading of messenger RNA	10–15 mg/kg IM per day, maximum daily dose of 1 g; usually only given for 6–8 mo of therapy but can be extended.	Observational studies only	Hearing loss, renal failure, abscess associated with injection sites	Overlapping toxicity with tenofovir	Should only be used in persons with limited treatment options and if hearing loss can be formally monitored
Bedaquiline[49–51]	Diarylquinoline that interferes with mycobacterial ATP synthase	400 mg/d for 14 d followed by 200 mg thrice weekly; for persons weighing 16–33 kg, recommendation is 200 mg/d followed by 100 mg thrice weekly; usually given for 24 wk but longer durations have been demonstrated to be safe	Phase IIB placebo-controlled RCT, observational studies; Phase III trial pending	Moderate QTcF prolongation, hepatotoxicity	Cannot be used with efavirenz; use with caution with other drugs that prolong the QTcF interval	Can routinely be given to children ages 6 y and older; Some cross-resistance with clofazimine moderated through an efflux pump
Clofazimine[52]	Rhimophenazine whose mechanism of action is not completely known	100 mg/d (some suggest a 2–4 wk loading dose of 200 mg/d for 14–28 d followed by 100 mg/d; 2–5 mg/kg/d for persons <34 kg	Non–placebo-controlled RCT, observational data	Skin hyper-pigmentation, moderate QTcF prolongation	Use with caution with other drugs that prolong the QTcF interval	Some cross-resistance with bedaquline moderated through an efflux pump

(continued on next page)

Table 4
(*continued*)

Medication	Mechanism of Action	Dosing Recommendations	Evidence to Support Use	Important Adverse Events	Drug–Drug Interactions	Comments
Cycloserine/terizidone	Inhibits mycobacterial cell wall biosynthesis	500–1000 mg/d; 15–20 mg/kg/d for persons <34 kg	Observational studies only	Psychosis, depression, anxiety, seizures		Cycloserine and terizidone can be used interchangeably, as there have been no studies showing differences in efficacy or safety of these 2 drugs
Delamanid[53–55]	Nitroimidazole that inhibits mycobacterial cell wall synthesis	100 mg twice daily (doses of 200 mg/d have been assessed after 8 wk of twice daily dosing); 50 mg twice daily in persons weighing 24–33 kg; 25 mg twice daily in persons weighing 7–15 kg	Phase IIB and III data, observational studies	Mild QTcF prolongation, generally well-tolerated.		Can routinely be given to children ages 3 y and older; can be given in combination with bedaquiline; Results of phase IIB trial showed improved efficacy when compared with placebo but phase III trial did not meet primary efficacy end point compared with placebo (although significant differences in efficacy were seen between delamanid and placebo in sensitivity analyses)

Ethambutol	Mechanism of action is not completely known	15–25 mg/kg/d	Observational studies only	Optic neuropathy	
Ethionamide/ prothionamide	Disruption of mycobacterial mycolic acid synthesis	15–20 mg/kg/d	Observational studies only	Nausea, vomiting, hypothyroidism	Ethionamide and prothionamide can be used interchangeably, as there have been no studies showing differences in efficacy or safety of these 2 drugs
Imipenem/ clavulanic acid	Inhibits mycobacterial cell wall synthesis	2 g twice daily IV with amoxicillin/ clavulanic acid (500 mg/125 mg) given 3 min before administration	Observational studies only	Seizures, rash, complications from long-term IV administration	Must be given with clavulanic acid (which is current only available in combination with amoxicillin)
Levofloxacin	Fluoroquinolone antibiotic that interferes with mycobacterial DNA gyrase	750–1500 mg/d; 15–20 mg/kg/d in persons weighing <34 kg	Observational studies only	Mild QTcF prolongation, tendinitis, Achilles tendon rupture	Dose optimization study shows higher doses are well-tolerated and may be more effective than doses lower than 1000 mg/d

(*continued on next page*)

Table 4
(continued)

Medication	Mechanism of Action	Dosing Recommendations	Evidence to Support Use	Important Adverse Events	Drug–Drug Interactions	Comments
Linezolid[56–58]	Oxazolidinone antibiotic that interferes with mycobacterial protein synthesis	Dosing recommendations unclear; most RR-TB patients receive 600 mg/d; dose reduction to 300 mg/d or 600 mg thrice weekly have been used in settings of linezolid-related toxicity; 15 mg/kg/d in children weighing <16 kg; 10 mg/kg/d in children weighing 16 kg or more.	Delayed-start RCT, observational studies	Bone marrow suppression, peripheral neuropathy, optic neuritis	Use with caution with other drugs that cause bone marrow suppression (ie, AZT) or that cause peripheral neuropathy	Multiple studies assessing optimal duration and length of treatment with linezolid.
Meropenem/clavulanic acid[59]	Inhibits mycobacterial cell wall synthesis	1 g thrice daily or 2 g twice daily with amoxicillin/clavulanic acid (500 mg/125 mg) given 3 min before administration	Phase IIA data (early bactericidal activity study), observational studies	Rash, complications from long-term IV administration		Must be given with clavulanic acid (which is current only available in combination with amoxicillin)

Moxifloxacin	Fluoroquinolone antibiotic that interferes with mycobacterial DNA gyrase	400 mg/d considered standard dose, 800 mg/d considered high-dose; 10–15 mg/kg/d in persons weighing <34 kg	Observational studies only	Moderate QTcF prolongation, tendinitis, Achilles' tendon rupture	May be more effective than other fluoroquinolones against strains with ofloxacin resistance
Para-aminosalicylic acid	May inhibit mycobacterial folate synthesis	8–12 g divided into 2 or 3 daily doses; 200–300 mg/kg given as 2 divided daily doses in persons weighing <34 kg	Observational studies only	Nausea, vomiting, diarrhea, hypothyroidism	Must be given with food, usually acidic
Pyrazinamide	Mechanism of action is not completely known	20–30 mg/kg/d in adults, 30–40 mg/kg/d in children	Observational studies only	Hepatotoxicity	

Abbreviations: ATP, adenosine triphosphate; AZT, azidothymidine; IM, intramuscular; IV, intravenous; QTcF, corrected QT interval using Fridericia formula; RCT, randomized controlled trial.

containing bedaquiline, as long as these were implemented under carefully monitored/operational research conditions.[33] One country that followed this model was South Africa, where an all-oral shorter (9- to 11-month) regimen containing bedaquiline (6 months), linezolid (2 months), high-dose isoniazid (4–6 months), and levofloxacin, clofazimine, pyrazinamide, and ethambutol (all for 9–11 months) was implemented under carefully monitored program conditions nationwide. The early results from more than 4000 patients who received this regimen showed high rates of treatment success (>80%) and were reviewed by the WHO in November 2019. Although the formal guideline recommendations are still pending, a rapid communication released by the WHO in December 2019 has now recommended an all-oral, bedaquiline-containing, shorter (9–11 months) regimen for a majority of people living with RR-TB.[34]

Extrapulmonary Forms of Rifampicin-Resistant Tuberculosis

In general, persons with extrapulmonary forms of RR-TB should receive the same treatment as those with pulmonary RR-TB, although some notable exceptions exist. Persons with osteoarticular and meningeal disease should be treated for a minimum of 12 months because this timing seems to be the minimal duration for these forms of TB, even when the strains are fully drug susceptible.[35] Regimen construction should also consider drug penetration into the affected tissue. Limited data on the central nervous system penetration of some of the newer and repurposed agents (including bedaquiline, delamanid, and clofazimine) are available, although studies are ongoing, and it is generally recommended that these drugs be used during the early phases of treatment given the presence of central nervous system inflammation. Drugs with excellent central nervous system penetration—including linezolid, pyrazinamide, ethionamide/prothioamide, cycloserine, and meropenem—should be given to people with documented or confirmed central nervous system disease.[36]

Highly Resistant Forms of Rifampicin-Resistant Tuberculosis

When RR-TB has additional resistance to other second-line medications, treatment outcomes may be further compromised, especially if there is resistance to highly effective second-line medications, most notably the fluoroquinolones.[37] In the past, the term "extensively drug-resistant TB" or "XDR TB" was used to denote strains of RR-TB with additional resistance to at least one of the second-line injectable agents (kanamycin, amikacin, or capreomycin) and at least 1 of the fluoroquinolones. This term came into clinical use after an outbreak of RR-TB in KwaZulu-Natal, South Africa, where resistance to both these categories of drugs was rapidly and almost uniformly fatal.[38] Later data suggest that resistance to the fluoroquinolones is what drives the poor outcomes, with little difference seen between people with injectable resistance and simple RR-TB.[39] The use of newer and repurposed medications—including bedaquiline, delamanid, and linezolid—has revolutionized the care of XDR TB, with some cohorts of patients living with XDR TB and treated with these medications having better outcomes than persons living with simpler RR-TB.[40]

Most RR-TB clinical trials exclude individuals with XDR TB from participation and thus there are limited formal data to optimize treatment recommendations for this type of TB. In general, the standard recommendation is that delamanid be used to build a 4- to 5-drug regimen if the fluoroquinolones cannot be used, and there are no longer concerns about synergistic QTc prolongation if bedaquiline and delamanid are given in combination.[41,42] Additionally, treatment duration should be 18 to 24 months. One single-arm, noncontrolled study among 109 people with XDR TB (or treatment intolerant/treatment nonresponsive RR-TB) used a 6-month regimen containing 3 drugs—including bedaquiline, high-dose linezolid (1200 mg/d) and the novel chemical entirety pretomanid—reported an 89% treatment success rate.[43] This study was known as the "Nix-TB" trial and its data were used to support the US Food and Drug Administration approval of pretomanid within a bedaquiline and high-dose linezolid containing regimen under the Limited Population Pathway for Antibacterial and Antifungal Drugs.[44] Although some in the TB community have hailed this 6-month, 3-drug combination as revolutionary, the high rates of treatment-related toxicity and the lack of a control arm in the study have led to many urging caution around its use.[45] In their December 2019 rapid communication, the WHO recommends the Nix-TB regimen only be used under research conditions.

Although there are several other ongoing or planned trials aimed at assessing the optimal treatment for persons with highly resistant forms of RR-TB, consensus around the optimal terms to use now that injectable agents are no longer recommended as part of standard or care for RR-TB does not seem to exist. Some have proposed redefining XDR TB as resistance to 2 or more of the WHO Group A agents, others have cautioned against premature development of a definition without a clear clinical implication.[46] For now, most people use the term fluoroquinolone-resistant RR-TB.

Access to Novel Therapeutic Regimens

Bedaquiline has been recommended by the WHO since 2013 and delamanid since 2014, but data show there has been limited global uptake of either of these drugs. Globally, a total of only 37,157 people have received bedaquiline since 2015 outside of clinical trials, and most of them (23,187 or 62.4%) are from South Africa. In terms of delamanid use, only 2940 people have received this drug outside of clinical trials since 2015.[47] The ability to benefit from scientific progress is considered a basic human right,[48] and the notable gap between the number of people in need of a new drug (estimated at >284,000 since 2015 using a very conservative estimate) and those who have received one is concerning (**Fig. 1**). The prices of bedaquiline and delamanid—which can exceed US$30,000 for a 6-month course—is a significant barrier to its use.[49] So too are issues with registration (ie, delamanid has not been registered in the United States and is only available via compassionate use), undue concerns about safety, and a contrary attitude expressed by many health care providers who often take care of patients with TB about "protecting the drug" (as opposed to protecting people living with RR-TB). Urgent action is needed to provide these therapeutic innovations to all persons living with RR-TB.[50]

Vulnerable Populations

There are multiple populations who are at increased risk for RR-TB and for poor outcomes who merit special attention when it comes to optimizing RR-TB treatment.[51] These include people living with human immunodeficiency virus, children, pregnant women, migrants, people who are incarcerated, and people who use/abuse substances. The special issues for each of these populations are summarized in **Table 5**.

Optimized Patient Support

The use of newer drugs and shorter regimens has revolutionized the treatment of RR-TB, but the relative acceptability of the innovative therapeutic strategies described in this section do not necessarily translate into absolute acceptability among people living with RR-TB. Treatment regimens are still long, associated with significant adverse events, and contain a high pill burden.[52] In addition, data from multiple studies have shown that persons with RR-TB face catastrophic costs and are more likely to be impoverished during and after treatment.[53] Thus, there is the need for significant social, economic, and psychological support during treatment.[54] In addition to

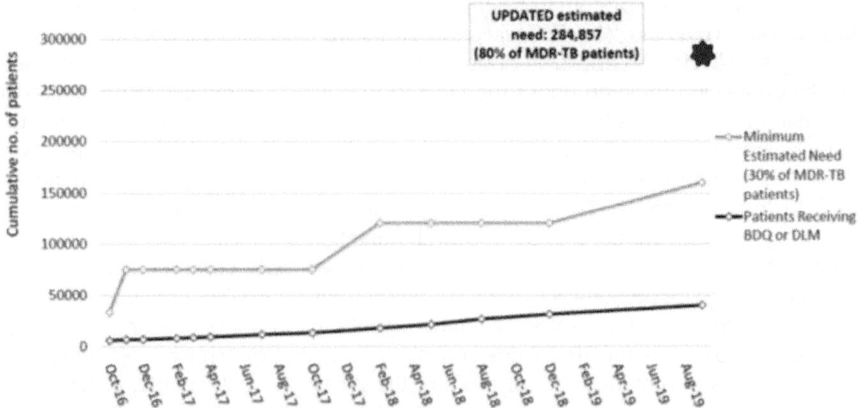

- **Calculation of minimum global estimated need for newer drugs: adjusted for yearly WHO Global TB Reports and based on 30% of those started on treatment requiring newer drug (cumulative)**
- **Updated estimated need in 2019 based on assumption that 80% of patients started on treatment would need bedaquiline for an all oral regimen in 2019**

Fig. 1. Global progress on access to bedaquiline and delamanid versus minimum estimated global need. (*Courtesy of* DR-TB STAT; with permission.)

this factor, current directly observed therapy–based approaches to adherence place a significant burden on people living with RR-TB and have denied people living with the disease access to treatment literacy and participatory decision making.[55]

The WHO has urged that "patient-centered" care be a pillar of the End TB strategy, but there are limited operational definitions about what this means and little accountability as to how it is provided. A human rights–based approach to RR-TB can help to ensure that people who are living with the disease are given the support they need to result in optimized treatment outcomes and is as central to the treatment of RR-TB as are the new drugs and regimens.[56]

Isoniazid-Resistant Forms of Tuberculosis

In 2017, the WHO issued new treatment recommendations on the management of isoniazid monoresistant forms of the disease (INHR-TB). INHR-TB is the most common form of drug-resistant TB and may account for 10% of the global TB burden.[57] Randomized controlled trial data to guide optimal treatment do not exist, and a recent meta-analysis done on programmatic data to inform the WHO guidelines found that more than 50 regimens were used worldwide to treat the disease.[58] The WHO has recommended that people with INHR-TB receive 6 months of therapy with daily levofloxacin, rifampicin, ethambutol, and pyrazinamide, but this is a conditional recommendation based on very low certainty in the estimated of effect.[59] With the imminent introduction of an expanded Xpert MTB/RIF cartridge that can detect INH resistance, it is likely clinicians will more commonly see this form of TB.[60] Several randomized trials on INHR-TB are being planned, but none have been started, meaning that there will not likely be evidence-based recommendations for another 5 to 7 years.

Treatment of Rifampicin-Resistant Tuberculosis Infection

Although much of this article has focused on the treatment of RR-TB disease, data on the treatment of RR-TB infection (or what is more commonly called "preventive

Table 5
Special populations and considerations for RR-TB treatment

Population	Considerations
People living with HIV	Outcomes vary by CD4 count with those who have fewer than 100 CD4 cells/μL having worse outcomes; Robust regimens containing bedaquiline, linezolid, a fluoroquinolone and clofazimine backbones should be used, especially given the high mortality rates seen with regimens that do not use these medications; Anitretorviral therapy should be administered within 2–8 wk of starting TB treatment, except in those with central nervous system disease; Need to consider overlapping drug toxicities and drug–drug interactions with various antiretroviral therapies (ie, efavirenz and bedaquiline cannot be co-administered, linezolid and azidothymidine should be used together with caution)
Children and adolescents[60,61]	Duration of therapy should be based on disease severity, and a majority of children can be successfully treated with 9- to 12-mo regimens; Bedaquiline can be routinely used in children ages 6 y and older and delamanid in children ages 3 y and older: use in younger children can be considered on a patient-by-patient basis; Child-friendly formulations should be used: pediatric formulations exist for levofloxacin, ethionamide, delamanid, and clofazimine; Injectable-containing regimens should be avoided; Children need to be included in TB trials, especially to establish dosing and safety; Different age groups will require different types of adherence support.
Pregnant women	Adequate therapy should be given as soon as possible to ensure best outcomes for woman and child; Evidence base for safety of most second-line drugs in pregnant women is lacking; bedaquiline seems to be most safe based on animal studies; Some drugs should NOT be given during pregnancy, including injectable agents; Breast feeding while on treatment is not contraindicated; Risk of transmission to neonate is low if mother is on effective therapy.
Migrants and refugees	Shorter durations of therapy may be more effective because many persons may become lost to follow-up during transfer; Coordination of care between countries and migratory centers is essential; Treatment should be provided in a way that is respectful of human rights, and persons should not be denied access to treatment or safe migration.
People who are incarcerated	Treatment should be provided in a way that is respectful of human rights; Shorter durations of therapy may be more effective because many persons may become lost to follow-up during transfer; Coordination of care between facilities and the general population is essential.

(*continued on next page*)

Table 5
(continued)

Population	Considerations
People who use/abuse substances	Harm reduction and enhanced adherence support needed in this population; Complete sobriety is NOT a prerequisite for TB treatment.
Persons with hepatitis B and/or C	Limited data on drug-drug interactions with Hepatitis C directly acting agents and TB drugs, but most second-line TB drugs seem to be safe and effective when co-administered; Most providers recommend treating TB first and then hepatitis, but this should be considered on a patient-by-patient basis. Potential for increased hepatotoxicity during treatment, so monitor liver function tests closely.
People living with diabetes mellitus	Good glycemic control essential to ensuring successful TB treatment outcomes; Adverse effects of TB drugs may be exacerbated in people on tuberculosis treatment, including peripheral neuropathy, optic neuropathy, and renal failure.

Abbreviation: HIV, human immunodeficiency virus.

therapy") exist. A meta-analysis of several observational cohorts found that, when fluoroquinolone-based preventive therapy is offered to close contacts of persons living with RR-TB, a 90% decrease in the development of TB is realized and the intervention is cost effective for health care systems.[61] In 2018, the WHO recommended that persons exposed to RR-TB in high-risk situations could receive treatment of infection (conditional recommendation with very low certainty in the estimate of effect).[62] The WHO does not recommend a specific regimen or duration of therapy, but rather emphasizes that the treatment should be based on the drug susceptibility data from the known source patient.

Most programs that offer treatment of RR-TB infection use fluoroquinolones, either alone or as part of combination therapy (with high-dose INH, ethambutol, and/or ethionamide) for a total of 6 months.[63,64] Delamanid was used in certain high-risk individuals with exposure to fluoroquinolone-resistant TB, as have short courses (1 month) of linezolid. Three ongoing randomized controlled trials for the treatment of RR-TB infection—including 2 that compare levofloxacin with placebo and one that compares delamanid with INH are being conducted; these results can be used to further refine recommendations on the treatment of RR-TB infection when they are available in 3 to 5 years' time.[65]

Drug-Resistant Tuberculosis Clinical Drug Development

The development of new and repurposed drugs to treat resistant TB is revolutionizing the treatment of drug-resistant TB. The breakthrough is the development of an all oral regimen, eliminating the need for difficult and toxic injectable agents. The main driver of this change was the discovery and development of the new drug bedaquiline. Initially discovered in the early 2000s,[66] bedaquiline development followed the traditional phase I and II trials, but has yet to be tested in a phase III trial. The pivotal phase II study that led to its FDA approval enrolled 160 patients who were randomly assigned to receive either 400 mg of bedaquiline once daily for 2 weeks, followed by 200 mg 3 times a week for 22 weeks (the standard dosing for bedaquiline), or placebo on top of a 5-drug regimen.[67] Patients in the bedaquiline group had significantly shorter time to culture conversion and higher rates of sputum culture conversion culture compared with placebo (83 vs 125 days [$P<.001$] and 79% vs 58% at 24 weeks [$P = .008$], respectively). Alarmingly, there were 10 deaths out of 79 patients (13%) in the bedaquiline group and 2 out of 81 patients (2%) in the placebo group. Nine of the 10 deaths occurred after completion of study drug (median, 49.1 weeks), and an association with QT prolongation was not found, and none were considered to be related to bedaquiline.[67] The deaths led to the addition of a black box warning regarding the increased risk of death as well as QTc prolongation.[68] The mortality difference was concerning, but bedaquiline use and study continued for difficult to treat MDR TB where the benefits far outweighed a truly unknown risk. Fortunately, data from these later studies did not reveal a significant mortality risk related to the use of bedaquiline.[69] Notably, a phase III study of bedaquiline has not yet been completed, but the RCT Stream Stage 2 trial of an all oral MDR regimen including bedaquiline is nearly enrolled, with results expected in 2021.[70]

The second major drug breakthrough was the development and 2014 European Medicines Agency approval of delamanid, a nitroimidazole, that has been studied in a phase III trial. In the trial, which randomized 511 patients to either delamanid or placebo + optimized background regimen, significant differences in treatment outcomes were not observed, with equal treatment success at 30 months of about 77%.[71] This surprising equivalency finding reflects improvement in MDR TB treatment and the importance of well-delivered treatment by directly observed therapy.

Another new nitroimidazole, pretomanid, was approved by the FDA in 2019 after a breakthrough study of XDR TB. The Nix-TB trial was a trial of pretomanid combined with bedaquiline and linezolid given for 6 to 9 months. Interim analysis data showed an 89% successful outcome in the first 45 patients enrolled.[72] If the results of this small study are validated, it will represent a breakthrough: a simple and short treatment of rifampin resistant TB.

The repurposing of drugs such as linezolid was critical for the advances made in MDR regimens. Extensive clinical trials of medications approved for indications other than TB treatment, such as linezolid, clofazimine, and the fluoroquinolones has made the development of new MDR combinations possible. Most of these drugs are associated with side effects, especially when given for long treatment durations, and work continues to optimize dosing and develop improved versions to minimize drug-related toxicity. An important example are the oxazolidinones such as linezolid, which has substantial hematologic and neuropathic side effects, and studies are ongoing to develop alternative dosing strategies to minimize toxicity.[70] Meanwhile, sutezolid is another promising oxazolidinone that early studies suggest may provide similar anti-TB activity as linezolid with minimal side effects.[73]

SUMMARY

The landscape of MDR TB has undergone major changes within recent years. We have seen rapid developments in diagnostic techniques with WGS based drug susceptibility prediction now in reach, an array of new drugs that transform treatment regimens to purely oral formulations, and a steady stream of multinational trials that inform us about most efficient combinations. Our hope is that the current momentum continues to keep the ambitious goal to end TB in 2030 in reach.

ACKNOWLEDGMENTS

K.M. Dousa received support from the Roe Green Center for Travel Medicine. R.A. Bonomo is supported by the National Institute of Allergy and Infectious Diseases of the National Institutes of Health (NIH) to R.A. Bonomo under Award Numbers R01AI100560, R01AI063517, and R01AI072219. R.A. Bonomo is also supported in part by funds and/or facilities provided by the Cleveland Department of Veterans Affairs, Award Number 1I01BX001974 to R.A. Bonomo from the Biomedical Laboratory Research & Development Service of the VA Office of Research and Development, and the Geriatric Research Education and Clinical Center VISN 10. The content is solely the responsibility of the authors and does not necessarily represent the official views of the NIH or the Department of Veterans Affairs. C.M. Bark reports research support from (NIH) under Award Number, R01AI147319-01.

REFERENCES

1. Shah NS, Auld SC, Brust JC, et al. Transmission of Extensively Drug-Resistant Tuberculosis in South Africa. N Engl J Med 2017;376(3):243–53.
2. Dheda K, Lenders L, Magombedze G, et al. Drug-Penetration Gradients Associated with Acquired Drug Resistance in Patients with Tuberculosis. Am J Respir Crit Care Med 2018;198(9):1208–19.
3. LoBue P. Extensively drug-resistant tuberculosis. Curr Opin Infect Dis 2009;22(2): 167–73.
4. Petersen E, Blumberg L, Wilson ME, et al. Ending the Global Tuberculosis Epidemic by 2030 - The Moscow Declaration and achieving a Major Translational Change in Delivery of TB Healthcare. Int J Infect Dis 2017;65:156–8.
5. Zumla A, Petersen E. The historic and unprecedented United Nations General Assembly High Level Meeting on Tuberculosis (UNGA-HLM-TB)-'United to End TB: an urgent global response to a global epidemic. Int J Infect Dis 2018;75: 118–20.
6. Reddy CL, Patterson RH, Caddell L, et al. Correction to: global surgery and the World Health Organization: indispensable partners to achieve triple billion goals. Can J Anaesth 2019;66(11):1425–6.
7. World Health Organization. Technical manual for drug susceptibility testing of medicines used in the treatment of tuberculosis 2018.
8. Chakravorty S, Simmons AM, Rowneki M, et al. The New Xpert MTB/RIF Ultra: improving detection of Mycobacterium tuberculosis and resistance to rifampin in an assay suitable for point-of-care testing. mBio 2017;8(4).
9. World Health Organization. The use of molecular line probe assays for the detection of resistance to second-line anti-tuberculosis drugs: policy guidance. World Health Organization; 2016. p. 9241516135.
10. World Health Organization. The use of molecular line probe assay for the detection of resistance to isoniazid and rifampicin: policy update 2016.
11. Daum LT, Rodriguez JD, Worthy SA, et al. Next-generation ion torrent sequencing of drug resistance mutations in Mycobacterium tuberculosis strains. J Clin Microbiol 2012;50(12):3831–7.
12. Koser CU, Bryant JM, Becq J, et al. Whole-genome sequencing for rapid susceptibility testing of M. tuberculosis. N Engl J Med 2013;369(3):290–2.
13. Walker TM, Kohl TA, Omar SV, et al. Whole-genome sequencing for prediction of Mycobacterium tuberculosis drug susceptibility and resistance: a retrospective cohort study. Lancet Infect Dis 2015;15(10):1193–202.
14. Consortium CR, the GP, Allix-Beguec C, et al. Prediction of Susceptibility to First-Line Tuberculosis Drugs by DNA Sequencing. N Engl J Med 2018;379(15): 1403–15.

15. Pankhurst LJ, Del Ojo Elias C, Votintseva AA, et al. Rapid, comprehensive, and affordable mycobacterial diagnosis with whole-genome sequencing: a prospective study. Lancet Respir Med 2016;4(1):49–58.
16. Miotto P, Tessema B, Tagliani E, et al. A standardised method for interpreting the association between mutations and phenotypic drug resistance in Mycobacterium tuberculosis. Eur Respir J 2017;50(6):1701354.
17. Colangeli R, Jedrey H, Kim S, et al. Bacterial Factors That Predict Relapse after Tuberculosis Therapy. N Engl J Med 2018;379(9):823–33.
18. Dheda K, Gumbo T, Maartens G, et al. The epidemiology, pathogenesis, transmission, diagnosis, and management of multidrug-resistant, extensively drug-resistant, and incurable tuberculosis. Lancet Respir Med 2017;5(4): 291–360.
19. Furin J, Cox H, Pai M. Tuberculosis. Lancet 2019;393(10181):1642–56.
20. South African National Department of Health. Interim clinical guidance for the implementation of injectable-free regimens for rifampicin-resistant tuberculosis in adults, adolescents, and children 2018.
21. World Health Organization. Rapid communication: key changes to treatment of multidrug- and rifampicin-resistant tuberculosis (MDR/RR-TB). Licence: CC BY-NC-SA 3.0 IGO.
22. Nahid P, Mase SR, Migliori GB, et al. Treatment of Drug-Resistant Tuberculosis. An Official ATS/CDC/ERS/IDSA Clinical Practice Guideline. Am J Respir Crit Care Med 2019;200(10):e93–142.
23. Dheda K, Chang KC, Guglielmetti L, et al. Clinical management of adults and children with multidrug-resistant and extensively drug-resistant tuberculosis. Clin Microbiol Infect 2017;23(3):131–40.
24. Milstein M, Brzezinski A, Varaine F, et al. (Re)moving the needle: prospects for all-oral treatment for multidrug-resistant tuberculosis. Int J Tuberc Lung Dis 2016; 20(12):18–23.
25. Collaborative Group for the Meta-Analysis of Individual Patient Data in MDR-TB treatment 2017, Ahmad N, Ahuja SD, et al. Treatment correlates of successful outcomes in pulmonary multidrug-resistant tuberculosis: an individual patient data meta-analysis. Lancet 2018;392(10150):821–34.
26. World Health Organization, 2019. WHO consolidated guidelines on drug-resistant tuberculosis treatment (No. WHO/CDS/TB/2019.7). World Health Organization.
27. Reid MJA, Arinaminpathy N, Bloom A, et al. Building a tuberculosis-free world: The Lancet Commission on tuberculosis. Lancet 2019;393(10178):1331–84.
28. Reuter A, Tisile P, von Delft D, et al. The devil we know: is the use of injectable agents for the treatment of MDR-TB justified? Int J Tuberc Lung Dis 2017; 21(11):1114–26.
29. World Health Organization. WHO treatment guidelines for multidrug-and rifampicin-resistant tuberculosis: 2018 Update. Pre-final text. Geneva: World Health Organization Document; 2018.
30. Loveday M, Reuter A, Furin J, et al. The STREAM trial: missed opportunities and lessons for future clinical trials. Lancet Infect Dis 2019;19(4):351–3.
31. Nunn AJ, Phillips PPJ, Meredith SK, et al. A Trial of a Shorter Regimen for Rifampin-Resistant Tuberculosis. N Engl J Med 2019;380(13):1201–13.
32. TB Online. Crisis of confidence in the WHO's ability to produce normative guidance for the treatment of RR/MDR-TB 2019. Available at: http://www.tbonline.info/posts/2019/6/7/crisis-confidence-whos-ability-produce-normative-g/.

33. Harries AD, Kumar AMV, Satyanarayana S, et al. How Can Operational Research Help to Eliminate Tuberculosis in the Asia Pacific Region? Trop Med Infect Dis 2019;4(1):47.
34. World Health Organization, Rapid Communication: Key changes to the treatment of drug-resistant tuberculosis. Geneva: WHO; 2019.
35. World Health Organization, Guidelines for the treatment of drug-susceptible tuberculosis and patient care, 2017 update. Geneva (Switzerland): World Health Organization; 2017 (WHO/HTM/TB/2017.05).
36. World Health Organization. Companion handbook to the 2016 WHO guidelines for the programmatic management of drug-resistant tuberculosis. Geneva (Switzerland): World Health Organization; 2016.
37. Chan ED, Strand MJ, Iseman MD. Multidrug-resistant tuberculosis (TB) resistant to fluoroquinolones and streptomycin but susceptible to second-line injection therapy has a better prognosis than extensively drug-resistant TB. Clin Infect Dis 2009;48(5):e50–2.
38. Gandhi NR, Moll A, Sturm AW, et al. Extensively drug-resistant tuberculosis as a cause of death in patients co-infected with tuberculosis and HIV in a rural area of South Africa. Lancet 2006;368(9547):1575–80.
39. Falzon D, Gandhi N, Migliori GB, et al. Resistance to fluoroquinolones and second-line injectable drugs: impact on multidrug-resistant TB outcomes. Eur Respir J 2013;42(1):156–68.
40. Schnippel K, Ndjeka N, Maartens G, et al. Effect of bedaquiline on mortality in South African patients with drug-resistant tuberculosis: a retrospective cohort study. Lancet Respir Med 2018;6(9):699–706.
41. Ferlazzo G, Mohr E, Laxmeshwar C, et al. Early safety and efficacy of the combination of bedaquiline and delamanid for the treatment of patients with drug-resistant tuberculosis in Armenia, India, and South Africa: a retrospective cohort study. Lancet Infect Dis 2018;18(5):536–44.
42. Dooley KE, Rosenkranz SL, Conradie F, et al. QT effects of bedaquiline, delamanid or both in MDR-TB patients: the deliberate trial. In: Conference on Retroviruses and Opportunistic Infections (CROI) (Vol. 5). 2019.
43. Conradie F, Diacon AH, Everitt D, et al. The NIX-TB trial of pretomanid, bedaquiline and linezolid to treat XDR-TB. In Conference on retroviruses and opportunistic infections (CROI). Seattle, Washington, 2017. p. 13-16.
44. Global Alliance for TB Drug Development. Pretomanid, Sponsor Briefing Document, Antimicrobial Drugs Advisory Committee, New York, June 6, 2019.
45. McKenna L, Furin J. Are pretomanid-containing regimens for tuberculosis a victory or a victory narrative? Lancet Respir ed 2019;7(12):999–1000.
46. Lange C, Chesov D, Furin J, et al. Revising the definition of extensively drug-resistant tuberculosis. Lancet Respir Med 2018;6(12):893–5.
47. Drug-resistant tuberculosis scale-up treatment action team. Country Updates; 2019. Available at: http://drtb-stat.org/country-updates/.
48. Frick M, Henry I, Lessem E. Falling short of the right to health and scientific progress: inadequate TB drug research and access. Health Hum Rights 2016; 18(1):9–24.
49. Schnippel K, Firnhaber C, Conradie F, et al. Incremental cost-effectiveness of bedaquiline for the treatment of rifampin-resistant tuberculosis in South Africa: model-based analysis. Appl Health Econ Health Policy 2018;16(1):43–54.
50. Cox V, Brigden G, Crespo RH, et al. Global programmatic use of bedaquiline and delamanid for the treatment of multidrug-resistant tuberculosis. Int J Tuberc Lung Dis 2018;22(4):407–12.

51. Stop TB Partnership. Data for action for tuberculosis for key, vulnerable, and under-served populations 2017.
52. Furin J, Loveday M, Hlangu S, et al. "A very humiliating illness": a qualitative study of patient-centered Care for Rifampicin-Resistant Tuberculosis in South Africa. BMC Public Health 2020;20(1):76.
53. Wingfield T, Boccia D, Tovar M, et al. Defining catastrophic costs and comparing their importance for adverse tuberculosis outcome with multi-drug resistance: a prospective cohort study, Peru. PLoS Med 2014;11(7):e1001675.
54. de Souza RA, Nery JS, Rasella D, et al. Family health and conditional cash transfer in Brazil and its effect on tuberculosis mortality. Int J Tuberc Lung Dis 2018; 22(11):1300–6.
55. Benbaba S, Isaakidis P, Das M, et al. Direct observation (DO) for drug-resistant tuberculosis: do we really DO? PLoS One 2015;10(12):e0144936.
56. Citro B, Lyon E, Mankad M, et al. Developing a human rights-based approach to tuberculosis. Health Hum Rights 2016;18(1):1–8.
57. Jenkins HE, Zignol M, Cohen T. Quantifying the burden and trends of isoniazid resistant tuberculosis, 1994-2009. PLoS One 2011;6(7):e22927.
58. Gegia M, Winters N, Benedetti A, et al. Treatment of isoniazid-resistant tuberculosis with first-line drugs: a systematic review and meta-analysis. Lancet Infect Dis 2017;17(2):223–34.
59. World Health Organization, 2018. WHO treatment guidelines for isoniazid-resistant tuberculosis: Supplement to the WHO treatment guidelines for drug-resistant tuberculosis (No. WHO/CDS/TB/2018.7).
60. Xie YL, Chakravorty S, Armstrong DT, et al. Evaluation of a Rapid Molecular Drug-Susceptibility Test for Tuberculosis. N Engl J Med 2017;377(11):1043–54.
61. Marks SM, Mase SR, Morris SB. Systematic Review, Meta-analysis, and Cost-effectiveness of Treatment of Latent Tuberculosis to Reduce Progression to Multidrug-Resistant Tuberculosis. Clin Infect Dis 2017;64(12):1670–7.
62. World Health Organization, 2018. Latent tuberculosis infection: updated and consolidated guidelines for programmatic management (No. WHO/CDS/TB/ 2018.4).
63. Malik AA, Fuad J, Siddiqui S, et al. TB Preventive Therapy for individuals exposed to drug-resistant tuberculosis: feasibility and safety of a community-based delivery of fluoroquinolone-containing preventive regimen. Clin Infect Dis 2019;70(9): 1958–65.
64. Cruz AT, Garcia-Prats AJ, Furin J, et al. Treatment of Multidrug-Resistant Tuberculosis Infection in Children. Pediatr Infect Dis J 2018;37(10):1061–4.
65. Reuter A, Hughes J, Furin J. Challenges and controversies in childhood tuberculosis. Lancet 2019;394(10202):967–78.
66. Andries K, Verhasselt P, Guillemont J, et al. A diarylquinoline drug active on the ATP synthase of *Mycobacterium Tuberculosis*. Science 2005;307(5707):223–7.
67. Diacon AH, Pym A, Grobusch MP, et al. Multidrug-resistant tuberculosis and culture conversion with bedaquiline. N Engl J Med 2014;371(8):723–32.
68. FDA. Sirturo (bedaquiline) tablets label. Washington, DC: Food and Drug Administration. 2012. Available at: http://www.accessdata.fda.gov/drugsatfda_docs/label/2012/204384s000lbl.pdf.
69. Mase S, Chorba T, Parks S, et al. Bedaquiline for the Treatment of Multidrug-Resistant Tuberculosis in the United States. Clin Infect Dis 2019;ciz914.
70. Everitt D. Phase, A., 3. study assessing the safety and efficacy of Bedaquiline Plus PA-824 Plus linezolid in subjects With drug resistant pulmonary tuberculosis. NCT02333799.

71. von Groote-Bidlingmaier F, Patientia R, Sanchez E, et al. Efficacy and safety of delamanid in combination with an optimised background regimen for treatment of multidrug-resistant tuberculosis: a multicentre, randomised, double-blind, placebo-controlled, parallel group phase 3 trial. Lancet Respir Med 2019;7(3):249–59.
72. FDA briefing document, June 6, 2019. 2019. Available at: https://www.fda.gov/media/127592/download.
73. Ignatius EH, Dooley KE. New Drugs for the Treatment of Tuberculosis. Clin Chest Med 2019;40(4):811–27.

Aminoglycoside Resistance

Updates with a Focus on Acquired 16S Ribosomal RNA Methyltransferases

Jun-Ichi Wachino, PhD[a,*], Yohei Doi, MD, PhD[b,c,d], Yoshichika Arakawa, MD, PhD[a,e]

KEYWORDS

- Aminoglycosides • 16S rRNA methyltransferases • Gram-negative bacteria
- Plazomicin

KEY POINTS

- Aminoglycoside-resistant gram-negative pathogens producing 16S ribosomal RNA (rRNA) methyltransferase (MTase) have emerged and spread globally.
- 16S rRNA MTase-producing gram-negative pathogens tend to show a multidrug-resistance profile against β-lactams and fluoroquinolones.
- 16S rRNA MTase producers resist the newly approved aminoglycoside, plazomicin.
- Treatment options are limited for infections caused by multidrug-resistant 16S rRNA MTase producers.

INTRODUCTION

The worldwide spread of antibiotic-resistant bacteria, collectively called the ESKAPE (*Enterococcus faecium*, *Staphylococcus aureus*, *Klebsiella pneumoniae*, *Acinetobacter baumannii*, *Pseudomonas aeruginosa*, and *Enterobacter* spp) pathogens, has become a major public health concern because of the shortage of effective antimicrobial agents available for treatment.[1] Increasing resistance to β-lactams (penicillins, cephems, monobactams, and carbapenems), fluoroquinolones, and aminoglycosides has become a serious clinical threat because of their heavy use in the treatment of gram-negative infections. Gram-negative bacteria have developed resistance to β-lactams, aminoglycosides, and fluoroquinolones through the production of various

[a] Department of Bacteriology, Nagoya University Graduate School of Medicine, 65 Tsurumai-cho, Showa-ku, Nagoya, Aichi 466-8550, Japan; [b] Division of Infectious Diseases, University of Pittsburgh School of Medicine, S829 Scaife Hall, 3350 Terrace Street, Pittsburgh, PA 15261, USA; [c] Department of Microbiology, Fujita Health University School of Medicine, Toyoake, Japan; [d] Department of Infectious Diseases, Fujita Health University School of Medicine, Toyoake, Japan; [e] Department of Medical Technology, Shubun University, Japan
* Corresponding author.
E-mail address: wachino@med.nagoya-u.ac.jp

Infect Dis Clin N Am 34 (2020) 887–902
https://doi.org/10.1016/j.idc.2020.06.002
id.theclinics.com

β-lactamases, aminoglycoside-modifying enzymes (AMEs)/16S ribosomal RNA (rRNA) methyltransferases (MTases), and substituting key amino acid residues in the QRDRs (quinolone resistance–determining regions) of DNA gyrase (GyrA) and topoisomerase IV (ParC), respectively.[2]

In the 1980s, the use of aminoglycosides became increasingly avoided because of ototoxicity and nephrotoxicity, and was subsequently replaced with β-lactams and fluoroquinolones, which had less toxicity and broader antibacterial spectra. However, with the rapid increase of β-lactam–resistant and fluoroquinolone-resistant bacteria, the clinical usefulness of aminoglycosides has now been revisited, together with an improvement in their safety through optimized dosing regimens, as an effective choice in the combined drug therapy against a range of resistant gram-negative bacterial infections.[3]

Streptomycin, produced by *Streptomyces griseus*, was the first clinically introduced aminoglycoside, reported by Jones and colleagues[4] in 1944, followed by neomycin, which was discovered from *Streptomyces fradiae* by Waksman and Lechevalier in 1949.[5] In 1957, Umezawa and colleagues[6] reported kanamycin from *Streptomyces kanamyceticus*, which proved to be effective in treating tuberculosis. Subsequently, gentamicin (1963) and tobramycin (1967) were identified from soil *Actinomycetes*.[7] Kasugamycin, composed of an inositol, an amino sugar, and an amidine carboxylic acid, was also discovered by Umezawa and colleagues,[8] in the 1960s, and this aminoglycoside was used in large amounts in agriculture to treat and prevent rice blast, but not in humans because of its toxicity. Semisynthetic aminoglycosides, such as amikacin (1972, kanamycin A–based), arbekacin (1973, kanamycin B/dibekacin-based), and isepamicin (1977, gentamicin B–based), which have potent activity against both gram-negative and gram-positive bacteria, were further developed.[7]

Clinically available aminoglycosides are structurally classified into 2 major classes: those with a 2-deoxystreptamine (2-DOS) core moiety and those without (eg, streptomycin) (**Fig. 1**). In addition, aminoglycosides with a 2-DOS core moiety are divided into subgroups, 4,5-disubstituted 2-DOS (neomycin, ribostamycin, paromomycin) and 4,6-disubstituted 2-DOS (kanamycin, gentamicin, tobramycin, amikacin, arbekacin, isepamicin), based on the substituent linkage position (see **Fig. 1**).

ACTION OF AMINOGLYCOSIDES AND AMINOGLYCOSIDE RESISTANCE MECHANISMS

Aminoglycosides with a 2-DOS core primarily bind to helix 44 of the 16S rRNA comprising bacterial 30S ribosomal subunits. Aminoglycoside binding causes various disruptions in protein synthesis: disturbing transfer RNA (tRNA) translocation, lowering translational fidelity, interfering with the ribosome subunit mobility, disturbing ribosome recycling, and interfering with the formation of intersubunit bridges.[9–14] Aminoglycosides also bind to, and may disturb protein synthesis at, helix 69 of the 23S rRNA in 50S ribosomal subunits.[12,14,15]

Bacteria resist aminoglycosides through a variety of intrinsic and acquired resistance mechanisms.[16] Base mutations within the A site of 16S rRNA, amino acid substitutions in ribosomal proteins, and activated efflux pumps are classic intrinsic aminoglycoside resistance mechanisms in pathogenic bacteria. Production of AMEs, either intrinsic or acquired, is the most common aminoglycoside resistance mechanism. AMEs are divided into 3 groups: acetyltransferase (AAC), phosphotransferase (APH), and adenylyltransferase (AAD or ANT). These AMEs modify NH_3 or OH groups at several positions in aminoglycosides, using cofactors, acetyl–coenzyme A or ATP, thereby deactivating them. The most clinically significant resistance mechanism is acquired 16S rRNA methyltransferase (MTase), because these confer high-

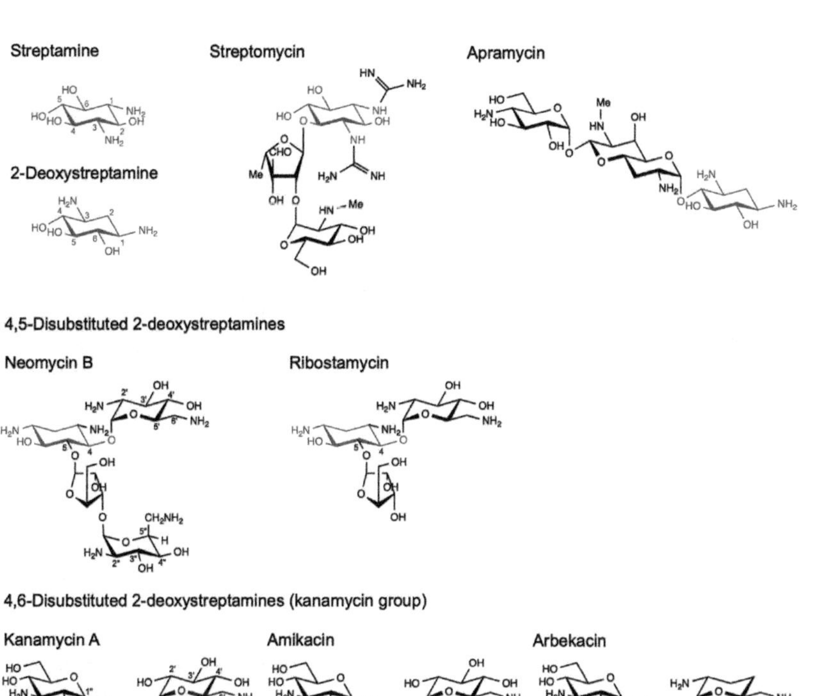

4,6-Disubstituted 2-deoxystreptamines (gentamicin group)

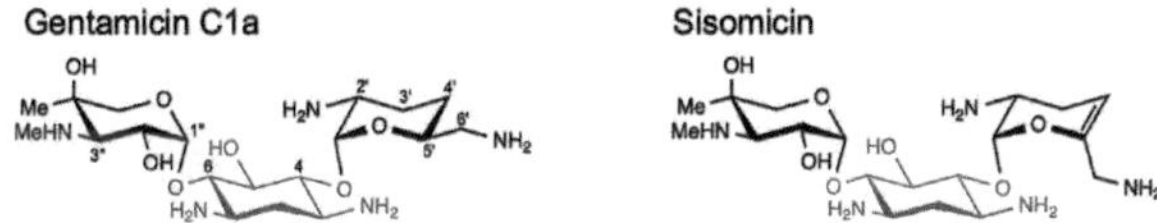

Fig. 1. Core elements of aminoglycosides and aminoglycoside structures.

level and broad-spectrum aminoglycoside resistance by adding a CH_3 group to specific residues within the A site of 16S rRNA using *S*-adenosylmethionine (SAM) as the cofactor (**Fig. 2**). The binding affinity of certain aminoglycosides to the CH_3-added 16S rRNA is predicted to be significantly reduced compared with that of the original 16S rRNA, resulting in high-level aminoglycoside resistance.

Globally Distributed N7-G1405 16S Ribosomal RNA Methyltransferases ArmA, RmtB, and RmtC

The 16S rRNA MTase gene *armA* was first identified together with $bla_{CTX\text{-}M3}$ on plasmid pCTX-M3 of *Citrobacter freundii* isolated in 1996, followed by documentation in 2007,[17] and was subsequently found on plasmid pIP1204 of *K pneumoniae* in 2000.[18] The *rmtB* and *rmtC* genes were found on the plasmids of *Serratia marcescens* and *Proteus mirabilis*, respectively, isolated in Japan in the first half of the 2000s.[19,20] Since then, these 3 16S rRNA MTases have been identified globally, primarily found in Enterobacterales, including *Escherichia coli*, *Klebsiella* spp, *Enterobacter* spp, *S marcescens*, *Citrobacter* spp, *Proteus* spp, and *Salmonella* spp, isolated from various sources, including humans, livestock, companion animals, and wastewater.[21,22]

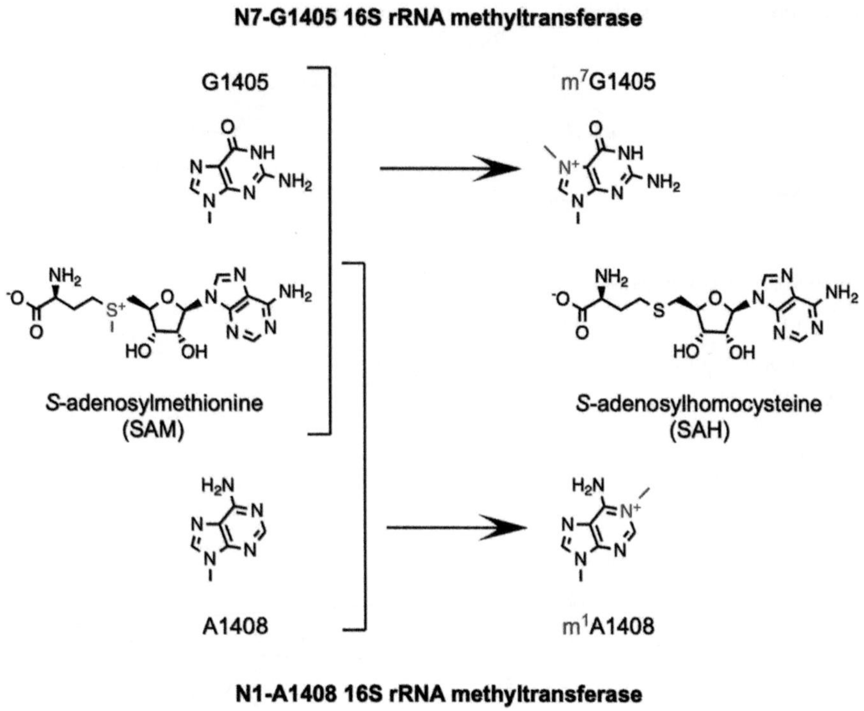

N7-G1405 16S rRNA methyltransferase

G1405 → m^7G1405

S-adenosylmethionine (SAM) → *S*-adenosylhomocysteine (SAH)

A1408 → m^1A1408

N1-A1408 16S rRNA methyltransferase

Fig. 2. Mechanisms of methylation of G1405 and A1408 residues in 16S rRNA by aminoglycoside resistance 16S rRNA MTases.

Regarding glucose-nonfermenting gram-negative bacteria, *armA* has mainly been identified in *A baumannii*, whereas *rmtB*/*rmtC* have rarely been found in that species.[23–26] So far, a few *P aeruginosa* clinical isolates have been reported to carry these 3 16S rRNA MTase genes.[25,27,28] The spread of these MTases has thus far been limited to gram-negative bacteria and has not reached clinically important pathogenic gram-positive bacteria, including *Staphylococcus* spp and *Enterococcus* spp, although the engineered introduction of these MTase genes could confer a high level of aminoglycoside resistance to *S aureus*, as well as in gram-negative bacteria.[29] One of the clinically concerning issues of these MTase producers is that they tend to also show resistance to β-lactams, fluoroquinolones, polymyxins, and fosfomycin in addition to aminoglycosides through various antimicrobial resistance genetic determinants; for example, β-lactamase genes (*bla*$_{SHV}$, *bla*$_{CTX-M}$, *bla*$_{KPC}$, *bla*$_{NDM}$, *bla*$_{CMY}$, *bla*$_{DHA}$, and *bla*$_{OXA}$), fluoroquinolone-resistance genes (*qnr*, *aac(6′)-Ib-cr*, *qep*, and nucleic mutations in QRDRs of *gyrA*/*parC*), colistin-resistance gene (*mcr*), and the fosfomycin-resistance gene (*fosA*).[21,22,30,31]

ArmA, RmtB, and RmtC 16S rRNA MTases can confer high-level resistance to 4,6-disubstituted 2-DOS (see **Fig. 1**). The levels of aminoglycoside resistance conferred by these MTases are high (eg, both amikacin and gentamicin have minimum inhibitory concentrations [MICs] ≥256 μg/mL) compared with those conferred by AMEs.[18–20] These increased MIC values are good indicators of the production of aminoglycoside-resistance 16S rRNA MTases relating to Enterobacterales, *Acinetobacter* spp, and *P aeruginosa*, and can be applied to the initial screening of 16S rRNA MTase producers (discussed later).

ArmA, RmtB, and RmtC 16S rRNA MTases share only modest amino acid identities with each other (up to 30%), but show high three-dimensional structural similarities (**Fig. 3**).[32,33] These MTases add a CH_3 group to the N7 position of G1405 in 16S rRNA, which causes steric hindrance to the substituent at 3″ position of ring III of 4,6-disubstituted 2-DOS, using SAM as a cofactor.[19,29,33] Moreover, although 16S rRNA MTases recognize the mature 30S ribosomal subunit consisting of 16S rRNA and ribosomal proteins, they do not methylate naked 16S rRNA alone, or mature 70S ribosomes.[29,33]

N7-G1405 MTases confer resistance to 4,6-disubstituted 2-DOS but not to 4,5-disubstituted 2-DOS or other aminoglycosides (eg, streptomycin and spectinomycin) (**Fig. 4**). The difference in specificity toward aminoglycosides can be explained based on the binding modes between aminoglycosides and 16S rRNA (see **Fig. 4**). The N7 position of the G1405 residue is closest to and oriented toward the substituent at 3″ position in the ring III of 4,6-disubstituted 2-DOS. The introduction of a CH_3 residue at the N7 position may lead to a steric clash and/or electrostatic repulsion against the side chain of ring III, leading to reduced binding affinities of aminoglycosides and resulting in increased 4,6-disubstituted 2-DOS resistance. In contrast, ring III and ring IV of 4,5-disubstituted 2-DOS are normally far away from the N7 position of G1405 (see **Fig. 4**), and the introduction of CH_3 by MTase does not disturb their binding, resulting in almost no change in the MIC values of 4,5-disubstituted 2-DOS (see **Fig. 4**). Other aminoglycosides, such as streptomycin, that bind to 16S rRNA without interacting with the G1405 position could still bind to 16S rRNA with m^7G1405 and show normal activity.

Sporadic N7-G1405 16S Ribosomal RNA Methyltransferases

Contrary to ArmA, RmtB, and RmtC, the spread of RmtA, RmtD, RmtE, RmtF, RmtG, and RmtH largely remain regional. RmtA has been reported in *P aeruginosa* clinical

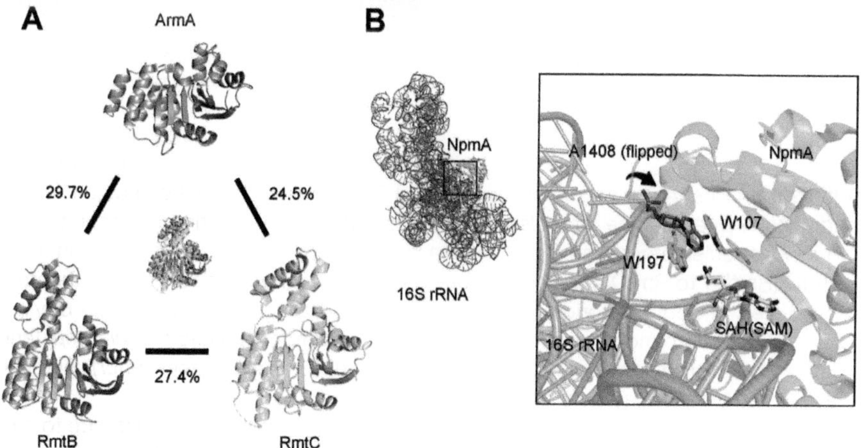

Fig. 3. (*A*) Three-dimensional structures of ArmA (*gray*), RmtB (*orange*), and RmtC (*light green*). These figures were rendered with Protein Data Bank (PDB) data (PDB identifier [ID], 3FZG, 3FRH, and 6PQB). The percentages indicate amino acid identities. (*B*) Binding mode between 16S rRNA (*orange*) and NpmA (*green*). The *S*-adenosyl-L-homocysteine (SAH) molecule is shown in yellow sticks and the A1408 residue in orange sticks. The 2 tryptophan residues (W107 and W197) of NpmA are shown in green sticks. This figure was rendered with PDB data (PDB ID, 4OX9).

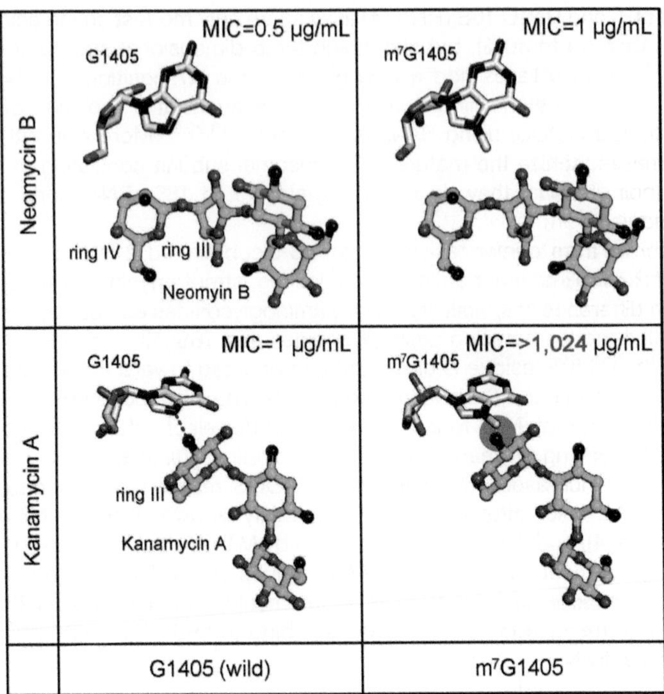

Fig. 4. Molecular models of binding mode between neomycin B/kanamycin A and wild G1405/m^{7}G1405 in 16S rRNA. These figures were rendered based on crystal structures (PDB ID, 2ESI and 2ET4). Basic residues and aminoglycoside molecules are depicted in silver and green sticks, respectively, and the orange dashed lines indicate hydrogen bonds. The red translucent circle indicates the predicted position of the steric clash between the residue and aminoglycoside. MIC values were cited from references.[20] (*From* Wachino J, Yamane K, Shibayama K, et al. Novel plasmid-mediated 16S rRNA methylase, RmtC, found in a *Proteus mirabilis* isolate demonstrating extraordinary high-level resistance against various aminoglycosides. *Antimicrob Agents Chemother* 2006;50(1):178-84 https://doi.org/10.1128/AAC.50.1.178-184.2006; with permission.)

isolates from East Asian countries, Japan, and South Korea.[34–36] Recently, an RmtA-producing *K pneumoniae* was also isolated in Switzerland, the first identification of RmtA in a species other than *P aeruginosa*.[37]

RmtD (RmtD1 to RmtD3) has mainly been found in *P aeruginosa* and Enterobacterales isolated in South America, Argentina, Chile, and Brazil. Notably, Tada and colleagues[38] and Urbanowicz and colleagues[39] reported RmtD3-producing clinical isolates of *P aeruginosa* from Myanmar and Poland, respectively, indicating that RmtD-group MTase may be starting to spread outside South America.

The number of reports for RmtE (RmtE1 to RmtE3) producers are also limited, 3 from the United States (all *E coli*),[40–43] 1 from China (*E coli*),[44] and the last 1, recently, from Myanmar (*P aeruginosa*).[45] *rmtE*-group genes have also been deposited in the GenBank from *A baumannii* and *Enterobacter cloacae* complex under accession numbers MH572011 and LC511997, respectively.

RmtF is the most prevalent MTase, after ArmA/RmtB/RmtC. The first identification of RmtF was in *K pneumoniae* isolates in La Réunion Island in 2011,[46] followed by Enterobacterales from India,[47–49] United Kingdom,[47,50] Nepal,[51] South Africa,[52]

United States,[53] Australia,[54] Egypt,[55] Switzerland,[56] and Ireland,[50] and *P aeruginosa* from Nepal.[57] One of the clinical risks associated with RmtF producers is that they frequently coproduce NDM-group metallo-β-lactamase, which confers carbapenem resistance.

RmtG producers (all *Klebsiella* spp), which often coproduce *Klebsiella pneumoniae* carbapenemase (KPC), have been reported from Chile,[58] United States,[59,60] Brazil,[61,62] India,[48] and Switzerland.[63] The sources of RmtH producers are limited, 1 in *K pneumoniae* from a patient who had been injured in Iraq,[64] and the other also in *K pneumoniae* from a newborn admitted to a hospital in Lebanon.[65] The enzymatic functions of RmtA, RmtD, RmtE, RmtF, RmtG, and RmtH are likely the same as those of ArmA, RmtB, and RmtC, in that they methylate the N7 position of G1405.[66]

N1-A1408 16S Ribosomal RNA Methyltransferase

NpmA was first identified in a clinical isolate of *E coli* (sequence type 131) in Japan.[67] This NpmA-producing *E coli* was identified through selection for high-level resistance to apramycin, a veterinary aminoglycoside. NpmA causes a flip of A1408 from h44 in 30S ribosomal subunits (see **Fig. 3**B)[68] and modifies the N1-A1408 position in 16S rRNA (and N1-G1408 in 16S rRNA[69]). The N1-A1408 position is proximal to ring I of 4,5-disubstituted, 4,6-disubstituted 2-DOS and apramycin (**Fig. 5**). Methylation at the N1 position of A1408 can confer broader aminoglycoside resistance than that of the N7-G1405 MTases because the spatial position of ring I remains the same regardless of the structures of aminoglycosides, at least for 4,5-disubstituted, 4,6-disubstituted 2-DOS and apramycin (see **Fig. 5**). Kanazawa and colleagues[70] recently reported that the introduction of a CH_3 group at the N1 position of A1408 prevents the formation of a pseudopair between the ring I of aminoglycosides and the A1408, especially the positively charged N1 atom that electrically prevents the binding of aminoglycosides carrying the NH_3^+ in ring I (eg, amikacin, gentamicin). Nevertheless, they modeled the mode of binding between aminoglycosides with a 6′-OH group in ring I (eg, paromomycin) and m^1A1408 and showed that this class of aminoglycoside might still be active against NpmA producers. The extent of MIC increase of paromomycin was, in fact, limited to only 4-fold by NpmA production (see **Fig. 5**). Therefore, 4,5-disubstituted 2-DOS with the ring I 6′-OH group may be a good starting point for designing the next generation of aminoglycosides that would be active against 16S rRNA MTase producers.[70]

The *E coli npmA* gene was flanked by 2 copies of IS*26* elements and located on 115-kb transferable IncF plasmids. Since the first report of *npmA* in 2007, reports of *npmA* are still rare compared with those of N7-G1405 MTase genes, such as *armA*, *rmtB*, and *rmtC*.[71,72] Notably, NpmA2, which has 1 amino acid difference compared with NpmA, was recently identified from *Clostridioides difficile* (discussed later).

Fitness Costs by 16S Ribosomal RNA Methyltransferase Production in Bacteria

ArmA/RmtB/RmtC are widespread, whereas reports of NpmA have been limited. To explore the difference, some researchers focused on the relationship between the fitness costs of aminoglycoside resistance 16S rRNA MTases and their distribution. Aminoglycoside-resistance 16S rRNA MTases modify the G1405 or A1408 positions, which are close to endogenously methylated residues, C1402 by RsmI and C1407 by RsmF, in *E coli*. Endogenous methylation at G1405 and A1408 may affect the normal process of housekeeping methylation at C1402 and C1407 positions and reduce optimal ribosomal function. G1405 methylation by ArmA production impeded the methylation of the C1402 position, but not C1407, and resulted in growth impairment.[73] In contrast, RmtC impedes methylation at C1407 but is not associated with

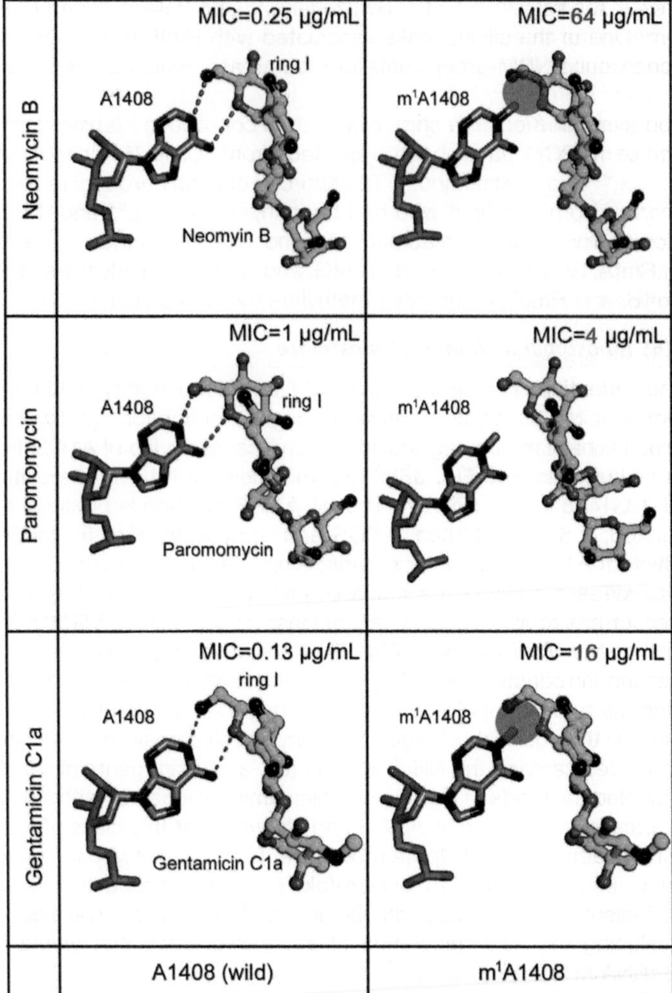

Fig. 5. Molecular models of binding mode between neomycin B/paromomycin/gentamicin C1a and wild A1408/m^{1}A1408 in 16S rRNA. The figures were rendered based on crystal structures (PDB ID, 2ET4, 5ZEM, 5ZEJ, and 2ET3). Basic residues and aminoglycoside molecules are depicted in orange and green sticks, respectively, and orange dashed lines indicate hydrogen bonds. The red translucent circle indicates the predicted position of the steric clash between the residue and aminoglycoside. MIC values were cited from references.[67] (*From* Wachino J, Shibayama K, Kurokawa H, et al. Novel plasmid-mediated 16S rRNA m1A1408 methyltransferase, NpmA, found in a clinically isolated *Escherichia coli* strain resistant to structurally diverse aminoglycosides. *Antimicrob Agents Chemother* 2007;51(12):4401-9; with permission.)

fitness cost.[74] Although NpmA interfered with the endogenous C1407 methylation, it does not affect cell fitness.[73] Ishizaki and colleagues[75] recently investigated the fitness cost incurred by NpmA production as well and showed low growth rate and cell survival for engineered *E coli* producing NpmA. Overall, aminoglycoside-resistance MTases might affect cell fitness cost, but it remains difficult to attribute the difference in the prevalence of N7-G1405 MTase (ArmA, RmtB, RmtC)/N1-A1408 MTase (NpmA) to the fitness costs their production incurs. NpmA confers a lower level of resistance to amikacin and gentamicin compared with N7-G1405 MTases, making it difficult to detect NpmA producers when using frank amikacin and gentamicin resistance as the screening criteria. Screening with apramycin resistance may facilitate identification of more N1-A1408 MTase producers.

Origin of Acquired 16S Ribosomal RNA Methyltransferase Gene

As described earlier, 9 types of acquired N7-G1405 MTases (ArmA, RmtA-RmtH) and N1-A1408 MTase, have thus far been identified in pathogenic gram-negative bacteria. Aminoglycoside-producing Actinomycetales innately possess aminoglycoside-resistance 16S rRNA MTase genes as a self-defense mechanism[22]; however, their G + C contents are high, indicating that they are unlikely the direct origin of 16S rRNA MTases of pathogenic bacteria, which have much lower G + C contents. Since the first report of N7-G1405 MTases early in the first decade of the 2000s, likely ancestor proteins have not been identified for any of the N7-G1405 MTases. However, Marsh and colleagues[76] recently reported that the potential origin of acquired N1-A1408 16S rRNA MTase gene *npmA* might be the chromosomally encoded 16S rRNA MTase gene carried by some *C difficile* strains. Near-identical nucleotide sequences (99%–100%) were observed between the acquired *npmA* in *E coli* and the chromosomal gene of *C difficile*. NpmA-producing *C difficile* showed a higher level of resistance to aminoglycosides compared with non–NpmA-producing *C difficile*, suggesting that NpmA is associated with aminoglycoside resistance in *C difficile*. However, aminoglycosides are not used in the treatment of *C difficile* infections, and susceptibility breakpoints for *C difficile* have not been defined either. The genetic environment of *E coli npmA* showed little similarity to those found in *C difficile*, whereas some *C difficile* isolates shared 99% genetic identity with each other within the 3-kb regions surrounding *npmA*. It is noteworthy that not every *C difficile* strain has *npmA* on its chromosome. The *npmA* gene found in some *C difficile* isolates might also have been derived from other bacteria.

Screening Methods for 16S Ribosomal RNA Methyltransferase Producers

N7-G1405 MTase producers show high-level resistance to 4,6-disubstitited 2-DOS, such as arbekacin, amikacin, and gentamicin. The MIC values of these 3 aminoglycosides for N7-G1405 MTase producers are mostly greater than 256 μg/mL, and no growth-inhibitory zone is observed around the disks containing these aminoglycosides by the disk diffusion test. Routine microdilution susceptibility testing performed in clinical microbiology laboratories does not generally include high concentrations of aminoglycosides. Thus, a practical approach for screening of potential N7-G1405 MTase producers would be to identify isolates resistant to both amikacin and gentamicin and subject them to manual susceptibility testing, which includes high concentrations of aminoglycosides. This screening strategy is applicable for Enterobacterales, *Acinetobacter* spp, and *P aeruginosa*. In contrast, it must be borne in mind that some nonfermenting gram-negative bacteria, *Pseudomonas* spp, *Burkholderia* spp, and *Stenotrophomonas maltophilia* and *Achromobacter xylosoxidans* innately show high levels of aminoglycoside resistance and should not be misidentified as aminoglycoside-resistance 16S rRNA MTase producers.

Because only N1-A1408 MTase producers have so far been detected, it is difficult to discuss screening methods for N1-A1408 MTase producers. In addition, in contrast with N7-G1405 MTase producers, resistance levels toward amikacin and gentamicin conferred by N1-A1408 MTases are similar to those conferred by AMEs. The most remarkable phenotype of N1-A1408 MTase producer is high-level apramycin resistance. The first *E coli* strain producing NpmA was identified through growth on agar plates containing 500 μg/mL apramycin, whereas almost all other tested clinical isolates could not grow on it (Wachino and colleagues, unpublished data, 2005). The only exception was AAC(3)-IV producers, which could also grow on agar plates containing higher concentration of apramycin.

New Aminoglycoside: Plazomicin

Plazomicin (PLZ), initially known as ACHN-490, is a new, semisynthetic, next-generation aminoglycoside (**Fig. 6**). PLZ is categorized as one of the essential medicines in the World Health Organization (WHO) model list in 2019.[77] This aminoglycoside was developed by Achaogen Co Ltd in 2009 by adding hydroxylaminobutyric acid to sisomicin at the 1 position and the 2-hydroxyethyl group at the 6′ position. PLZ was approved in 2018 by the Food and Drug Administration (FDA) for the treatment of complicated urinary tract infections and acute pyelonephritis. PLZ was designated to avoid modification by a variety of clinically relevant AMEs, thus its effectiveness is expected to be greater than conventional aminoglycosides for aminoglycoside-resistant pathogens producing AMEs (see **Fig. 6**).

PLZ has shown high potency in in vitro susceptibility testing against gram-negative bacteria.[78] The susceptibility percentage of *E coli*, *K pneumoniae*, *Klebsiella aerogenes*, *Klebsiella oxytoca*, *E cloacae* complex, and *S marcescens* to PLZ ranged from 97.6% to 100%, and the MIC_{90} (MIC required to inhibit the growth of 90% of organisms) values of PLZ for these Enterobacteriaceae were 0.5 to 1 μg/mL, which is less than the clinical breakpoint of 2 μg/mL approved by FDA.[78] Overall, PLZ was as potent as or superior to other aminoglycosides, including amikacin, gentamicin, and tobramycin. Compared with these Enterobacteriaceae, PLZ was less active against *P mirabilis* and *Morganella morganii*, with 44.3% and 66.7% susceptibility, respectively, and MIC_{90} values of 4 μg/mL for both, similar or inferior to amikacin, gentamicin, and tobramycin.[78] Compared with Enterobacterales, glucose-nonfermenting gram-negative pathogens, including *P aeruginosa* and *A baumannii*, were less susceptible to PLZ, with MIC_{90} values of 16 and 8 μg/mL, respectively.[78] The activity of PLZ was also significantly lower against *S maltophilia*, with an MIC_{90} value of greater than 64 μg/mL,[78] although this organism also showed natural resistance to other aminoglycosides. It is also noteworthy that PLZ is highly active against ESBL-producing *E coli* and *K pneumoniae*, carbapenemase-producing Enterobacteriaceae, and colistin-resistant Enterobacteriaceae, with susceptibility rates of greater than 90%.[78]

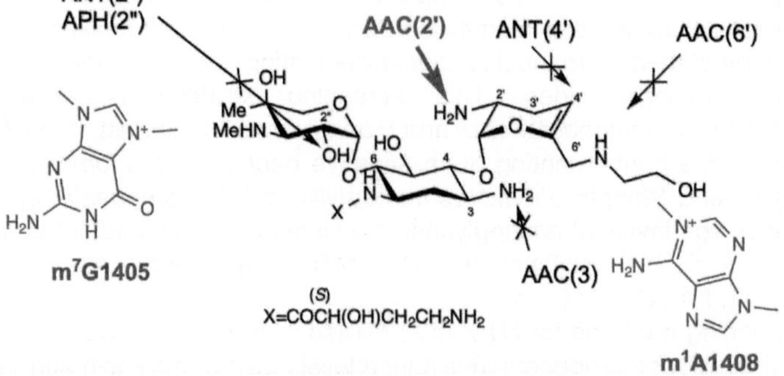

Fig. 6. Structure of plazomicin and modification targets of AMEs.

Mechanisms of Plazomicin Resistance

PLZ showed potent activity against clinically relevant AME-producing bacteria, as expected, but a small portion of the tested Enterobacterales strains were highly resistant to PLZ.[79] All these resistant bacteria were reported to be 16S rRNA MTase producers. PLZ has the same ring III structure as sisomicin, whose MIC values are very high for N7-G1405 MTase producers. Thus, it is reasonable that N7-G1405 MTase producers show cross-resistance to PLZ (MIC>256 μg/mL) (see **Fig. 6**). N1-A1408 MTase producers also confer PLZ resistance (MIC>256 μg/mL),[80] probably through the 2-hydroxyethyl group at the 6′ position of ring I interfering with m^1A1408 (see **Fig. 6**).

Cox and colleagues[80] recently reported the detailed behavior of various AMEs toward PLZ. As expected, production of most AMEs tested, including AAC(3)-Ia, AAC(3)-II, AAC(3)-IV, AAC(6′)-Ib, AAC(6′)-Ib-cr, AAC(6′)-Ie-APH(2″)-Ia, AAC(6′)-Ii, ANT(2″)-Ia, ANT(4′)-Ia, APH(2″)-IIa(-Ib), APH(2″)-IVa(-Id), APH(3′)-IIIa, APH(3″)-Ia, APH(4)-Ia, APH(6)-Ia, and APH(9)-Ia in engineered *E coli* BW25113 strain (originally PLZ MIC 2 μg/mL) conferred no or only slight resistance (2-fold to 4-fold increase in MIC) to PLZ. In contrast, only AAC(2′)-Ia showed a 16-fold increase in PLZ MIC. Cox and colleagues[80] modeled the complex structure of AAC(2′)-Ia and PLZ and confirmed the binding mode between them. AAC(2′)-Ia production is likely one of the causes for PLZ resistance, as observed in organisms such as *Providencia stuartii* that possess chromosomally encoded *aac(2′)-Ia* genes.

SUMMARY

Gram-negative bacteria with high-level aminoglycoside resistance caused by the production of 16S rRNA MTases have spread globally and across a variety of environments since their first identification in the early 2000s, and new variants of the 16S rRNA MTase have since emerged. This development is further complicated by the fact that 16S rRNA MTase producers often carry other clinically relevant resistance genes, including carbapenemase genes (eg, bla_{NDM} and bla_{KPC}) and colistin-resistance genes (*mcr*). The threat of 16S rRNA MTase in the emergence and spread of extensive drug resistance and pandrug resistance among pathogenic gram-negative bacteria therefore should not be underestimated.

ACKNOWLEDGMENTS

This research was supported by the Japan Society for the Promotion of Science (Grant-in-Aid for Scientific Research C). The work by Y. Doi was supported by grants from the National Institutes of Health (R01AI104895, R21AI135522).

CONFLICT OF INTEREST

The authors declare no conflicts of interest associated with this article.

REFERENCES

1. Mulani MS, Kamble EE, Kumkar SN, et al. Emerging strategies to combat ESKAPE pathogens in the era of antimicrobial resistance: a review. Front Microbiol 2019;10:539.
2. Blair JM, Webber MA, Baylay AJ, et al. Molecular mechanisms of antibiotic resistance. Nat Rev Microbiol 2015;13(1):42–51.

3. Serio AW, Keepers T, Andrews L, et al. Aminoglycoside revival: review of a historically important class of antimicrobials undergoing rejuvenation. EcoSal Plus 2018;8(1). https://doi.org/10.1128/ecosalplus.ESP-0002-2018.
4. Jones D, Metzger HJ, Schatz A, et al. Control of gram-negative bacteria in experimental animals by streptomycin. Science 1944;100(2588):103–5.
5. Waksman SA, Lechevalier HA. Neomycin, a new antibiotic active against streptomycin-resistant bacteria, including tuberculosis organisms. Science 1949;109(2830):305–7.
6. Umezawa H, Ueda M, Maeda K, et al. Production and isolation of a new antibiotic: kanamycin. J Antibiot (Tokyo) 1957;10(5):181–8.
7. Becker B, Cooper MA. Aminoglycoside antibiotics in the 21st century. ACS Chem Biol 2013;8(1):105–15.
8. Umezawa H, Hamada M, Suhara Y, et al. Kasugamycin, a new antibiotic. Antimicrob Agents Chemother (Bethesda) 1965;5:753–7.
9. Hirokawa G, Kiel MC, Muto A, et al. Post-termination complex disassembly by ribosome recycling factor, a functional tRNA mimic. EMBO J 2002;21(9):2272–81.
10. Rodnina MV, Wintermeyer W. Fidelity of aminoacyl-tRNA selection on the ribosome: kinetic and structural mechanisms. Annu Rev Biochem 2001;70:415–35.
11. Ogle JM, Ramakrishnan V. Structural insights into translational fidelity. Annu Rev Biochem 2005;74:129–77.
12. Wasserman MR, Pulk A, Zhou Z, et al. Chemically related 4,5-linked aminoglycoside antibiotics drive subunit rotation in opposite directions. Nat Commun 2015;6: 7896.
13. Garneau-Tsodikova S, Labby KJ. Mechanisms of resistance to aminoglycoside antibiotics: overview and perspectives. Medchemcomm 2016;7(1):11–27.
14. Halfon Y, Jimenez-Fernandez A, La Rosa R, et al. Structure of *Pseudomonas aeruginosa* ribosomes from an aminoglycoside-resistant clinical isolate. Proc Natl Acad Sci U S A 2019. https://doi.org/10.1073/pnas.1909831116.
15. Wang L, Pulk A, Wasserman MR, et al. Allosteric control of the ribosome by small-molecule antibiotics. Nat Struct Mol Biol 2012;19(9):957–63.
16. Davies J, Wright GD. Bacterial resistance to aminoglycoside antibiotics. Trends Microbiol 1997;5(6):234–40.
17. Golebiewski M, Kern-Zdanowicz I, Zienkiewicz M, et al. Complete nucleotide sequence of the pCTX-M3 plasmid and its involvement in spread of the extended-spectrum β-lactamase gene $bla_{\text{CTX-M-3}}$. Antimicrob Agents Chemother 2007;51(11):3789–95.
18. Galimand M, Courvalin P, Lambert T. Plasmid-mediated high-level resistance to aminoglycosides in *Enterobacteriaceae* due to 16S rRNA methylation. Antimicrob Agents Chemother 2003;47(8):2565–71.
19. Doi Y, Yokoyama K, Yamane K, et al. Plasmid-mediated 16S rRNA methylase in *Serratia marcescens* conferring high-level resistance to aminoglycosides. Antimicrob Agents Chemother 2004;48(2):491–6.
20. Wachino J, Yamane K, Shibayama K, et al. Novel plasmid-mediated 16S rRNA methylase, RmtC, found in a *Proteus mirabilis* isolate demonstrating extraordinary high-level resistance against various aminoglycosides. Antimicrob Agents Chemother 2006;50(1):178–84.
21. Doi Y, Wachino JI, Arakawa Y. Aminoglycoside resistance: the emergence of acquired 16S ribosomal RNA methyltransferases. Infect Dis Clin North Am 2016; 30(2):523–37.

22. Wachino J, Arakawa Y. Exogenously acquired 16S rRNA methyltransferases found in aminoglycoside-resistant pathogenic Gram-negative bacteria: an update. Drug Resist Updat 2012;15(3):133–48.
23. Wachino JI, Jin W, Kimura K, et al. Intercellular transfer of chromosomal antimicrobial resistance genes between *Acinetobacter baumannii* strains mediated by prophages. Antimicrob Agents Chemother 2019;63(8). https://doi.org/10.1128/AAC.00334-19.
24. Yamane K, Wachino J, Doi Y, et al. Global spread of multiple aminoglycoside resistance genes. Emerg Infect Dis 2005;11(6):951–3.
25. Tada T, Miyoshi-Akiyama T, Kato Y, et al. Emergence of 16S rRNA methylase-producing *Acinetobacter baumannii* and *Pseudomonas aeruginosa* isolates in hospitals in Vietnam. BMC Infect Dis 2013;13:251.
26. Bado I, Papa-Ezdra R, Delgado-Blas JF, et al. Molecular characterization of carbapenem-resistant *Acinetobacter baumannii* in the intensive care unit of Uruguay's University Hospital identifies the first *rmtC* gene in the species. Microb Drug Resist 2018;24(7):1012–9.
27. Gurung M, Moon DC, Tamang MD, et al. Emergence of 16S rRNA methylase gene *armA* and cocarriage of bla_{IMP-1} in *Pseudomonas aeruginosa* isolates from South Korea. Diagn Microbiol Infect Dis 2010;68(4):468–70.
28. Mohanam L, Menon T. Emergence of *rmtC* and *rmtF* 16S rRNA methyltransferase in clinical isolates of *Pseudomonas aeruginosa*. Indian J Med Microbiol 2017;35(2):282–5.
29. Wachino J, Shibayama K, Kimura K, et al. RmtC introduces G1405 methylation in 16S rRNA and confers high-level aminoglycoside resistance on Gram-positive microorganisms. FEMS Microbiol Lett 2010;311(1):56–60.
30. Lupo A, Saras E, Madec JY, et al. Emergence of $bla_{CTX-M-55}$ associated with *fosA*, *rmtB* and *mcr* gene variants in *Escherichia coli* from various animal species in France. J Antimicrob Chemother 2018;73(4):867–72.
31. Bartoloni A, Sennati S, Di Maggio T, et al. Antimicrobial susceptibility and emerging resistance determinants (bla_{CTX-M}, *rmtB, fosA3*) in clinical isolates from urinary tract infections in the Bolivian Chaco. Int J Infect Dis 2016;43:1–6.
32. Nosrati M, Dey D, Mehrani A, et al. Functionally critical residues in the aminoglycoside resistance-associated methyltransferase RmtC play distinct roles in 30S substrate recognition. J Biol Chem 2019. https://doi.org/10.1074/jbc.RA119.011181.
33. Schmitt E, Galimand M, Panvert M, et al. Structural bases for 16 S rRNA methylation catalyzed by ArmA and RmtB methyltransferases. J Mol Biol 2009;388(3):570–82.
34. Yokoyama K, Doi Y, Yamane K, et al. Acquisition of 16S rRNA methylase gene in *Pseudomonas aeruginosa*. Lancet 2003;362(9399):1888–93.
35. Yamane K, Doi Y, Yokoyama K, et al. Genetic environments of the *rmtA* gene in *Pseudomonas aeruginosa* clinical isolates. Antimicrob Agents Chemother 2004;48(6):2069–74.
36. Jin JS, Kwon KT, Moon DC, et al. Emergence of 16S rRNA methylase *rmtA* in colistin-only-sensitive *Pseudomonas aeruginosa* in South Korea. Int J Antimicrob Agents 2009;33(5):490–1.
37. Poirel L, Schrenzel J, Cherkaoui A, et al. Molecular analysis of NDM-1-producing enterobacterial isolates from Geneva, Switzerland. J Antimicrob Chemother 2011;66(8):1730–3.

38. Tada T, Shimada K, Mya S, et al. A new variant of 16S rRNA Methylase, RmtD3, in a clinical isolate of *Pseudomonas aeruginosa* in Myanmar. Antimicrob Agents Chemother 2018;62(1). https://doi.org/10.1128/AAC.01806-17.
39. Urbanowicz P, Izdebski R, Baraniak A, et al. *Pseudomonas aeruginosa* with NDM-1, DIM-1 and PME-1 β-lactamases, and RmtD3 16S rRNA methylase, encoded by new genomic islands. J Antimicrob Chemother 2019;74(10):3117–9.
40. Lee CS, Hu F, Rivera JI, et al. *Escherichia coli* sequence type 354 coproducing CMY-2 cephalosporinase and RmtE 16S rRNA methyltransferase. Antimicrob Agents Chemother 2014;58(7):4246–7.
41. Lee CS, Li JJ, Doi Y. Complete sequence of conjugative IncA/C plasmid encoding CMY-2 β-lactamase and RmtE 16S rRNA methyltransferase. Antimicrob Agents Chemother 2015;59(7):4360–1.
42. Davis MA, Baker KN, Orfe LH, et al. Discovery of a gene conferring multiple-aminoglycoside resistance in *Escherichia coli*. Antimicrob Agents Chemother 2010;54(6):2666–9.
43. Li B, Pacey MP, Doi Y. Chromosomal 16S ribosomal RNA Methyltransferase RmtE1 in *Escherichia coli* sequence type 448. Emerg Infect Dis 2017;23(5): 876–8.
44. Xia J, Sun J, Li L, et al. First report of the IncI1/ST898 conjugative plasmid carrying *rmtE2* 16S rRNA Methyltransferase gene in *Escherichia coli*. Antimicrob Agents Chemother 2015;59(12):7921–2.
45. Tada T, Hishinuma T, Watanabe S, et al. Molecular characterization of multidrug-resistant *Pseudomonas aeruginosa* isolates in Hospitals in Myanmar. Antimicrob Agents Chemother 2019;63(5). https://doi.org/10.1128/AAC.02397-18.
46. Galimand M, Courvalin P, Lambert T. RmtF, a new member of the aminoglycoside resistance 16S rRNA N7 G1405 methyltransferase family. Antimicrob Agents Chemother 2012;56(7):3960–2.
47. Hidalgo L, Hopkins KL, Gutierrez B, et al. Association of the novel aminoglycoside resistance determinant RmtF with NDM carbapenemase in *Enterobacteriaceae* isolated in India and the UK. J Antimicrob Chemother 2013;68(7):1543–50.
48. Filgona J, Banerjee T, Anupurba S. Incidence of the novel *rmtF* and *rmtG* methyltransferases in carbapenem-resistant *Enterobacteriaceae* from a hospital in India. J Infect Dev Ctries 2015;9(9):1036–9.
49. Rahman M, Prasad KN, Pathak A, et al. RmtC and RmtF 16S rRNA Methyltransferase in NDM-1-Producing *Pseudomonas aeruginosa*. Emerg Infect Dis 2015; 21(11):2059–62.
50. Taylor E, Sriskandan S, Woodford N, et al. High prevalence of 16S rRNA methyltransferases among carbapenemase-producing *Enterobacteriaceae* in the UK and Ireland. Int J Antimicrob Agents 2018;52(2):278–82.
51. Tada T, Miyoshi-Akiyama T, Dahal RK, et al. Dissemination of multidrug-resistant *Klebsiella pneumoniae* clinical isolates with various combinations of carbapenemases (NDM-1 and OXA-72) and 16S rRNA methylases (ArmA, RmtC and RmtF) in Nepal. Int J Antimicrob Agents 2013;42(4):372–4.
52. Rubin JE, Peirano G, Peer AK, et al. NDM-1-producing *Enterobacteriaceae* from South Africa: moving towards endemicity? Diagn Microbiol Infect Dis 2014;79(3): 378–80.
53. Lee CS, Vasoo S, Hu F, et al. *Klebsiella pneumoniae* ST147 coproducing NDM-7 carbapenemase and RmtF 16S rRNA methyltransferase in Minnesota. J Clin Microbiol 2014;52(11):4109–10.

54. Sidjabat HE, Townell N, Nimmo GR, et al. Dominance of IMP-4-producing *Enterobacter cloacae* among carbapenemase-producing *Enterobacteriaceae* in Australia. Antimicrob Agents Chemother 2015;59(7):4059–66.
55. Gamal D, Fernandez-Martinez M, Salem D, et al. Carbapenem-resistant *Klebsiella pneumoniae* isolates from Egypt containing bla_{NDM-1} on IncR plasmids and its association with *rmtF.* Int J Infect Dis 2016;43:17–20.
56. Mancini S, Poirel L, Tritten ML, et al. Emergence of an MDR *Klebsiella pneumoniae* ST231 producing OXA-232 and RmtF in Switzerland. J Antimicrob Chemother 2018;73(3):821–3.
57. Tada T, Shimada K, Satou K, et al. *Pseudomonas aeruginosa* Clinical Isolates in Nepal Coproducing Metallo-β-Lactamases and 16S rRNA Methyltransferases. Antimicrob Agents Chemother 2017;61(9). https://doi.org/10.1128/AAC.00694-17.
58. Poirel L, Labarca J, Bello H, et al. Emergence of the 16S rRNA methylase RmtG in an extended-spectrum-β-lactamase-producing and colistin-resistant *Klebsiella pneumoniae* isolate in Chile. Antimicrob Agents Chemother 2014;58(1):618–9.
59. Bueno MF, Francisco GR, O'Hara JA, et al. Coproduction of 16S rRNA methyltransferase RmtD or RmtG with KPC-2 and CTX-M group extended-spectrum β-lactamases in *Klebsiella pneumoniae.* Antimicrob Agents Chemother 2013; 57(5):2397–400.
60. Hu F, Munoz-Price LS, DePascale D, et al. *Klebsiella pneumoniae* sequence type 11 isolate producing RmtG 16S rRNA methyltransferase from a patient in Miami, Florida. Antimicrob Agents Chemother 2014;58(8):4980–1.
61. Ramos PI, Picao RC, Almeida LG, et al. Comparative analysis of the complete genome of KPC-2-producing *Klebsiella pneumoniae* Kp13 reveals remarkable genome plasticity and a wide repertoire of virulence and resistance mechanisms. BMC Genomics 2014;15:54.
62. Passarelli-Araujo H, Palmeiro JK, Moharana KC, et al. Molecular epidemiology of 16S rRNA methyltransferase in Brazil: RmtG in *Klebsiella aerogenes* ST93 (CC4). An Acad Bras Cienc 2019;91(suppl 1):e20180762.
63. Mancini S, Poirel L, Corthesy M, et al. *Klebsiella pneumoniae* co-producing KPC and RmtG, finally targeting Switzerland. Diagn Microbiol Infect Dis 2018;90(2): 151–2.
64. O'Hara JA, McGann P, Snesrud EC, et al. Novel 16S rRNA methyltransferase RmtH produced by *Klebsiella pneumoniae* associated with war-related trauma. Antimicrob Agents Chemother 2013;57(5):2413–6.
65. Beyrouthy R, Robin F, Hamze M, et al. IncFIIk plasmid harbouring an amplification of 16S rRNA methyltransferase-encoding gene *rmtH* associated with mobile element IS*CR2*. J Antimicrob Chemother 2017;72(2):402–6.
66. Correa LL, Witek MA, Zelinskaya N, et al. Heterologous expression and functional characterization of the exogenously acquired aminoglycoside resistance methyltransferases RmtD, RmtD2, and RmtG. Antimicrob Agents Chemother 2016; 60(1):699–702.
67. Wachino J, Shibayama K, Kurokawa H, et al. Novel plasmid-mediated 16S rRNA m1A1408 methyltransferase, NpmA, found in a clinically isolated *Escherichia coli* strain resistant to structurally diverse aminoglycosides. Antimicrob Agents Chemother 2007;51(12):4401–9.
68. Dunkle JA, Vinal K, Desai PM, et al. Molecular recognition and modification of the 30S ribosome by the aminoglycoside-resistance methyltransferase NpmA. Proc Natl Acad Sci U S A 2014;111(17):6275–80.

69. Zelinskaya N, Witek MA, Conn GL. The pathogen-derived aminoglycoside resistance 16S rRNA methyltransferase NpmA possesses dual m1A1408/m1G1408 specificity. Antimicrob Agents Chemother 2015;59(12):7862–5.
70. Kanazawa H, Baba F, Koganei M, et al. A structural basis for the antibiotic resistance conferred by an N1-methylation of A1408 in 16S rRNA. Nucleic Acids Res 2017;45(21):12529–35.
71. Yeganeh Sefidan F, Mohammadzadeh-Asl Y, Ghotaslou R. High-level resistance to aminoglycosides due to 16S rRNA methylation in *Enterobacteriaceae* isolates. Microb Drug Resist 2019. https://doi.org/10.1089/mdr.2018.0171.
72. Zhao Z, Lan F, Liu M, et al. Evaluation of automated systems for aminoglycosides and fluoroquinolones susceptibility testing for Carbapenem-resistant *Enterobacteriaceae*. Antimicrob Resist Infect Control 2017;6:77.
73. Lioy VS, Goussard S, Guerineau V, et al. Aminoglycoside resistance 16S rRNA methyltransferases block endogenous methylation, affect translation efficiency and fitness of the host. RNA 2014;20(3):382–91.
74. Gutierrez B, Escudero JA, San Millan A, et al. Fitness cost and interference of Arm/Rmt aminoglycoside resistance with the RsmF housekeeping methyltransferases. Antimicrob Agents Chemother 2012;56(5):2335–41.
75. Ishizaki Y, Shibuya Y, Hayashi C, et al. Instability of the 16S rRNA methyltransferase-encoding *npmA* gene: why have bacterial cells possessing npmA not spread despite their high and broad resistance to aminoglycosides? J Antibiot (Tokyo) 2018;71(9):798–807.
76. Marsh JW, Pacey MP, Ezeonwuka C, et al. *Clostridioides difficile*: a potential source of NpmA in the clinical environment. J Antimicrob Chemother 2019; 74(2):521–3.
77. World Health Organization Model List of Essential Medicines, 21st List, 2019. Geneva: World Health Organization; 2019. Licence: CC BY-NC-SA 3.0 IGO.
78. Saravolatz LD, Stein GE. Plazomicin: a new aminoglycoside. Clin Infect Dis 2019. https://doi.org/10.1093/cid/ciz640.
79. Castanheira M, Deshpande LM, Woosley LN, et al. Activity of plazomicin compared with other aminoglycosides against isolates from European and adjacent countries, including *Enterobacteriaceae* molecularly characterized for aminoglycoside-modifying enzymes and other resistance mechanisms. J Antimicrob Chemother 2018;73(12):3346–54.
80. Cox G, Ejim L, Stogios PJ, et al. Plazomicin retains antibiotic activity against most aminoglycoside modifying enzymes. ACS Infect Dis 2018;4(6):980–7.

The Role of Antibiotic Stewardship and Telemedicine in the Management of Multidrug-Resistant Infections

Thomas M. File Jr, MD, MSc[a,b,*], Robin L.P. Jump, MD, PhD[c,d], Debra A. Goff, PharmD, FCCP[e]

KEYWORDS

• Antimicrobial stewardship • Antimicrobial resistance • Antibiotics • Telemedicine

KEY POINTS

- The primary goal of antimicrobial stewardship is to optimize clinical outcomes while minimizing unintended consequences of antimicrobial use, including toxicity, the selection of pathogenic organisms, and the emergence of resistance.
- Antimicrobial stewardship is an important modifiable factor to address the public health crisis of antimicrobial resistance.
- The advent of secure electronic networks has led to the advances in the use of telemedicine to support antimicrobial stewardship programs in settings with limited resources.

INTRODUCTION

Antimicrobial resistance is a public health crisis. Inappropriate antimicrobial use is the most important modifiable factor in tackling this crisis. In addition to selection for antimicrobial resistance, unnecessary antimicrobial use can be associated with several untoward effects: adverse effects such as *Clostridioides difficile* infection (CDI); increased health care costs; and disruption of normal microbiome (which can adversely affect immunity). Although principles of appropriate use have been

Funding: None.
[a] Infectious Disease Division, Antimicrobial Stewardship Program, Summa Health, 75 Arch Street Suite 506, Akron, OH 44304, USA; [b] Internal Medicine, Infectious Disease Section, Northeast Ohio Medical University (NEOMED), Rootstown, OH, USA; [c] Department of Medicine, Case Western Reserve University, Cleveland, OH, USA; [d] Geriatric Research, Education and Clinical Center (GRECC), VA Northeast Ohio Healthcare System, 10701 East Boulevard, 111C(O), Cleveland, OH 44016, USA; [e] Department of Pharmacy, College of Pharmacy, The Ohio State University Wexner Medical Center, 368 Doan Hall, Columbus, OH 43210, USA
* Corresponding author. Infectious Disease Division, Antimicrobial Stewardship Program, Summa Health, 75 Arch Street Suite 506, Akron, OH 44304.
E-mail address: filet@summahealth.org

Infect Dis Clin N Am 34 (2020) 903–920
https://doi.org/10.1016/j.idc.2020.05.002 id.theclinics.com
0891-5520/20/

encouraged since the introduction of antimicrobials, abiding by them is now more urgent than ever. The good news is that there is a solution to this problem. Since their inception, antimicrobial stewardship programs (ASPs) have been proven highly successful in improving antibiotic use.[1] A 2018 CDC survey of more than 4900 acute-care hospitals found that more than 85% reported adhering to all 7 of the agency's core elements of hospital antibiotic stewardship programs.[2] ASP can improve patient outcomes, reduce adverse events (including CDI), reduce readmission rates, and even reduce antibiotic resistance. In addition, the recent use of telemedicine can extend the impact of ASP to areas and institutions with limited resources.

The discovery of potent antimicrobial agents was one of the greatest contributions to medicine in the twentieth century. When introduced, they had an immediate and dramatic impact on the outcomes of infectious diseases (ID), making once-lethal infections readily curable. Unfortunately, the emergence of antimicrobial-resistant pathogens now threatens these advances. Many procedures—cancer chemotherapy, organ and bone marrow transplants, and other surgeries (joint replacements, Caesarian sections, and many more)—are made possible by safe and effective antibiotics. Unfortunately, there are already patients every day who contract infections that cannot be treated with currently available antimicrobials. It is certainly tragic for a patient who is cured of cancer but only to die due to a resistant infection.

RESISTANCE AND NEED FOR ANTIMICROBIAL STEWARDSHIP

The primary goal of ASP is to optimize clinical outcomes while minimizing unintended consequences of antimicrobial use, including toxicity, the selection of pathogenic organisms (including *C difficile*), and the emergence of resistance.[3] Thus, the appropriate use of antimicrobials is an essential part of patient safety and deserves careful oversight and guidance. There is strong association between antimicrobial use and emergence of resistance. Observational studies associate greater antibiotic prescribing with greater rates of antibiotic resistance.[4,5] Thus, overuse or inappropriate use of antimicrobials are primary drivers for antimicrobial resistance. However, according to CDC, 20% to 50% of all antibiotics prescribed in US acute care hospitals are either unnecessary or inappropriate.[6]

The Centers for Disease Control estimates that antibiotic-resistant organisms cause at least 2.8 million illnesses resulting in more than 35,000 deaths annually.[7] These are conservative estimates, and the true burden is likely even greater. As stated in the report on Antimicrobial Resistant Threats, "Untreatable or pan-resistant infections are no longer a future threat—they are a reality." Around the world, including in the United States, people are dying from infections for which effective antibiotics are not available. In fact, many experts, including at CDC, believe we are already in a "postantibiotic" era.

The increasing prevalence of bacterial resistance has been a major driver of ASP initiatives. The National Action Plan for Combating Antibiotic-Resistant Bacteria was issued in 2015 and called for the Centers for Medicare and Medicaid Services to issue a Condition of Participation requiring hospitals to establish ASPs based on recommendations from the Centers for Disease Control.[8] The establishment of ASPs has now been a standard for hospital accreditation by The Joint Commission (TJC) since 2017. New antimicrobial stewardship standards from TJC for ambulatory care centers will also go into effect January 2020.[9] Criteria for the TJC standards are largely based on CDC's 2014 core elements of ASP, which have been recently revised (**Table 1**).[2] Further, the Centers for Medicare and Medicaid Services (CMS) have implemented mandates for all participating hospitals and long-term care settings to establish

Table 1
Summary of center for disease control and prevention core elements of Hosp antibiotic stewardship (2019)

Hospital Leadership Commitment	Dedicate necessary human, financial, and information technology resources.
Accountability	Appoint a leader or co-leaders, such as a physician and pharmacist, responsible for program management and outcomes.
Pharmacy Expertise (previously " Drug Expertise"):	Appoint a pharmacist, ideally as the co-leader of the stewardship program, to help lead implementation efforts to improve antibiotic use.
Action	Implement interventions, such as prospective audit and feedback or preauthorization, to improve antibiotic use.
Tracking	Monitor antibiotic prescribing, impact of interventions, and other important outcomes, such as *Clostridioides difficile* infection (CDI) and resistance patterns
Reporting	Regularly report information on antibiotic use and resistance to prescribers, pharmacists, nurses, and hospital leadership.
Education	Educate prescribers, pharmacists, nurses, and patients about adverse reactions from antibiotics, antibiotic resistance, and optimal prescribing.

Adapted from https://www.cdc.gov/antibiotic-use/core-elements/hospital.html?CDC_AA_refVal=https%3A%2F%2Fwww.cdc.gov%2Fantibiotic-use%2Fhealthcare%2Fimplementation%2Fcore-elements.html Accessed December 7 2019.

antibiotic stewardship programs.[10] These requirements, which make expert and coordinated interventions to improve the use of antimicrobial drugs mandatory in virtually all US hospitals and long-term care settings, will help curb inappropriate use of some of our most valuable medicines, reducing risks to patients and averting increased health care costs.

COLLABORATE FOR SUCCESS

Control of antimicrobial resistance with an effective stewardship programs requires a multifactorial collaborative effort including physicians and pharmacists as the core members along with infection control, nurses, microbiology, administration, information technology, quality control, and other key stakeholders.

An ID physician is a key core member of an effective ASP.[11] Smaller facilities may formulate an effective program with other physicians who have a strong knowledge of appropriate antimicrobial use. Hospitalists can be effective physician members of a stewardship program given their presence in inpatient care and their frequent use of antimicrobials.[12] As discussed later in further detail, telemedicine can connect antibiotic stewardship-trained physicians and pharmacists with settings with limited resources, enhancing the growth and development of ASPs led by professionals without ID training.

ID specialists optimize treatment in the inpatient setting by recommending appropriate antibiotic choices, duration of therapy, and route of delivery. Existing evidence suggests that when recommendations by an ID specialist are followed, patients are more often correctly diagnosed, have shorter lengths of stay, receive more appropriate therapies, have fewer complications, and may use fewer antibiotics overall.[13,14] A good example of the beneficial effect of ID consultation is *Staphylococcus aureus* bacteremia, where consultation is associated with a better diagnostic workup and reduces complications and mortality.[13]

Pharmacists, preferably with advanced training in ID, are also essential members of an ASP. The American Society of Health System Pharmacists states "Pharmacist have a responsibility to take prominent roles in ASP, in part, from pharmacists' understanding of and influence over antimicrobial use within the health system."[12] One role of the pharmacists is to ensure the optimal use of antimicrobials by assuring the right indication and dose at the right time by the right route of administration for the right duration. Once appropriate therapy has been initiated, pharmacists can optimize therapy by applying pharmacokinetic pharmacodynamic principles such as extended-infusion β-lactam therapy. As shown in one study, patients who received extended-infusion cefepime for the treatment of multidrug-resistant (MDR) *Pseudomonas aeruginosa* infections had a lower mortality compared with those who receive standard 30-minute infusions (3% vs 20%, $P = .03$).[15]

Time to effective antimicrobial therapy is important to optimize patient outcomes. Pharmacists play a key role in applying microbiology rapid diagnostic test (RDT) results. One of the first studies to evaluate using an RDT for *S aureus* bacteremia in conjunction with ID pharmacist intervention showed mean time to optimal antimicrobial therapy was 1.7 days shorter ($P = .002$) post-RDT implementation.[16] Two collateral benefits were observed: pharmacists were able to advocate and obtain ID consults in many cases and the mean hospital costs were $21,387 less per patient in the post-RDT group.

Ongoing education to the medical staff is another important role. The emergence of new resistance enzymes such as carbapenem-resistant *Enterobacteriaceae* (CRE), New Delhi metallo-β-lactamase, and *Klebsiella pneumoniae* carbapenemases (KPC) creates an "alphabet-soup" of confusion for non-ID physicians. Pharmacists should provide timely education and guidance to health care providers for each new antimicrobial and emerging MDR organisms (MDROs). The impact of MDROs on patient care extends beyond optimizing drug therapy. It also affects infection control.

Even with ASPs, the most effective antimicrobials are of little value if health care providers do not wash their hands and thereby contribute to the spread of infection between patients. The need for meticulous attention to the fundamentals of infection control should not be understated. This was demonstrated in the 2011 KPC-producing *K pneumoniae* (KPC-*K pneumoniae*) outbreak at the National Institutes for Health.[17] Despite isolation measures implemented at the beginning of hospitalization, silent transmission spawned a cluster that led to infections in 8 patients, 6 of whom died of infection. Multidisciplinary meetings to keep everyone informed included physicians, nurses, pharmacists, infection preventionists, respiratory therapists, housekeepers, nutritionists, hospital administration, patient and environmental safety, and other staff. These meetings, which stressed unwavering attention to basic infection prevention and control principles, were a critical aspect for quelling the outbreak.

As part of the ASP team, infection control preventionists play an important role in preventing the spread of MDRO. One of the most successful examples is Israel's nationwide intervention aimed at containing the spread of CRE. Following the implementation of national guidelines that included carrier isolation, cohorting, and active surveillance, nosocomial CRE acquisition in acute care declined from a monthly high of 55.5 to an annual low of 4.8 cases per 1000,000 patient-days ($P<.001$).[18]

The microbiologist provides essential data for ASPs. Hospital and unit-specific antibiograms help guide appropriate empirical antimicrobial therapy. New rapid molecular diagnostic tests (RDT) are "game changing" in the management of patients. This new technology allows for the identification of organisms in hours versus 3 to 4 days using traditional methods. Multiple studies have documented the positive impact on patient care when RDT are used in conjunction with ASP.[19] Improvement in time to optimal therapy, shorter length of stay, and lower mortality has been reported.

COST OF RESISTANCE AND IMPACT OF ANTIMICROBIAL STEWARDSHIP PROGRAM

Cost is the "elephant in the room" for ASP. Hospital administration often expect ID physicians to oversee ASP without any financial compensation. Pharmacists who are not ID trained are asked to perform stewardship intervention in addition to their current responsibilities without additional training, mentoring, or compensation. Without buy-in from hospital administration and without appropriate financial support for ASP, it is unlikely hospitals can implement successful and sustainable stewardship.

Frequently ASPs will recommend 2 or more antibiotics to treat patients infected with MDROs. The collateral damage from exposure to multiple antibiotics is the development of CDI. An infection control survey of 571 US hospitals asked questions related to CDI prevention and found the use of ASP to prevent CDI is lacking in 48% of hospitals.[20]

New expensive antibiotics are often the most appropriate option but the silo budget mentality in hospitals place tremendous pressure on the pharmacy department to use the least expensive antimicrobials. This "penny wise, pound foolish" approach has negative impact on clinical outcomes. Over the past few years several new, more effective, and less toxic antimicrobial agents have been developed and approved for use to treat MDRO including CRE infections (ceftazidime-avibactam, ceftolozane-tazobactam, meropenem-vaborbactam, imipenem-cilastin-relebactam, cefiderocol, plazomicin, eravacycline, and fosfomycin). However, despite evidence that their use is associated with better outcomes, one study found these newer agents were prescribed in only 35% of such infections.[21] Another study found among 132 hospitals identified, the median time to use any new agent was 398 days.[22] Use of new agents likely has been constrained by concerns over cost. Thus, patients may be regrettably deprived of better drugs because of the cost. ASP must not be perceived as primarily about reducing costs but rather toward optimal clinical outcomes. Older antibiotics with high toxicity, such as colistin, are still being used in many cases instead of new antibiotics. Colistin can cause severe kidney damage, sometimes requiring dialysis.

EVIDENCE OF STEWARDSHIP ON IMPACT OF ANTIMICROBIAL RESISTANCE

There are 2 core strategies that provide the foundation for an ASP. These strategies are not mutually exclusive[3]:

1. Prospective audit with intervention and feedback. Prospective audit of antimicrobial use with direct interaction and feedback to the prescriber, performed by either an ID physician or a clinical pharmacist with ID training, can result in reduced inappropriate use of antimicrobials.
2. Formulary restriction and preauthorization. Formulary restriction and preauthorization requirements can lead to immediate and significant reductions in antimicrobial use and cost and may be beneficial as part of a multifaceted response to a nosocomial outbreak of infection.

Several methods of improving prescribing of antimicrobial agents by ASPs have been evaluated and include antimicrobial avoidance or discontinuation when not warranted (eg, avoid antibacterial agents for viral respiratory infections); appropriateness of initial antimicrobial choices and doses that can be optimized by following existing guidelines; monitoring for drug-bug mismatches (eg, when the pathogen is resistant in vitro to the initially prescribed antimicrobial); reducing unnecessary prolongation of duration; and deescalation to a more narrow antimicrobial regimen from the empirical choice once a culture reveals the pathogen. No single intervention can solve the problem.

Data are variable as to the impact each of the strategies have on reducing antimicrobial resistance. Antibiotic stewardship strategies have evolved over time. The application of the science of behavior change has been an important addition to ASP.[20,23] To influence behaviors of prescribers it is first necessary to study how and why health care professionals behave the way they do.[24]

The best strategies for the prevention and containment of antimicrobial resistance are not definitively established. Often multiple interventions have been made simultaneously, making it difficult to assess the benefit attributable to any one specific intervention. However, a comprehensive program that includes active monitoring of resistance, fostering of appropriate antimicrobial use, and collaboration with an effective infection control program to minimize secondary spread of resistance is considered to be optimal.

A Cochrane review evaluated 89 studies from 19 countries to determine effective interventions to improve antimicrobial prescribing practices for hospital inpatients.[25] Most of the interventions (80/95, 84%) targeted the choice of antibiotic prescribed (drug selected, timing of first dose or route of administration). The remaining 15 interventions aimed to change exposure of patients to antibiotics by changing the decision to treat or the duration of treatment. Twelve studies evaluated antimicrobial resistance as an outcome. Interventions to change antimicrobial prescribing were associated with a decrease in CDI, resistant gram-negative bacteria, methicillin-resistant *S aureus*, and vancomycin-resistant enterococci. The meta-analysis indicated that restrictive interventions tended to have a more immediate effect on reducing resistance of the restricted agent, but prospective audit and feedback seemed to be more effective for a long-term effect.

Several systematic reviews of ASP's impact have been published since 2016. Schuts and colleagues[26] reviewed 145 studies and found that 6 process interventions (empirical therapy according to guidelines, deescalation of therapy, intravenous to oral switch, therapeutic drug monitoring, use of a list of restricted antibiotics, and bedside consultation) showed some benefit on one or more of 4 predetermined outcomes (clinical outcomes, adverse effects, cost, and bacterial resistance rates). Resistance rates were reduced in association with restrictions on antibiotics. A more recent systematic review of 146 studies found that hospital ASPs have a significant value with beneficial clinical and economical impacts.[27] Most of the studies showed a decrease in length of stay (85%) and antibiotic expenditure (92%); antimicrobial resistance was not assessed in most studies. In another recent review, Schweitzert and colleagues[28] found the overall quality of antimicrobial stewardship studies is low. Most studies do not report clinical and microbiological outcome data. Studies conducted in the community setting were associated with better quality. These limitations should inform the design of future stewardship evaluations so that a robust evidence base can be built to guide clinical practice.

Table 2 lists the effect of several different studies on antimicrobial resistance.[29–45] The studies listed assessed various interventions, which include antimicrobial restriction, deescalation; reduction of duration, and various forms of comprehensive antimicrobial stewardship programs with protocol adherence and audit and feedback. Robust evidence has shown that the prevalence of bacteria resistant to a specific antimicrobial decreases following restricted use of that antimicrobial. An unintended consequence, however, may be development of resistance to alternative agents used in place of restricted agents—"squeezing the balloon."[46]

Although there is a general perception that "deescalation" is appropriate and is a primary principle of antimicrobial stewardship and although prior national guidelines and numerous papers contend that "deescalation" is beneficial for patients and the health system (e.g., reduction of cost and resistance), there is very little high-level evidence to support this. As stated in a Cochrane review of antimicrobial deescalation for adults with sepsis, "There is no adequate or direct evidence on whether deescalation of antimicrobial agents is effective and safe for adults with sepsis...Appropriate studies are needed to investigate the potential benefits proposed by de-escalation treatment."[25] Subsequent to this Cochrane Review, Leone and colleagues[35] reported the first randomized controlled trial (RCT) to specifically assess deescalation, defined as narrowing the spectrum of the initial antimicrobial therapy, in patients with sepsis in the intensive care unit (ICU).[37] Of 116 patients included in the analysis, 59 were randomly assigned to the deescalation group and 57 in the continuation of appropriate antimicrobial therapy group. Pneumonia was the cause of infection in 58% and 40% patients in the deescalation and continuation arms, respectively ($P = .06$). Deescalation was associated with an increased number of antimicrobial days (the primary study outcome) as well as risk of superinfection; but there was no mention of an effect on resistance. The investigators concluded that deescalation was not noninferior to the continuation of appropriate empirical antimicrobial therapy. There was no impact on mortality or length of ICU stay. Despite the RCT design there were several limitations of the study, which included nonblinding; misbalance of type of infection (more lung infections in the deescalation arm); nonreporting the number of cases of health care–associated versus ventilator-associated pneumonia; and nonreporting of "appropriateness" of initial antimicrobial therapy. Furthermore, in a post hoc analysis of the 56 patients with pneumonia there was no difference in outcomes measured. In light of the absence of mortality difference and the presence of "serious" flaws of this RCT, the authors believe deescalation should remain recommended for the potential benefits to reduce antimicrobial use and resistance. The best use of deescalation is discontinuation of unnecessary antimicrobial therapy.

Many of the programs described in these studies combined some form of restriction (eg, reserved specific antimicrobials for ID or ICU use) with a prospective audit and feedback process. Several used computer systems to identify various bug-drug relationships or for implementation of specific protocols for a particular syndrome (eg, pneumonia or urinary tract infection).

Duration of therapy is important, as each additional day of unnecessary antibiotics increases a patients' risk of acquiring CDI. Recent evidence suggests that "shorter therapy is better."[47] One example is the appropriate duration of therapy for intraabdominal infections. Traditionally duration of antimicrobial therapy has been 7 to 14 days. A shorter course could decrease the risk of antimicrobial resistance. A recent study in patients with complicated intraabdominal infection and adequate source control found that the outcomes after short-course antibiotic therapy (approximately 4 days) were similar to those after a longer course of antibiotics (approximately 8 days).[48]

USE OF NEW ANTIMICROBIALS

After an extended period in which few new systemic antibiotics were approved for use in the United States, the last few years have seen an increase in newly approved antimicrobials, and government policies and professional society advocacy are

Table 2
Antimicrobial stewardship interventions: impact on resistance as an outcome

Study (Reference #)/Design	Intervention	Resistance Outcome Assessed	Finding
De Man et al,[29] 2000/Cross-over study in 2 neonatal ICUs; same hospital	Antimicrobial restriction: During the first 6 mo of the study unit A used an amoxicillin and cefotaxime regimen, whereas unit B used a penicillin and tobramycin regimen. During the second 6 mo the units switched antibiotics	Colonization of cefotaxime- or tobramycin-resistant GNR at 6 mo	68% reduction in days of colonization with resistant bacteria
Lewis et al,[30] 2012/Interrupted time analysis	*Restriction of ciprofloxacin*	Rate of ciprofloxacin-resistant *Pseudomonas*	Significant decreasing trend observed in the percentage and the rate of isolates of *P aeruginosa* that were resistant to antipseudomonal carbapenems and ciprofloxacin.
White et al,[31] 1997/Observational	*ABX restriction*; pre- and postimplementation of restriction of amikacin, ceftazidime, ciprofloxacin, fluconazole, ofloxacin	Susceptibility of gram-negative blood isolates	Reduced resistance $P<.01$
Singh et al,[32] 2000/RCT	*Duration* and use of monotherapy vs standard duration based on CPIS	Antimicrobial resistance and superinfection	Less resistance or superinfection with intervention (15% vs 37%; $P = 0.017$)
Chastre et al,[33] 2003/RCT	*Duration:* 7 d vs 14 d for VAP	Resistance, mortality, recurrence	Multidrug-resistant pathogens developed less with 8-d therapy ($P = .04$)
Kim et al,[34] 2012/Prospective	*Deescalation/RCT for initial therapy of VAP; deescalation based on culture*	Development of antimicrobial resistance	Nonsignificant more MRSA in deescalation arm; no difference in GNR

Leone et al,[35] 2014/Prospective RCT	*Deescalation of patients with sepsis*	Development of superinfection	Increased superinfection in deescalation arm but no mention of resistance effect
Dortch et al,[36] 2011/Prospective, observational	*Antibiotic stewardship protocols;* observed effect	Rate of MDR gram-negative bacilli during implementation	MDR GNB decreased from 37.4% to 8.5%
Nowak et al,[37] 2012/Observational, pre-, and postanalysis	*ASP Intervention*	Rates of infections due to common nosocomial pathogens caused by resistant pathogens	Rates of MRSA, *C difficile,* and VRE decreased
DiazGranados et al,[38] 2012/ Prospective audit	*Audit for ASP in ICU; baseline compared with intervention*	ID physician and ID pharmacist-recommendations and rounds	Lower rates of resistance (*P* = .033). Audit and feedback were independently associated with appropriate antimicrobial selection and prevention of resistance
Wang et al,[39] 2019 Retrospective, observational	*Multiaspect intervention measures were implemented by clinical pharmacists advising on antibacterial prescription and training*	Number of antibiotic prescriptions and resistance of *E coli*, *K. pneumoniae*, and *P aeruginosa*	Proportion of antibiotic prescriptions decreased. Resistant rates of *E coli* and *P aeruginosa* to FQ decreased, whereas resistance rates of *E coli* and *K. pneumoniae* to carbapenems increased
Stulz et al,[40] 2019 Observational	*Implementation of prospective audit and feedback program*	Observance of meropenem susceptibility	Meropenem use decreased over 62%; noncystic fibrosis *P aeruginosa* susceptibility to meropenem increases from 89% to 98% (*P*<.001)
Hernandez-Santiago et al,[41] 2019 Segmented regression analysis	*Examined associations between antimicrobial stewardship and prescribing of fluoroquinolones, cephalosporins, and co-amoxiclav and resistance among community-associated coliform bacteremia*	Observance of resistance rates	There was a significant reduction of resistance to fluoroquinolones and cephalosporins

(*continued on next page*)

Table 2
(continued)

Study (Reference #)/Design	Intervention	Resistance Outcome Assessed	Finding
Hecker et al,[42] 2019 Quasi-experimental	*Quasi-experimental study to determine impact of reducing treatment of asymptomatic bacteriuria and health care–associated pneumonia*	Measured fluoroquinolone use and susceptibility of isolates	Reduced use of FQ; FQ susceptibility increased significantly in *P. aeruginosa*, but not in *E coli* or *Klebsiella* spp.
Abbarra et al,[43] 2019 prescriptive review	*Restriction and postprescription review and feedback*	Measured consumption of ABX and resistance rates of *P aeruginosa*	A shift toward the consumption of low ecological impact antibiotics in an ICU. Rates of resistant *P. aeruginosa* and of AmpC-hyperproducing group 3 Enterobacteriaceae decreased simultaneously.
Lee et al,[44] 2018 Retrospective	*Restriction of FQ by ASP at large academic medical center*	Measured susceptibility of 5 gram-negative bacteria to FQ	A stewardship-driven FQ restriction program stopped overall declining FQ susceptibility rates for all species except *E coli*. For 3 species (ie, *Acinetobacter* spp, *E cloacae*, and *P aeruginosa*), susceptibility rates improved after implementation, and this improvement has been sustained over a 10-year period.

Kinnear et al,[45] 2019 Retrospective	*ASP interventions*	Measured daptomycin prescriptions and VRE	The proportion of patients experiencing an increase in daptomycin MIC during an infection declined from 14.6% (7/48 patients) in 2014 to 1.9% (1/54 patients) in 2017. Hospital-wide resistance to daptomycin also decreased in the postintervention period, but this was not maintained. This study shows that an antimicrobial stewardship–guided intervention reduced daptomycin use and improved individual level outcomes but had only transient impact on the hospital-level trend.

Abbreviations: GNR, gram-negative rods; ICU, intensive care unit; MRSA, methicillin-resistant *Staphylococcus aureus*; RCT, randomized controlled trial; VAP, ventilator-associated pneumonia.

combining to increase the development of additional agents. Several approvals have focused on gram-positive infections (dalbavancin, oritavancin, tedizolid) and gram-negative infections (ceftolozane-tazobactam and ceftazidime-avibactam, delafloxacin, eravacycline, omadacycline, fosfomycin, cefiderocol, imipenem-cilistatin-relebactam and plazomicin). The appropriate use of these new agents will be facilitated by effective stewardship.

Return on investment is a key factor in limited uptake of new antibiotics and threatens development of new drugs to treat MDROs. Antibiotics are typically taken for a short duration and used in a limited fashion—only when necessary—to preserve their effectiveness. Nearly all large pharmaceutical companies have left the antibiotic development field. The small companies that are responsible for most of the antibiotic innovation are struggling to stay in business. Indeed, 2 companies, Achaogen and Melinta, which developed important new antibiotics have had to file for bankruptcy.

The CMS reimbursement system can make it challenging for patients to access new antibiotics even when they are clinically appropriate. The Diagnosis Related Group (DRG) payment is too low to cover the costs of new antibiotics, making it difficult in many instances for new antibiotics to be added to hospital formularies or prescribed even when they are medically the best choice for the patient. In addition to harming patient care, this scenario also makes it extremely difficult for antibiotic developers—primarily small companies—to earn a return on their investment. A potential solution is to carve new antibiotics out of the DRG, allowing them to be reimbursed separately and making them more accessible to patients who need them. This is the basis of the Developing an Innovative Strategy for Antimicrobial Resistant Microorganisms (DISARM) Act, which aims to ensure that these drugs are not overused or misused.[49] DISARM would require hospitals receiving higher payments for antibiotics to establish ASPs and to report their antibiotic use and resistance data to CDC National Health care Safety Network (NHSN). The stewardship requirement is aligned with a Medicare Condition of Participation finalized by CMS in September 2019. The NHSN reporting mechanism would allow evaluation of the impact of new reimbursement policy on antibiotic utilization and resistance.

Many clinicians accept at face value the misperception that use of newer agents is not in accordance with practicing stewardship; this idea represents a false dichotomy. In reality the concepts of use of new drugs and stewardship can be very compatible. There has been a common perception in the past that as new agents became available, we were going to restrict them and never use them because we wanted to save them. But that may not be best for our patients. We have patients who are at high risk and so are good candidates for use of these new agents as initial therapy. Appropriate selection and timely administration of initial therapy is critically important and has a major impact on outcomes, including risk for death. Given the effectiveness of newer—and sometimes more expensive—agents against pathogens that have developed resistance to established agents, the use of newer agents in appropriately selected patients is compatible with good clinical care and antimicrobial stewardship. Oversight of treatment of newer agents by ASPs can assure appropriate use. As stated in the past by Dennis Maki, "The development of new antibiotics without having mechanisms to ensure their appropriate use is much like supplying your alcoholic patient with finer brandy."[50]

The development of rapid molecular tests able to quickly identify or rule out the presence of MDROs will also be of great value in helping clinicians individualize newer antimicrobial therapy to optimal effect. Diagnostic stewardship is critical in improving patient care and combating antibiotic resistance. Ordering the wrong tests, ordering tests at the wrong time, or interpreting tests incorrectly can result in delayed diagnosis or wrong diagnosis that can affect lives. For example, there is a strong link between overtesting nursing home patients with urine cultures and unnecessary antibiotic use, which can lead to CDI and other adverse events as well as resistance.

TELEMEDICINE AND ANTIMICROBIAL STEWARDSHIP

The number of ID-trained physicians and pharmacists is insufficient to meet the need for ASPs, particularly when considering long-term care settings.[51] The advent of secure electronic networks has led to advances in the use of telemedicine to support ASP in settings with limited resources, which includes insufficient access to professional with ID expertise, and effectively extends the reach of ID experts. Telemedicine ASPs, a rapidly developing field, can be broadly divided into asynchronous and synchronous approaches, with most programs using elements of both.

Asynchronous programs involve a "store and forward" approach in which a request is placed via a shared electronic medical record or dedicated Web application that an ID expert receives and responds to using the same platform. This approach has the advantage of permitting greater flexibility for both the individuals placing and those responding to the requests to do so as their schedule permits. Further, the responding provider has an opportunity to review the medical record and literature if needed. In Massachusetts, a telemedicine program for a 212-bed long-term acute care hospital (LTACH) that involved sending daily reports detailed the use of specific broad-spectrum antibiotics sent to off-site ID physicians and pharmacists who, in turn, communicated nonbinding recommendations to LTACH clinicians via secure email.[52] The LTACH clinicians accepted approximately 50% of recommendations, and the program achieved a significant and sustained reduction in both total antibiotic use and in rates of CDI. For a remote hospital in Brazil, a well-established telemedicine program that reviewed antibiotic prescriptions led to a decrease in prescriptions for fluoroquinolones, carbapenems, and polymyxins, with a concomitant decrease in the rates of cultures positive for carbapenem-resistant *Acinetobacter* spp.[53] As typical for antibiotic stewardship interventions, the decrease in the rates of pathogens achieved by these telemedicine programs were achieved over at least a 2-year time frame. Electronic consults, or e-consults, in which a clinician requests an ID opinion via the electronic medical record, serve to increase the breadth and volume of questions asked of ID experts and may, in time, also serve to reduce inappropriate antibiotic use and decrease the prevalence of MDROs.[54]

Synchronous programs use technology to permit a multidisciplinary team of professionals to discuss cases in real time. Especially when used with video-capable systems, this approach has the advantage of face-to-face communication, discussion of local practice patterns, and bidirectional education, all of which lead to team building and robust professional relationships. In southeastern Washington, a pharmacist-led ASP team that included the chief medical officer, director of pharmacy, infection preventionist, and microbiologist enlisted services from an off-site ID physician for weekly teleconference rounds.[55] The program reported an increase in antimicrobial stewardship interventions accompanied by a decrease in the rate of CDI in the 13-month assessment period. A telemedicine ASP program implemented at 2 rural Veterans Affairs Medical Centers (VAMCs) addressed patients from both the acute and long-term care units during weekly videoconferences that involved an off-site ID physician. Providers accepted approximately two-thirds of the recommendations made during the telemedicine sessions, leading to a significant decrease in overall antibiotic use.[56] Interviews with the team members at the rural VAMCs revealed that participants valued the multidisciplinary aspects of the sessions and believed that it improved their antimicrobial stewardship efforts and patient care.

Direct-to-consumer telemedicine for hospitalized patients may also help improve antimicrobial stewardship. A program in South Dakota found that ID consultations via telemedicine found a decrease in the days of intravenous antibiotic therapy as well as hospital length of stay for patients evaluated for neutropenic fever, bacterial pneumonia, and bacteria wound infections.[57] A similar program in Pennsylvania found that length of stay decreased following implementation of an ID telemedicine program, with a nonsignificant trend toward a decrease in antibiotic use.[58]

SUMMARY

In light of the serious threat of emerging antimicrobial-resistant pathogens, it is crucial that ASPs be put into practice now to provide for optimal patient outcomes and preserve antimicrobials for future use. Strategies for improving antibiotic use and evidence for best practices in antibiotic stewardship will continue to evolve. The specific types of interventions implemented by institutions will depend on local circumstances, resources, and capabilities, with telemedicine as a potential means to expand ASPs to resource-challenged settings. Nevertheless, it is vital that health care settings have ASP so that patients, both present and future, will continue to have the benefit of life-saving antimicrobials.

ACKNOWLEDGMENTS

This work was supported in part by funds and facilities provided by the Geriatric Research Education and Clinical Center (GRECC) at the VA Northeast Ohio Healthcare System, Cleveland, Ohio. The findings and conclusions in this document are those of the authors, who are responsible for its content, and do not necessarily represent the views of the VA or of the United States Government.

CONFLICT OF INTEREST

None of the authors have relevant conflicts of interest to disclose. Dr T.M. File: TF's institution has received research grants from Nabriva and Pfizer; he has served on scientific advisory boards for Merck, GlaxoSmith Kline, Melinta and MotifBio and participated on a DSMB for Shionogi and Paratek. Dr R.L.P. Jump: RJ is the Principal Investigator on research grants from the Pfizer and Accelerate; she has also participated in advisory boards for Pfizer and Merck. Dr D.A. Goff: DG is the Principal Investigator on research grants from Pfizer and Merck; she is on the CARBx advisory board and attended advisory boards for OpGen.

REFERENCES

1. File TM Jr, Srinivasan A, Bartlett JB. Antimicrobial stewardship: importance for patient and public health. Clin Infect Dis 2014;59(S3):S93–6.
2. Available at: https://www.cdc.gov/antibiotic-use/core-elements/hospital.html?CDC_AA_refVal=https%3A%2F%2Fwww.cdc.gov%2Fantibiotic-use%2Fhealthcare%2Fimplementation%2Fcore-elements.html Accessed December 7, 2019.
3. Dellit TH, Owens RC, McGowan JE Jr, et al. Infectious Diseases Society of America and the Society for Healthcare Epidemiology of America guidelines for developing an institutional program to enhance antimicrobial stewardship. Clin Infect Dis 2007;44:159–77.

4. Neuhauser MM, Weinstein RA, Rydman R. Antibiotic resistance among gram negative bacilli in US intensive care units: implications for fluoroquinolone use. JAMA 2003;289(7):885–8.
5. Costelloe C, Metcalfe C, Lovering A. Effect of antibiotic prescribing in primary care on antimicrobial resistance in individual patients: systematic review and meta-analysis. BMJ 2010;340:c2096.
6. Antibiotic prescribing and use in hospitals and long term care. Available at: https://www.cdc.gov/antibiotic-use/healthcare/. Accessed December 23, 2019.
7. Centers for Disease Control and Prevention. Antibiotic resistance threats in the US 2019. Available at: https://www.cdc.gov/drugresistance/pdf/threats-report/2019-ar-threats-report-508.pdf. Accessed December 6, 2019.
8. Available at: https://obamawhitehouse.archives.gov/the-press-office/2015/03/27/fact-sheet-obama-administration-releases-national-action-plan-combat-ant. Accessed June 1, 2015
9. Antimicrobial stewardship in ambulatory health care: R3 report: requirement, rationale, reference: The Joint Commission, Issue 23 [Internet]. 2019 [cited November 1, 2019]. Available at: https://www.bing.com/search?q=joint+commission+standard+for+ambulatory+care&form=APMCS1&PC=APMC#. Accessed December 23, 2019.
10. Available at: https://www.federalregister.gov/documents/2019/09/30/2019-20736/medicare-and-medicaid-programs-regulatory-provisions-to-promote-program-efficiency-transparency-and. Accessed December 23, 2019
11. Ostrowsky B, Banerjee R, Bonomo RA, et al. Infectious diseases physicians: leading the way in antimicrobial stewardship. Clin Infect Dis 2018;66:995–1003.
12. ASHP statement on the pharmacist's role in antimicrobial stewardship and infection prevention and control. Am J Health Syst Pharm 2010;67:575–7.
13. Robinson JO, Pozzi-Langhi S, Phillips M, et al. Formal infectious diseases consultation is associated with decreased mortality in Staphylococcus aureus bacteraemia. Eur J Clin Microbiol Infect Dis 2012;31(9):2421–8.
14. Nilhom H, Holmsrand L, Ahl J. An audit-based infections disease specialist-guided antimicrobial stewardship program profoundly reduced antibiotic use without negatively affecting patient outcomes. Open Forum Infect Dis 2015;2(2):ofv042.
15. Bauer KA, West JE, O'Brien JM, et al. Extended-infusion cefepime reduces mortality in patients with Pseudomonas aeruginosa infections. Antimicrobial Agents Chemother 2013;57(7):2907–12.
16. Bauer KA, West JE, Balada-Llasat JM, et al. An antimicrobial stewardship program's impact with rapid polymerase chain reaction methicillin-resistant Staphylococcus aureus/S. aureus blood culture test in patients with S. aureus bacteremia. Clin Infect Dis 2010;51(9):1074–80.
17. Palmore TN, Henderson DK. Managing transmission of carbapenem-resistant Enterobacteriaceae in healthcare settings: a view from the trenches. Clin Infect Dis 2013;57(11):1593–9.
18. Schwaber MJ, Carmeli Y. An ongoing national intervention to contain the spread of carbapenem-resistant Enterobacteriacieae. Clin Infect Dis 2014;58:697–703.
19. Bauer KA, Perez KK, Forrest GN, et al. Review of rapid diagnostic tests used by antimicrobial stewardship programs. Clin Infect Dis 2014;59(Suppl 3):S134–45.
20. Saint S, Fowler KE, Krein SL, et al. Clostridium difficile infection in the United States: A national study assessing preventive practices used and perceptions of practice evidence. Infect Control Hose Epidemilo 2015;36:969–71.

21. Clancy CJ, Potoski BA, Buehrle D, et al. Estimating the treatment of carbapenem-resistant enterobacteriaceae infections in the United States using antibiotic prescription data. Open Forum Infect Dis 2019;6(8):ofz344.
22. Schultz L, Kim S, Haetsell A, et al. Antimicrobial stewardship during a time of rapid antimicrobial development: Potential impact on industry for future investment. Diagn Microbiol Infect Dis 2019;95(3):114857.
23. Donisi V, Sibani M, Carrara E, et al. Emotional, cognitive and social factors of antimicrobial prescribing: can antimicrobial stewardship intervention be effective without addressing psycho-social factors? J Antimicrob Chemother 2019; 74(10):2844–7.
24. Charani E, Ahmad R, Rawson TM, et al. The differences in antibiotic decision-making between acute surgical and acute medical teams: an ethnographic study of culture and team dynamics. Clin Infect Dis 2019;69(1):12–20.
25. Davey P, Brown E, Charani E, et al. Interventions to improve antibiotic prescribing practices for hospital inpatients. Cochrane Database Syst Rev 2013;(4):CD003543.
26. Schuts EC, Hulscher M, Mouton JW, et al. Current evidence on hospital antimicrobial stewardship objectives: a systematic review and meta-analysis. Lancet Infect Dis 2016;16:847–56.
27. Nathwani D, Varghese D, Stephens J, et al. Value of hospital antimicrobial stewardship programs: a systematic review. Antimicrob Resist Infect Control 2019; 8:35.
28. Schweitzert VA, van Heijl I, van Werkhoven CH, et al. The quality of studies evaluating antimicrobial stewardship interventions: a systematic review. Clin Microbiol Infect 2019;25:555–61.
29. de Man P, Verhoeven BAN, Verbrugh HA, et al. An antibiotic policy to prevent emergence of resistant bacilli. Lancet 2000;355:973–8.
30. Lewis GJ1, Fang X, Gooch M, et al. Decreased resistance of Pseudomonas aeruginosa with restriction of ciprofloxacin in a large teaching hospital's intensive care and intermediate care units. Infect Control Hosp Epidemiol 2012;33(4): 368–73.
31. White AC Jr, Atmar RL, Wilson J. Effects of requiring prior authorization for selected antimicrobials: expenditures, susceptibilities, and clinical outcomes. Clin Infect Dis 1997;25:230–9.
32. Singh N, Rogers P, Atwood CW, et al. Short-course empiric antibiotic therapy for patients with pulmonary infiltrates in the intensive care unit. A proposed solution for indiscriminate antibiotic prescription. Am J Respir Crit Care Med 2000;162: 505–11.
33. Chastre J, Wolff M, Fagon JY, et al. Comparison of 8 vs 15 days of antibiotic therapy for ventilator-associated pneumonia in adults: a randomized trial. JAMA 2003;290(19):2588–98.
34. Kim JW, Chung J, Choi SH, et al. Early use of imipenem and vancomycin followed b de-escalation versus conventional antimicrobials without de-escalation for patients with HAP in a medical ICU: a randomize trial. Crit Care 2012;16:R28.
35. Leone M, Bechis C, Baumstarck K, et al. De-escalation versus continuation of empirical antimicrobial treatment in severe sepsis: a multicenter non-blinded randomized noninferiority trial. Intensive Care Med 2014;40:1399–408.
36. Dortch MJ, Fleming SB, Kauffmann RM, et al. Infection reduction strategies including antibiotic stewardship protocols in surgical and trauma intensive care units are associated with reduced resistant gram-negative healthcare-associated infections. Surg Infect (Larchmt) 2011;12(1):15–25.

37. Nowak MA, Nelson RE, Breidenbach JL, et al. Clinical and economic outcomes of a prospective antimicrobial stewardship program. Am J Health Syst Pharm 2012; 69:1500–8.
38. Diaz Granados CA. Prospective audit for antimicrobial stewardship in intensive care: impact on resistance and clinical outcomes. Am J Infect Control 2012;40: 526–9.
39. Wang J, Uy X, Shou J, et al. Impact of antimicrobial stewardship managed by clinical pharmacists on antibiotic use and drug resistance in a Chinese hospital, 2010-2016: a retrospective observational study. BMJ Open 2019;9:e026072.
40. Stulz JS, Arnold SR, Shelton CM, et al. Antimicrobial stewardship impact on Pseudomonas aeruginosa susceptibility to meropenem at a tertiary pediatric institution. Am J Infect Control 2019;47:1513–5.
41. Hernandez-Santiago V, Davey PG, Nathwani D, et al. Changes in resistance among coliform bacteraemia associated with a primary care antimicrobial stewardship intervention: A population-based interrupted time series study. PLoS Med 2019;16:e1002825.
42. Hecker MT, Son AH, Murphy NN, et al. Impact of syndrome-specific stewardship interventions on use of and resistance to fluoroquinolones: an interrupted time series analysis. Am J Infect Control 2019;47:869–75.
43. Abbarra S, Pitsch A, Jochmans S, et al. Impact of a multimodal strategy combining a new standard of care and restriction of carbapenems, fluroquinolones, and cephalosporins on antibiotic consumption and resistance of Pseudomonas aeruginosa in a French intensive care unit. Inter J Antimicrob Agents 2019;53:416–22.
44. Lee RA, Scully MC, Camins BC, et al. Improvement of gram-negative susceptibility to fluoroquinolones after implementation foa pre-authorization fluoroquinolone use; a decade-long experience. Infect Control Hosp Epidemiol 2018;39:1419–24.
45. Kinnear CL, Patel TS, Young CL, et al. Impact of an antimicrobial stewardship intervention on within-and between-patient daptomycin resistance in vancomycin-resistance *Enterococcus faecium*. Antimicrobial Agents Chemother 2019;63:e01800–18.
46. Rahal JJ, Urban C, Segal-Maurer S. Nosocomial antibiotic resistance in multiple gram-negative species: experience at one hospital with squeezing the resistance balloon at multiple sites. Clin Infect Dis 2002;34(4):499–503.
47. Spellberg B, Rice LB. Duration of antibiotic therapy: shorter is better. Ann Intern Med 2019;171(3):210–1.
48. Sawyer RG, Claridge JA, Nathens AB, et al. Trial of short-course antimicrobial. Therapy for intraabdominal infection. N Engl J Med 2015;372:1996–2005.
49. Available at: https://cc.bingj.com/cache.aspx?q=disarm+act+2019&d=4990417076293973&mkt=en-US&setlang=en-US&w=ag5TKbDgNBndYR_qJdQytr0USGITvgSx. Accessed December 24, 2019
50. Fishman N. Antimicrobial stewardship. Am J Med 2006;119:S53–61.
51. Stenehjem E, Hyun DY, Septimus E, et al. Antibiotic stewardship in small hospitals: barriers and potential solutions. Clin Infect Dis 2017;65(4):691–6.
52. Beaulac K, Corcione S, Epstein L, et al. Antimicrobial stewardship in a long-term acute care hospital using offsite electronic medical record audit. Infect Control Hosp Epidemiol 2016;37(4):433–9.
53. dos Santos RP, Deutschendorf C, Carvalho O, et al. Antimicrobial stewardship through telemedicine in a community hospital in Southern Brazil. J Telemed Telecare 2013;19(1):1–4.

54. Strymish J, Gupte G, Afable MK, et al. Electronic consultations (E-consults): advancing infectious disease care in a large veterans affairs healthcare system. Clin Infect Dis 2017;64(8):1123–5.
55. Yam P, Fales D, Jemison J, et al. Implementation of an antimicrobial stewardship program in a rural hospital. Am J Health Syst Pharm 2012;69(13):1142–8.
56. Wilson BM, Banks RE, Cnich CJ, et al. Changes in antibiotic use following implementation of a telehealth stewardship pilot program. Infect Control Hosp Epidemiol 2019;40:810–4.
57. Assimacopoulos A, Alam R, Arbo M, et al. A brief retrospective review of medical records comparing outcomes for inpatients treated via telehealth versus in-person protocols: is telehealth equally effective as in-person visits for treating neutropenic fever, bacterial pneumonia, and infected bacterial wounds? Telemed J E Health 2008;14:762–8.
58. Monkowski D, Rhodes LV, templer S, et al. A retrospective cohort study to assess the impact of an inpatients infectious disease telemedicine consultation service on hospital and patient outcomes. Clin Infect Dis 2019. https://doi.org/10.1093/cid/ciz293.

Emerging Issues in Antifungal Resistance

John R. Perfect, MD[a,*], Mahmoud Ghannoum, PhD[b]

KEYWORDS

• Fungi • Drug resistance • Invasive fungal disease • Antifungal agents

KEY POINTS

- Invasive fungal diseases continue to cause substantial mortality in the enlarging immunocompromised population.
- It is fortunate that the field has moved past amphotericin B deoxycholate as the only available antifungal drug but clearly, despite new classes of antifungal agents, both primary and secondary drug resistance in molds and yeasts abound.
- From the rise of multiple-drug–resistant *Candida auris* to the agrochemical selection of environmental azole-resistant *Aspergillus fumigatus*, it is and will be critical to understand antifungal drug resistance and both prevent and treat it with new strategies and agents.

INTRODUCTION

This review attempts to frame the issues around antifungal drug resistance. From its epidemiology, mechanisms, measurements, and clinical significance, invasive fungal diseases (IFDs) and their resistance to treatment have never been more important with the enlarging, fragile immunocompromised patient populations. With only 3 major classes of antifungal drugs for IFDs and at times their poor fungicidal activity, failures of treatment continue to abound. How to recognize, measure, and respond to antifungal drug resistance will be necessary for improvement of managing patients with severe underlying diseases. Unlike bacteria, fungi possess no clinically relevant drug-resistant plasmids or transposons that are passed from strain to strain. As discussed, however, these eukaryotic pathogens have dynamic genomes and stealth tools to resist and survive under the stresses of the human host immunity and treatment with antifungal drugs. Antifungal drug resistance must be overcome in the clinics, and this effort begins with knowledge of what it is.

J.R. Perfect Conflicts: Consultant/Research Grants: Merck, Pfizer, Astellas, Scynexis, F2G, Appili, Matinas, Amplyx, and Cidara.

[a] Trent Drive, Hanes House, Duke University Medical Center, Durham, NC 27710, USA; [b] Center for Medical Mycology, Case Western Reserve University, University Hospitals Cleveland, Cleveland, OH 44106, USA

* Corresponding author.

E-mail address: Perfe001@mc.duke.edu

Infect Dis Clin N Am 34 (2020) 921–943
https://doi.org/10.1016/j.idc.2020.05.003

DEFINITION OF DRUG RESISTANCE

The mainstay measurement of defining whether a strain isolated from a patient with IFD is susceptible or resistant to a given antifungal agent is the in vitro minimum inhibitory concentration (MIC) and associated interpretive breakpoint for the different drugs. To aid clinicians in managing patients with IFDs, over the past 2 decades, the Clinical and Laboratory Standards Institute (CLSI), previously National Committee for Clinical Laboratory Standards, and various associated working groups have established standardized susceptibility testing methods with interpretive breakpoints for both yeasts and molds[1,2] for a vast majority of clinically available antifungals (fluconazole, voriconazole, echinocandins, and so forth). In certain cases (such as rare yeasts and molds), however, no interpretive breakpoints are available. To address this gap, CLSI established epidemiologic cutoff values (ECVs), defined as the MIC or minimal effective concentration that separates a population into isolates with and those without acquired or mutational resistance based on their phenotypic MIC value.[3,4] ECV represents an alternative value to determine whether an isolate is wild type (ie, possibly susceptible) with respect to its in vitro response to a given antifungal agent. The usefulness of an ECV to guide patient management lies in its ability to predict a given isolate's possible resistance to an antifungal agent that has been demonstrated to possess some inhibition against the species but for which there are not enough data to establish specific clinical breakpoints. It is important to stress, however, that the predictability of therapeutic success/failure in response to the administration of a specific antifungal agent depends, in addition to the MIC value for the infecting strain, on host factors, such as the clinical status of a patient (eg, immunocompromised state), presence of foreign material (eg, indwelling catheter), and location of infection.[5,6]

More than 2 decades ago, Rex and colleagues[7] suggested that in vitro antifungal susceptibility testing was approaching the 90-60 rule that was appreciated in antibacterial susceptibility testing. In this rule, 90% of susceptible isolates responded to therapy and 60% of resistant isolates had a successful outcome. It may not be as exact in IFDs because the underlying disease so vividly controls outcome, but the general principle continues to hold today, that, with serious IFDs, an MIC evaluation of the fungal pathogen provides clinicians with important but not perfect insights to drug resistance.

EPIDEMIOLOGY OF FUNGAL DRUG RESISTANCE

In 1999, Ghannoum and Rice[8] wrote a review that compared the status of antifungals with antibacterials by focusing on their modes of action and mechanisms of resistance. At that time, most of the attention was devoted to the study of antibiotic resistance in bacteria. In contrast, the study of antifungal drug resistance lagged behind. In the past 2 decades, however, IFDs are now recognized as serious infections with high associated morbidity and mortality with significant clinical impact and cost to the health care system. Additionally, although early resistance studies were focused around those caused by *Candida albicans* largely due to mucosal disease in human immunodeficiency virus, an increase in resistant fungal infections caused by non-*albicans Candida* spp (eg, *C glabrata*),[9] molds including *Aspergillus*,[10,11] *Lomentospora* (formerly *Scedosporium*) *prolificans*, and *Fusarium solani* were noted. An increase in these fungal infections in the immunosuppressed population was accompanied by a simultaneous increase in issues around primary antifungal resistance.[12,13]

Until recently, the pattern of antifungal drug resistance was limited to resistance to 1 antifungal class (ie, although a fungal strain may be resistant to an azole, it was susceptible to an echinocandin). This changed in 2009 with the emergence of *C auris* and

C glabrata.[14] The specific emergence of the multidrug-resistant *C auris* represented a paradigm shift in the way antifungal drug resistance was considered. Although for years multidrug resistance was confined to antibacterials, this example was a fungal species that had both susceptible and multidrug-resistant strains. To face this emerging health threat, the Centers for Disease Control and Prevention (CDC) strongly encouraged all US-based laboratories that identify *C auris* to notify their state/local public health authorities as well as the CDC as a reportable fungal infection. The recent epidemiology clearly demonstrates that resistance to antifungals represents a serious threat for IFD management. With the rise of echinocandins as first-line therapy for invasive candidiasis, cancer units and intensive care units began to see echinocandin-resistant *Candida* spp, and at its peak 1 medical center reported 14% of bloodstream isolates with the haploid yeast *C glabrata* were resistant to echinocandins both in vitro and in vivo.[15] Finally, the threat of antifungal resistance even in superficial fungal infections continues to evolve as is evidenced by recent reports coming out of India and Japan[16] as well as the United States (Barbara Elewski and Mahmoud Ghannoum, unpublished data, 2019) of resistant *Trichophyton* spp isolated from cutaneous infections. These discoveries emphasize the need for vigilance and close monitoring of antifungal resistance patterns and new antifungal agents.

ANTIFUNGAL DRUG TARGETS AND SPECIFIC MECHANISMS OF RESISTANCE

Antifungal Targets

Historically, fungal membrane sterols and fungal cell walls represented fungal inhibition targets. Azoles, polyenes, and allyamines targeted the former, whereas echinocandins interfered with the latter. The pyrimidine pathway in its nucleic acid formation was an additional fungal target inhibited by flucytosine. The initial promise of this specific antifungal agent was diminished, however, by its high prevalence of primary and secondary resistance for many fungal species. The resultant emergence of resistance to high-use azoles has intensified the search for new compounds that are active against drug-resistant fungi, and echinocandins have seen increases in the clinical appearance of resistant strains. To respond to the unmet need for new antifungal agents, several pharmaceutical/biotech companies initiated research and development programs aimed at developing new antifungal drugs with new targets or better agents within old classes. These efforts led to several investigational drugs, such as isavuconazole, which inhibits ergosterol synthesis (approved by the Food and Drug Administration [FDA] for the treatment of invasive aspergillosis and invasive mucormycosis), and oteseconazole (VT-1161), an orally administered inhibitor of cytochrome (CYP [cytochrome P450])51. This compound circumvents one of the main limitations of the azole class of antifungals, which is drug-drug interactions. To overcome this problem, chemists substituted the triazole metal-binding group with a tetrazole that binds less avidly to both Cyp51 enzyme (the active site) and mammalian CYP enzymes. In addition, the portion of the drug that is recognized by amino acids of the substrate-binding site within this enzyme also was modified. These alterations resulted in molecules with more specific inhibition of fungal Cyp51 compared with mammalian CYP enzymes, thereby reducing drug-drug interactions.[17,18]

Other investigational antifungals under development include rezafungin and ibrexafungerp, both of which inhibit the enzyme 1,3-beta-D-glucan synthase critical for fungal cell wall synthesis. The former was structurally modified to confer a long half-life (>80 hours),[19] which may allow for less-frequent intravenous dosing (eg, once or twice weekly). Ibrexafungerp, structurally different from other echinocandins, has the ability to be absorbed via the gastrointestinal tract, thus making it the only orally available glucan synthase inhibitor. Potentially, it could be used in echinocandin-resistant yeast and mold infections.[20]

Unlike the antifungals, discussed previously, several other investigational antifungals under development target new fungal sites. For example, olorofim inhibits the oxidoreductase enzyme, dihydroorotate dehydrogenase, which is important for pyrimidine biosynthesis.[21] Fosmanogepix targets glycosylphosphatidylinositol-anchored proteins by inhibiting inositol acyltransferase,[22] thus preventing the maturation of these proteins. Finally, an allylamine compound that is still in early development is T-2307. This compound causes collapse of fungal mitochondrial membrane potential and is preferentially taken up by fungal cells compared with mammalian cells via transporter-mediated systems.[23] Readers interested in a more in-depth discussion of the mechanisms of action of different antifungal agents are referred to the following review by Perfect.[24]

Specific Mechanisms of Resistance

Azole resistance in Candida species

It is now well established that azole resistance resides mainly in non-*albicans* species, which is a reflection of the change in the epidemiology of *Candida* species infections. In the early 1990s, yeast infections were caused mainly by *C albicans.* The incidence of invasive candidiasis, however, now is commonly due to non-*albicans* species, such as *C glabrata*, *C parapsilosis*, and *C tropicalis*. This change in the epidemiology of *Candida* infections has been a direct correlation to the increase in azole resistance among non-*albicans* species seen around the world.[25,26] Because the ergosterol pathway is shared by these yeast species, the observed resistance is too often pan-azole (ie, a strain with elevated MIC to fluconazole usually has elevated MICs to the other members of this class of antifungal agents). An exception is *C krusei*, in which its 14α-demethylase is poorly inhibited specifically by fluconazole.[27]

Table 1 summarizes the different mechanisms underlying azole resistance in *Candida* spp. As can be seen, azole-resistant strains either exhibit a modification in the quality/quantity of target enzyme, reduced access to the fungal target, or some combination of these mechanisms.

Mechanisms underlying azole resistance in *C auris* were investigated recently by Lockhart and colleagues[33] and other investigators,[34] who identified Erg11 amino acid substitutions (eg, F126T, Y132F, and K143R) in clinically resistant strains of *C auris* from South Africa, Venezuela, India, and Pakistan. These substitutions were associated with elevated azole MICs. In contrast, a wild-type *ERG11* genotype was reported in 4 of 5 isolates exhibiting low-fluconazole MICs (1–2 μg/mL).[35] Moreover, expression of alleles encoding I466M, Y501H, or other clade-defined amino acid differences yielded susceptible MICs. These studies demonstrate that *C auris* shares mechanisms of azole resistance similar to other *Candida* spp, namely, specific *ERG11* mutations leading to reduced susceptibility to this class of compounds.

Echinocandin-resistant Candida

Mutations in the *FKS* gene, which encodes 1,3-beta-glucan synthase, the target of echinocandins, represent the main underlying mechanism of echinocandin resistance in *Candida*. This underlying resistance mechanism is conferred by limited amino acid substitutions in the Fks subunits of the glucan synthase.[36] In a majority of *Candida* spp, these mutations occur in 2 highly conserved hot-spot regions of FKS1[37,38] incorporating Phe641–Pro649 and Arg1361 residues. Equivalent regions of FKS2 occur in *C glabrata*. The amino acid substitutions decrease sensitivity of the target enzyme

Table 1
Azole resistance mechanisms in *Candida* species**

Mechanism	Caused by	Remarks
Alteration in drug target (14α-demethylase)	Mutations that alter drug binding but not binding of the endogenous substrate	Target is active (ie, can catalyze demethylation) but has a reduced affinity toward azoles
Alteration in sterol biosynthesis	Lesions in the D5(6)-desaturase	Results in accumulation of 14α-methyl fecosterol instead of ergosterol
Transcription factor; regulatory control	UpC is a Zn (II)-Cys6 transcription factor that regulates ERG and transporter genes expression	Overexpression of UpC increases fluconazole resistance; absence of UpC makes strains hypersusceptible
Reduction in the intercellular concentration of target enzyme	Change in membrane lipid and sterols; overexpression of specific drug efflux pumps (CDR1, PDR5, and BENr)	Poor penetration across the fungal membrane; active drug efflux
Overexpression of antifungal drug target	Increased copy number of the target enzyme	Results in increased ergosterol synthesis; contributes to cross-resistance between fluconazole and itraconazole

**References in support of these mechanisms.[27–32]

inhibition to an antifungal echinocandin by up to 3000-fold,[39] with 100-fold increase in MIC values. The most important changes in *C glabrata* are at amino acid Ser645 and for *C albicans*, amino acid changes at Fks 1 Ser645 and at Fks 2 Ser663 cause the most frequent and pronounced resistance phenotype.[40] As observed previously with azole-resistant strains, echinocandin-resistant isolates tend to lose some virulence attributes making them less pathogenic than the wild-type strains[41] but they still can cause disease.

RNA interference–dependent epimutation, a novel broad antifungal resistance mechanism in molds such as mucor

Recently, Calo and colleagues[42] described a novel antifungal drug resistance to FK506 and rapamycin developed through a transient mechanism evoked via RNA interference (RNAi)-dependent epimutations in *Mucor circinelloides*. Epimutations, selected by drug exposure, silence the drug target gene, which is re-expressed. This resistance phenotype is temporary as susceptibility to the drug is restored following passage of the strain in the absence of drug. The silencing process, which occurs via core RNAi pathway proteins, involves generation of small RNAs against the target gene attributable to extensive DNA methylation leading to gene silencing. In a subsequent study, epimutants that conferred resistance to the antifungal 5-fluoroorotic acid were isolated, confirming that epimutation may play a broad antifungal resistance role in *Mucor*,[43] which is known to be frequently resistant to antifungal agents. Moreover, the transient nature of epimutation provides the fungus with rapid, facile reversion and flexible responses for adaptation to stressful environments.

THE CLINICAL MICROBIOLOGY LABORATORY VALUE IN DRUG RESISTANCE DETERMINATION

The recent changes in antifungal resistance patterns highlighted by the emergence of the multidrug-resistant *C auris* and reports about resistant dermatophytes from India/Japan and the authors' own experience in the United States emphasize the need for increased vigilance and call for resistance monitoring of local hospitals to ensure that any evolving changes are not missed. It is prudent to call for performing antifungal susceptibility, particularly in cases of patients failing therapy, but many clinicians should consider in vitro susceptibility testing for all yeasts and molds causing serious IFDs. To achieve these goals, it is important that physicians and clinical laboratory personnel form close relationships for the benefit of complex patients The clinical microbiology laboratory provides a much-needed expertise in antifungal resistance determination in several ways that could help in the management of patients with IFDs, in particular those who are not responding to treatment. First, accurate diagnosis of the yeasts or molds identity can allow clinicians to predict drug susceptibility. Second, MIC data may provide therapeutic direction if isolate is susceptible or resistant to a given drug based on the CLSI interpretive breakpoints. In cases of such breakpoints not available, MICs can point treating clinicians to ECVs. As discussed previously, these values can guide patient management because of their ability to predict for a given isolate possible resistance to an antifungal agent with the absence of interpretive breakpoints. Reference mycology laboratories, due to their involvement in research and development of experimental antifungal agents, also can point the clinician to sponsors developing new agents and provide a possible compassionate use route into a management strategy of a devastating IFD that is not responding to currently available therapies.

THE EMERGING THREAT OF *CANDIDA AURIS*

C auris is a confirmed multidrug-resistant pathogen with global influence. It has been noted by the CDC as well as the World Health organization, Pan American Health Organization, and National Institute of Communicable Diseases of South Africa[44,45] as a drug-resistant threat. A majority of reported *C auris* infections have been nosocomial[46–48] and many strains are reported to be resistant to fluconazole, amphotericin B, and echinocandins, with variable resistance to members of the 3 major classes of clinically available antifungal agents. Some strains are resistant to all currently available antifungal agents, with limited treatment options.[49,50] Due to its relatively recent emergence, precise epidemiologic analysis of *C auris* transmission is ongoing and theories to its multicontinental emergence in 4 specific clades range from the increased use of systemic antifungal agents to a newly generated hypothesis regarding global warming.[51] Given the potential of *C auris* for high resistance to current therapies and as an infection control nuisance, identification of efficacious management options remain a critical gap in the current knowledge base regarding control of this growing threat.

Due to its ability to colonize cutaneous niches and fomites and the nosocomial infectious route with its high pathogenicity with subsequent high mortality, *C auris* is considered a severe public health threat.[45,49,52] The proposed human contact transmission typical of *C auris* is atypical of most other types of candidal infections that usually arise from a patient's commensal arsenal. Also unusual is the persistence exhibited by *C auris* on hardware surfaces, such as medical implants (ie, catheter surfaces...silicon elastomer) and structural surfaces (tables, chairs, handrails, and other fomites) found in hospitals.[53,54] The significance of hospitals as transmission routes should not be understated. The World Health Organization has reported that the highest prevalence of nosocomial infections occurs in intensive care units and in acute surgical and orthopedic wards. Infection rates are higher among patients with increased susceptibility because of old age, underlying diseases, or chemotherapy.[55] Among the most common routes of transmission for nosocomial infections are environmental surfaces in health care facilities and contact with health care workers.[56] Given that *C auris* appears to readily colonize various material surfaces, it was hypothesized that colonization may occur via biofilm formation; however, studies have demonstrated that *C auris* forms a less robust biofilm compared with *C albicans* on these surfaces.[57–59] Nevertheless, the ability to form biofilms by *C auris* has been suggested to account for some of the resistance to common antifungal therapies.[58,59]

In addition to general resistance to antifungal agents, *C auris* appears to evoke less innate immune defenses from infected hosts because neutrophil-mediated phagocytosis/killing of *C auris* was less robust compared with that of *C albicans*.[60] The precise mechanism(s) underlying this inability of neutrophils to efficiently attack *C auris*, its evasion of phagocytosis, and the general immune response to *C auris* infection are in need of further definitive studies.

One inherent problem in addressing *C auris* infection is the likely underestimate of its damage. Identification of *C auris* is complicated and often misdiagnosed, given its close genetic relationship to *C haemulonii*. Therefore, identification of *C auris* is challenging and a majority of isolates are misidentified by commercially available systems (VITEK, API 20 C AUX, and so forth); thus, molecular DNA sequencing methods are most precise in differentiating *C auris* from other *Candida* spp, and the actual current rates of *C auris* infection worldwide are likely to be under-reported.

Due to the overwhelming evidence regarding the high level of pathogenicity of *C auris*, it is clear that development of further measures to control and/or eradicate this yeast is necessary. The correct approach, however, depends on developing a strategy that will decolonize affected individuals. Several new therapeutics being developed to treat *C auris*, including ibrexafungerp,[57] fosmanogepix,[61] and rezafungin.[62] They are capable of killing *C auris* in systemic preclinical animal models but they fail to clear the skin. Thus, other more rigorous measures must be sought that show greater promise for cutaneous yeast clearance.

Finally, the CDC recommends that all *C auris* isolates should be tested for antifungal susceptibility using CLSI guidelines. Because there currently are no established *C auris*–specific susceptibility breakpoints, clinical microbiology laboratories should determine whether an isolate is susceptible or resistant to a given antifungal based on breakpoints established for closely-related *Candida* spp as well as on the expert opinion of a medical mycologist.[63] The CDC encourages all US laboratory staff who identify *C auris* to notify their state or local public health authorities and CDC at candidaauris@cdc.gov.

ASPERGILLUS RESISTANCE TO DRUGS

The primary treatment of invasive aspergillosis generally includes a triazole, but over the past decade the identification of azole-resistance *Aspergillus fumigatus* strains has increased in those with chronic pulmonary aspergillosis or those at risk for infection and exposed to locations in which the environment has been heavily exposed to agricultural azole fungicides.[64,65] For instance, the Netherlands has been identified particularly for their triazole-resistant strains in both the agricultural environment and concordantly certain high-risk patient populations,[65] but it may become a worldwide problem.[11]

An in vitro phenotypic assessment for drug resistance using established in vitro susceptibility testing has determined a breakpoint MIC at 2 μg/mL for voriconazole with isolates over this MIC considered to be clinically resistant.[66] Many of the isolates show specific mutations in the azole target Cyp5IA gene, such as TR_{34}/L98H or TR_{46}/YI2IF/T289A.[67] Approximately 80% of isolates appear to possess a pan-triazole–resistant phenotype (itraconazole, voriconazole, isavuconazole, and posaconazole).[67] This is easy to understand because the target of the triazole is the Cyp5IA enzyme but approximately 20% of isolates of *A fumigatus* appear to possess uncharacterized resistance mutation outside the target gene or are possibly mixed infections. The clinical relevance of this azole resistance phenotype has recently been validated in a multicenter retrospective cohort study.[66] It showed that triazole-resistant *Aspergillus* strains compare to triazole-susceptible ones have a 21% to 25% increased mortality and, after 10 days of inappropriate therapy, even switching to appropriate therapy did not improve outcome. These results have caused hospitals in regions with high-frequency environmental triazole resistance to consider switching from empirical triazole prophylaxis and treatment to either combination antifungal therapy or liposomal amphotericin B when the incidence of azole-resistant *A fumigatus* has risen to 10% or above in frequency.[10,68] The exact recommendation for treatment remains controversial, however, in these areas of high-level azole resistance.

Cryptic species of *Aspergillus* can have variable drug resistance. For instance, *A terreus* and to some extent *A flavus* have a polyene-resistant phenotype, and other species like *A calidoustus* and *A lentulus* can be pan-resistant to current antifungal agents.

Therefore, it seems clear that, when available, in vitro susceptibility testing should be performed on *Aspergillus* isolates from deep or sterile body sites and, similarly, proper identification of all *Aspergillus* isolates to species level helps predict antifungal susceptibility and helps select initial antifungal regimen. In seriously ill patients and those with a known environmental epidemiology of resistance, clinicians may choose initial combination therapy.

CRYPTOCOCCUS NEOFORMANS AND *CRYPTOCOCCUS GATTII* ANTIFUNGAL RESISTANCE

Methods for in vitro susceptibility testing for both *Cryptococcus neoformams* and *Cryptococcus gattii* have been standardized and ECVs to azoles have been established. By molecular techniques, most relapsed isolates represent the primary isolate rather than the appearance of a new isolate.[69] It is true that there may be some correlation between MICs and clinical resistance but there are so many factors in cryptococcal meningoencephalitis failures, including the host and the plasticity of the cryptococcal genome, that there has not yet been created a specific robust therapeutic MIC breakpoint for azoles against *Cryptococcus*.[5,70,71] Some resistance guidelines have suggested that a greater than 3-fold rise in MIC of a persistent or relapse isolate compared with original isolate to the antifungal drug[72] or with a single MIC, such as flucytosine greater than or equal to 128 μg/mL or fluconazole at greater than or equal to 16 μg/mL, there might be consideration of a drug-resistant strain. The 16-μg/mL fluconazole MIC is always a difficult MIC to consider if it is resistant, but most clinicians increase fluconazole dosing when faced with this specific MIC. Frequently, voriconazole follows fluconazole MICs except for generally lower MICs but occasionally strains are less resistant to posaconazole and itraconazole. For instance, a Y145F alteration in ERGII gene makes a strain resistant to fluconazole and voriconazole but very susceptible to posaconazole and itraconazole.[73] Most primary cryptococcal isolates do not show drug-resistant phenotypes,[74] but, with drug exposure through treatments, these yeasts can change rapidly and increase their resistance.

Many mechanisms for drug resistance in *Cryptococcus* are known.[75] First, flucytosine resistance is well known in that it is a mutation in the pyrimidine pathway (cytosine permease, cytosine deaminase, and uracil phosphoribosyltransferase [FURI])[76,77] and occurs at a rate of 1 in 10^{6-7} colonies, so this drug cannot be used as monotherapy for meningitis. Second, occasionally in severely immunosuppressed patients with substantial polyene exposure, a strain develops amphotericin B resistance,[78] through a mutation in the ergosterol pathway.[79] Fluconazole resistance has a variety of mechanisms. Details of azole tolerance and heteroresistance in cryptococcus are discussed later. Drug resistance, however, has been described by overexpression and duplication of the target ERGII gene encoding the 14α-demethylase protein in ergosterol synthesis, mutations in the ERGII gene (ie G3445, Y145F, and G484S),[80] and through augmentation of drug efflux pumps (Afrl, Afr2, and Mdrl) through mutations or duplications with Afr1 as the major efflux pump, but others (Afr2 and Mdrl) can be additive.[81] Also, expression of these efflux pumps in *Cryptococcus* can occur with agrochemical exposures leading to resistant strains.[82]

Although *Cryptococcus gattii* has been less studied than *Cryptococcus neoformans*, it is likely to have similar mechanisms for drug resistance. There are some in vitro studies that suggest *Cryptococcus gattii* in general might have higher MICs.[83] This not always is consistent, however, and as yet all clinical data suggest that these 2 species can be treated with similar antifungal drugs and regimens.

THE CONCEPT AND REALITY OF TOLERANCE AND HETERORESISTANCE IN *CANDIDA* AND *CRYPTOCOCCUS*

Much of antifungal drug resistance revolves around formalized MICs and described clinical breakpoints for efficacy. Yeast growth versus no growth, however, with some drugs is not quite as simplistic. There is the ability to quantify yeast growth above the MIC of fluconazole. For instance, tolerance is defined as slow growth of subpopulations of yeast cells that can overcome the azole drug stresses more efficiently than the rest of the yeast population and can be observed for each strain. The growth inversely correlates with intracellular drug accumulation. In elegant and important studies, Rosenberg and colleagues,[84] with *C albicans*, measured each strain's quantitative tolerance to fluconazole exposure. They found a correlation between more azole-tolerant strains and persistent candidemia under azole therapy. For years, MIC measurements have been the marker for resistant strains and clinicians tend to minimize or ignore tolerance cells or trailing growth above the MIC. These yeast cells generally are not quantitated by the clinical laboratories; yet, frequently patients respond to fluconazole treatment in a fungistatic manner. These trailing growth yeast cells are sensitive to environmental conditions and importantly it has been shown that the slow-growing tolerant population of yeast cells frequently can be eliminated by the use of combination therapy with different mechanisms of action. This ability to utilize combination therapy, such as fluconazole with flucytosine or inhibitors of Hsp90, calcineurin, or TOR, to help eliminate the slow-growing cell populations constituting the trailing endpoint is likely an important goal. This subpopulation of tolerant yeast cells has been shown to be important for treatment success[84] and has not yet been measured for individual strains in the clinics. The quantitation of tolerance for certain antifungal agents for each strain may have importance to clinicians and in the future may be reported like MICs.

In sum, tolerance is a phenomenon for yeast exposure to azoles: (1) it is a subpopulation effect, and the size of the subpopulation is stable within a strain but may vary between strains; (2) it is due to slow yeast growth during drug stress; (3) exact mechanisms are not certain but correlate with drug levels; (4) it is dependent on stress response pathways; (5) it is mechanistically distinct from direct resistance; and (6) it has therapeutic relevance.

A second mechanism used by yeasts to protect themselves from an azole exposure is heteroresistance.[85–88] This is a different concept from tolerance in that these subpopulations of yeasts grow as well as resistant yeast cells above the MIC for the strain. The demonstration of heteroresistance to fluconazole has been elegantly described in *C neoformans*. In early studies by Sionov and colleagues,[89,90] it was reported that heteroresistant yeast colonies were observed above the MIC but these colonies did not have the same stable resistance seen as true resistant strains. On subculture, these yeast subpopulations without azole exposure reverted back to susceptible yeast subpopulations.

In a series of elegant experiments, it was shown that under stress the plasticity of the cryptococcal genome was remarkable and that this subpopulation was aneuploidy with duplication of chromosomes[91]; particularly enriched was chromosome I containing the ERGII gene, encoding the 14α-demethylase target for fluconazole and the AFR1 gene, which encodes a drug efflux pump. These features allowed the fungus to survive the azole antifungal activity. Also, it has been shown mechanistically that an apoptosis pathway controlled by the AFR1 gene may suppress the heteroresistant yeast growth and when *AIF 1* is inactivated or reduced heteroresistant colonies are more common.[92] These subpopulations clearly increased their resistance to fluconazole and grow well above the MICs but they also were unstable and without selection they would remove the extrachromosomal material and then show susceptible MICs. Importantly, these investigators showed the development of high level heteroresistance populations during the stress of infection in mice treated with fluconazole. These findings suggested potential clinical relevance to heteroresistance mechanisms. Stone and colleagues[86] proved this relevance with experiments in which yeasts were cultured directly onto fluconazole plate in patients with cryptococcal meningitis treated with fluconazole monotherapy. They clearly demonstrated these frequent heteroresistant colonies growing in the presence of fluconazole and mechanistically confirmed the dynamic ploidy changes in these heteroresistant colonies with frequent duplications of chromosome I in the isolates. They also found that under azole stress all their clinical strains could produce heteroresistant colonies. Importantly and similar to tolerant yeast populations, they were able to rapidly eliminate these heteroresistant populations if patients were treated with both fluconazole and another agent, such as flucytosine, in combination. Further results clearly explain the poor clinical response to fluconazole monotherapy[93] and support the potential importance of combination therapy for cryptococcal meningoencephalitis if fluconazole is considered in primary induction therapy.[94] The recent Antifungal Combination for Treatment in Africa study in cryptococcal meningitis supports the use of fluconazole plus flucytosine by examining cerebrospinal fluid (CSF) yeast cultures and outcomes.[95] Heteroresistance and its mechanisms clearly show how yeasts like *Cryptococcus* use their dynamic genetic machinery to respond to stresses on a real-time basis.[86,96]

Both the tolerant subpopulations of *C albicans* and the heteroresistant colonies of *Cryptococcus neoformans* represent transient events allowing yeasts to survive in the presence of high concentrations of an azole. They are not the stable mechanisms of target mutations and alterations or development of efflux pumps and standard MICs do not precisely measure them. They have been clearly shown, however, to have clinical relevance that needs to be considered in the composite resistance phenotype and both measured and understood with each infecting strain as a reason for monotherapy failure.

CLINICAL RESISTANCE

When reports show that invasive fungal infections have such high mortality rates, which can range from 20% to 50% for certain fungi, it suggests substantial antifungal drug resistance and, although specific primary and secondary antifungal drug resistance does occur and develop, that a majority of patients with an invasive mycosis develop what is called "clinical resistance" that cannot be detected by in vitro susceptibility testing or a comparative animal model study. Clinical resistance is not as precise as an in vitro susceptibility testing breakpoint but it is important and can occur under multiple circumstances.[97] The following 9 factors specifically define the clinical resistance phenotype:

- First, an incorrect diagnosis can cause resistance to therapy. This may manifest itself when another unsuspected and untreated pathogen also is producing disease. The most common scenario, however, in the immunocompromised population for the clinical resistance phenotype is the immune reconstitution inflammatory syndrome. It is associated with prominent signs and symptoms of uncontrolled inflammation without a specific test to precisely identify it. It can be confused with failure to control fungal growth.[98]
- Second, the net state of a patient's immunosuppression is so negative that antifungal agents cannot overcome the lack of an effective host immune response. For example, treatment of invasive aspergillosis in neutropenic patients fails if host leukocytes do not return to an acceptable level. Similarly, during the acquired immunodeficiency syndrome pandemic before antiretroviral therapy, cryptococcal meningitis treatment had a miserable success rate without treatment of the immunosuppressive condition. Utilization of correct antifungal agents can push infection in the right direction but requires a competent or improving host response for cure.
- Third, the inoculum of fungus in the host may become a critical factor in resistance to treatment. For instance, multiple studies have confirmed the importance of early antifungal therapy for candidemia and improved outcome.[99,100] Similarly, in cryptococcal meningitis, a higher burden of yeasts in the subarachnoid space at the beginning of therapy can predict treatment failure.[101]
- Fourth, the intrinsic pathogenicity or virulence of the fungal strain may produce a resistance to treatment that is not directly appreciated in antifungal susceptibility testing. This area of strain diversity and virulence attributes continues to be actively investigated in this age of whole-genome sequencing. Genetic factors within the fungus controlling outcome, however, are starting to be determined. For example, the natural creation of a recombinant *Cryptococcus gattii* strain produced a more virulent strain that helped produced a widespread outbreak in the US Pacific Northwest/Canada[102]; recent work suggests that certain cryptococcal genotypes have been correlated with increased host mortality.[103]
- Fifth, the impact of pharmacokinetics/pharmacodynamics can be utilized in understanding drug resistance. There have been multiple studies that have shown the importance of voriconazole use and therapeutic drug monitoring for a successful outcome.[104,105] Drug-resistant infections occur from poor drug absorption to host genetic differences in drug metabolism, causing reduced drug exposures. The importance of drug exposure to infection resistance must be

emphasized. Ideally, this is measured by achieving the highest drug area under the curve/MIC ratio for the azoles in treatment of invasive candidiasis.[6] Furthermore, in the era of polypharmacy, drug-drug interactions and direct drug toxicity can be major reasons for therapeutic failures and thus apparent drug resistance. From the added direct nephrotoxicity of the polyenes to drug-drug interactions impacting antifungal drug metabolism (eg, rifampin and azoles) to synergistic drug toxicity through QTc prolongation (azoles plus amiodarone),[106] antifungal drug toxicities and interactions play out daily on the clinical potential for antifungal treatment resistance.

- Sixth, the site of infection may have a major influence on drug resistance. For example, in central nervous system (CNS) fungal infections, it is encouraged to use azoles like fluconazole and voriconazole, which have higher CNS penetration[107] than the less CNS penetrating (lipophilic) azole agents or echinocandins. Furthermore, fungal cystitis is better treated with fluconazole, which is excreted in the urine over the other extended-spectrum azoles and echinocandins, which have poor urinary excretion. Another important site is the foreign body. The foreign body represents an ideal location for fungi to stick and form a biofilm. For instance, infected central venous catheters with hardware for attachment of fungi within biofilms produce a fungal community that is not easy to eliminate. Frequently, echinocandins and/or lipid formulations of amphotericin B are favored for treatment because these antifungal agents appear to have better impact on fungi in the biofilm state.[108] In this community, however, fungi frequently can be recalcitrant to direct antifungal therapies. The best way to care for a patient with hardware and biofilm organisms is simply to remove the hardware from the body. Numerous retrospective trials involving candidemia have shown high treatment failure and mortality without hardware removal of the catheter in catheter-related infections, but this strategy remains a contentious area because some catheters are not easy to remove and surely success has occurred with systemic antifungal therapy and catheter(s) remaining in place.[109] As a major potential area in clinical drug resistance research, a robust prospective, randomized trial of treatment of candidemia with or without catheter removal would be a major therapeutic advance.
- Seventh, the length of treatment can be a factor in drug resistance. This can occur in 2 ways. First, the patient and/or clinician becomes disengaged with the long treatment regimens and starts to reduce courses before clearance of infection is complete. Second, clinicians simply get nervous about persistent cultures and call treatment failures too early. For instance, 10% to 20% of patients have positive blood cultures at 4 days of treatment when either amphotericin B or an echinocandin is used in treatment of candidemia despite eventual successful management.[110] Many clinicians, however, consider failure with this length of persistent positive blood cultures. Many infectious diseases do not have precise lengths of therapy and, in fungal infections, this lack of careful studies for best lengths of therapy can manifest at the bedside as apparent drug resistance.
- Eighth, disseminated fungal infections live in the new age clinical world of "mibs, mabs, and nibs." These new anticancer and anti-inflammatory agents have in some patients produced collateral damage of IFDs. From the ibrutinib story with invasive CNS aspergillosis and cryptococcosis[111] to the anti–tumor necrosis factor and anti-CD52 therapies with associated IFDs, the ability to successfully manage IFDs while receiving these immunosuppressants is compromised. As is known from the old age of corticosteroids and calcineurin inhibitors, continuing full-dose immunosuppressants produces clinical resistance. On the other hand,

dropping these immunosuppressants too quickly can lead to immune reconstitution inflammatory syndrome. The pendulum of immunosuppression is a major factor in clinical resistance to IFDs and clinicians must be sure to identify the conundrum and balance it at the bedside.

- Ninth, a critical clinical resistance factor to successful management of IFDs is the successful management of the underlying disease. The underlying disease represents the barometer that measures failures or successes of most IFD management. The clinical resistance must be approached by either prevention of IFDs in high-risk patients or better control of underlying diseases when IFDs occur.

RESPONSE TO ANTIFUNGAL DRUG RESISTANCE—COMBINATION AGENTS AND NEW AGENTS WITH DIFFERENT FORMULATIONS, KINETICS OR TARGETS

With 3 major classes (polyenes, azoles, and echinocandins) and 2 minor classes (flucytosine and allylamine-terbinafine) of antifungal agents for IFDs, there always has been some consideration of combination antifungal agents for treatment regimens.[112,113] The rationale for combination antifungal drug agents includes reducing risk for antifungal resistance; potential for lower doses of agents to reduce significant side effects, either additive or synergistic antifungal activity to increase potency of therapy to reduce lengths of treatment; and, finally, widening the spectrum of empirical antifungal regimens. The challenges of antifungal combination therapy evaluation are substantial but their use in clinical practice frequently occurs.[114] The combination of amphotericin B or its lipid formulations plus flucytosine is the regimen of choice for induction therapy for cryptococcal meningitis. This regimen has 2 important features for its rationale. First, it is a potent fungicidal regimen, which improves the rapid killing of yeasts in CNS.[115,116] Second, it actually prevents the development of drug resistance. It has been known for years that *Cryptococcus* frequently can mutate within the pyrimidine pathway at a rate of $1 \times 10^{6-7}$ colony-forming units (CFUs), and cryptococcal infections can present with more than 1×10^{6} CFUs of yeasts in the CSF. This selection of a flucytosine-resistant clone during monotherapy is reasonable to predict. This has been the experience of flucytosine monotherapy, with frequent failures due to development of drug resistance of the strain. On the other hand, the use of flucytosine in combination with amphotericin B or fluconazole has made the development of flucytosine-resistant relapse strains rare.[115,116] Also, as discussed previously regarding tolerance phase for *C albicans* and heteroresistance for *Cryptococcus neoformans* under stress, the use of combination therapy with different mechanisms of action make these 2 growth phases neutralized in their impact on drug resistance.[86,94,95,117]

In mold infections, the prime example has been consideration of combination therapy for invasive aspergillosis. In some early animal studies, there was concern that azoles and polyenes both working on fungal cell membranes together could antagonize their individual actions.[118] It seemed that giving azoles first made the polyene less active. Twenty-years later, there seems to be no clinical evidence that this combination for IFDs is antagonistic in humans. On the other hand, the most common combination for invasive aspergillosis has been voriconazole (cell membrane target) and echinocandin (cell wall target). Unlike the combination for cryptococcal meningitis, the azole/echinocandin combination remains an alternative regimen. However, 3 areas support its use. First, in a large randomized study of invasive aspergillosis in heme-oncology patients who were diagnosed with probable aspergillosis by biomarkers, the combination produced better outcome than voriconazole monotherapy.[119] Second, in areas where there is high-level azole resistance in *A fumigatus* in the environment, initial therapy with combination of drugs is considered until susceptibility testing has been performed.[66] Third, there has been improved outcome reported for combination therapy as a salvage regimen.[120] Finally, there are cases where combination therapy is started when identification of the fungus and its general susceptibility results are still unknown. Even when known, combination therapy may be continued because of primary antifungal resistance to all classes of the fungus and the IFD is so serious that attempts to attack the fungus by several mechanisms are considered necessary.[121,122]

The second approach to antifungal drug resistance is to develop new antifungal drugs with different mechanism of antifungal activity. Both humans and fungi use similar eukaryotic machinery, so, despite a plethora of targets, there needs to be substantial selectivity toward the fungal target to avoid host toxicity. Some investigators have voiced skepticism about finding new antifungal agents because approximately 80% of antifungal targets in the literature turnout to be false positives with little potential to develop target-based inhibitors with desirable features.[123] The need for better antifungals is clearly documented and, despite the small number of patients with IFDs in the world to help Big Pharma acquire profits, the GAIN (Generating Antibiotic Incentives Now) Act, the Orphan Drug Act, and the Fast Track designation by the FDA for antifungal drug development have given an important economic boost, and there has been substantial promising early antifungal drug development. For instance, novel pathways and fungal targets have been investigated, such as pathways through calcineurin, Hsp90, sphingolipid synthesis, RAS and trehalose, have yielded interesting targets and inhibitors for future development.[124–128] The merger of molecular biology, structural biology, robust animal models, and in vitro screens has allowed a robust foundation for basic identification, validation, and inhibitor discovery available and active today. These targets likely are unique and able to be attacked in current drug-resistant strains.[24]

The antifungal field has progressed even further than targets and inhibitors and now has multiple agents in early clinical trials. The current drugs in study are as follows. (1) Olorofim (F2G) is a member of the new orotomide class that targets dihydroorotate dehydrogenase, which is critically involved in fungal pyrimidine biosynthesis.[21] It has potent anti-*Aspergillus* activity, including against azole-resistant strains and other molds and endemic mycoses, and is in clinical trials. It recently received FDA breakthrough status for refractory and primary resistance to available agents. (2) Fosmanogepix (Amplyx) is an inhibitor glycosyl phosphatidyl inositol synthesis within the fungal cell wall.[129] It has broad-spectrum antifungal activity against yeasts and molds. It also is in clinical studies for several fungal infections. (3) The allylamine T-2307 (Appili) is selectively transported into fungal cells and specifically inhibits the mitochondrial membrane potential.[130] With different targets, it appears that these 3 classes will provide excellent antifungal activity against current drug-resistant strains.

There are 5 drugs that use current target(s) but have unique features with which they could improve success in management of resistant IFDs. (1) Rezafungin is a very-long-acting echinocandin in clinical studies and attempts to optimize the long half-life to get better Pharmacokinetic/Pharmacodynamic (PK/PD) relationships in the clinic.[131] (2) SUBA-itraconazole (Mayne) is a new nanotechnology formulation of itraconazole.[132] It substantially improves the drug exposure compared with current formulations of itraconazole. This formulation is now FDA approved. (3) Cochleated amphotericin B formulation (Matinas) has a goal of treating IFDs orally with a product that allows systemic exposure to amphotericin B through the oral route.[133] (4) Ibrexafungerp (Scynexis-078) is a triterpene 1,3-beta-glucan synthase inhibitor and not an echinocandin. It has value in its oral bioavailability and there is not necessarily cross-resistance to the echinocandins. Therefore, this drug is being tested in clinical trials for both echinocandin-susceptible and echinocandin-resistant yeast and mold infections[134] (5) VT-1598 (Mycovia) is a broad-spectrum azole with a long half-life.[135] Importantly, it has been engineered so that much of the troublesome azole-drug interactions have been eliminated, which has the potential to reduce failures occurring within a patient's polypharmacy environment. Although this drug is still in early animal trials, a similar agent, oteseconazole, already has positive findings in the treatment of superficial fungal infections.[136]

Finally, there are creative studies to meet the demand of treating resistant IFDs, from adoptive transfer of activated immune cells[137] to biphasic molecules attaching antifungals to host cells/proteins to deliver the pay load at the site of infection.[138] There also are antibody studies to augment killing of fungi[139] or direct delivery of an antifungal compound to the fungal surface.[140] Finally, there is the development of fungal vaccines.[141]

SUMMARY

IFDs continue to cause substantial mortality in the enlarging immunocompromised population. It is fortunate that the field has moved past amphotericin B deoxycholate as the only available antifungal drug but clearly, despite new classes of antifungal agents, both primary and secondary drug resistance in molds and yeasts abound. From the rise of multiple-drug–resistant *C auris* to the agrochemical selection of environmental azole-resistant *A fumigatus*, it is and will be critical to understand antifungal drug resistance and both prevent and treat it with new strategies and agents. The challenges are clear; the tools are here; and its fear must be controlled.

REFERENCES

1. Clinical and Laboratory Standards Institute Reference Method for Broth Dilution Antifungal Susceptibility Testing of Yeast; approval standard. Wayne (PA): 2008. 3rd edition: M27-A23.
2. Clinical and Laboratory Standards Institute. Reference method for Broth Dilution Antifungal Susceptibility Testing for Filamentos Fungi (Moulds) that cause invasive and cutaneous fngal infections. Wayne (PA): 2017. 3rd edition. M38.
3. Lockhart SR, Ghannoum MA, Alexander BD. Establishment and use of epidemiological cutoff values for molds and yeasts by use of the clinical and laboratory standards institute M57 standard. J Clin Microbiol 2017;55(5):1262–8.
4. Clinical and Laboratory Standards Institute. Principles and procedures for the developmennt of epidemiological cutoff values for antiifungal susceptibility testing. Wayne (PA): 2016.
5. Witt MD, Lewis RJ, Larsen RA, et al. Identification of patients with acute AIDS-associated cryptococcal meningitis who can be effectively treated with fluconazole: the role of antifungal susceptibility testing. Clin Infect Dis 1996;22:322–8.
6. Rex JH, Rinaldi MG, Pfaller MA. Resistance of Candida species to fluconazole. Antimicrob Agents Chemother 1995;39:1–8.
7. Rex JH, Pfaller MA. Has antifungal Susceptibility testing come of age? Clin Infect Dis 2002;35:982–9.
8. Ghannoum MA, Rice LB. Antifungal agents: mode of action, mechanisms of resistance, and correlation of these mechanisms with bacterial resistance. Clin Microbiol Rev 1999;12(4):501–17.
9. Vallabhaneni S, Cleveland AA, Farley MM, et al. Epidemiology and risk factors for echinocandin nonsusceptible candida glabrata bloodstream infections:

data from a large multisite population-based candidemia surveillance program, 2008-2014. Open Forum Infect Dis 2015;2(4):ofv163.
10. Verweij PE, Chowdhary A, Melchers WJ, et al. Azole resistance in Aspergillus fumigatus: can we retain the clinical use of mold-active antifungal azoles? Clin Infect Dis 2016;62(3):362–8.
11. Rivero-Menendez O, Alastruey-Izquierdo A, Mellado E, et al. Triazole resistance in Aspergillus spp.: a worldwide problem? J Fungi (Basel) 2016;2(3).
12. Lackner M, Hagen F, Meis JF, et al. Susceptibility and diversity in the therapy-refractory genus scedosporium. Antimicrob Agents Chemother 2014;58(10): 5877–85.
13. Walsh TJ, Groll A, Hiemenz J, et al. Infections due to emerging and uncommon medically important fungal pathogens. Clin Microbiol Infect 2004;10(Suppl 1): 48–66.
14. Lockhart SR, Etienne KA, Vallabhaneni S, et al. Simultaneous emergence of multidrug-resistant Candida auris on 3 continents confirmed by whole-genome sequencing and epidemiological analyses. Clin Infect Dis 2017;64(2): 134–40.
15. Alexander BD, Johnson MD, Pfeiffer CD, et al. Increasing echinocandin resistance in Candida glabrata: clinical failure correlates with presence of FKS mutations and elevated minimum inhibitory concentrations. Clin Infect Dis 2013; 56(12):1724–32.
16. Monod M. Antifungal resistance in dermatophytes: emerging problem and challenge for the medical community. J Mycol Med 2019;29(4):283–4.
17. Hoekstra WJ, Garvey EP, Moore WR, et al. Design and optimization of highly-selective fungal CYP51 inhibitors. Bioorg Med Chem Lett 2014;24(15):3455–8.
18. Warrilow AG, Parker JE, Price CL, et al. The investigational drug VT-1129 is a highly potent inhibitor of cryptococcus species CYP51 but only weakly inhibits the human enzyme. Antimicrob Agents Chemother 2016;60(8):4530–8.
19. Sandison T, Ong V, Lee J, et al. Safety and pharmacokinetics of CD101 IV, a novel echinocandin, in healthy adults. Antimicrob Agents Chemother 2017; 61(2) [pii:e01627-16].
20. Pfaller MA, Messer SA, Motyl MR, et al. Activity of MK-3118, a new oral glucan synthase inhibitor, tested against Candida spp. by two international methods (CLSI and EUCAST). J Antimicrob Chemother 2013;68(4):858–63.
21. Oliver JD, Sibley GE, Beckmann N, et al. F901318 represents a novel class of antifungal drug that inhibits dihydroorotate dehydrogenase. Proc Natl Acad Sci U S A 2016;113(45):12809–14.
22. Miyazaki M, Horii T, Hata K, et al. In vitro activity of E1210, a novel antifungal, against clinically important yeasts and molds. Antimicrob Agents Chemother 2011;55(10):4652–8.
23. Nishikawa H, Yamada E, Shibata T, et al. Uptake of T-2307, a novel arylamidine, in Candida albicans. J Antimicrob Chemother 2010;65(8):1681–7.
24. Perfect JR. The antifungal pipeline: a reality check. Nat Rev Drug Discov 2017; 16(9):603–16.
25. Pfaller MA, Messer SA, Moet GJ, et al. Candida bloodstream infections: comparison of species distribution and resistance to echinocandin and azole antifungal agents in Intensive Care Unit (ICU) and non-ICU settings in the SENTRY Antimicrobial Surveillance Program (2008-2009). Int J Antimicrob Agents 2011; 38(1):65–9.
26. Yapar N. Epidemiology and risk factors for invasive candidiasis. Ther Clin Risk Manag 2014;10:95–105.

27. Orozco AS, Higginbotham LM, Hitchcock CA, et al. Mechanism of fluconazole resistance in Candida krusei. Antimicrob Agents Chemother 1998;42(10): 2645–9.
28. Cowen LE, Sanglard D, Howard SJ, et al. Mechanisms of antifungal drug resistance. Cold Spring Harb Perspect Med 2014;5(7):a019752.
29. Sokol-Anderson ML, Brajtburg J, Medoff G. Sensitivity of Candida albicans to amphotericin B administered as single or fractionated doses. Antimicrob Agents Chemother 1986;29(4):701–2.
30. White TC. Increased mRNA of ERG16, CDR, and MDR1 correlate with increases in azole resistance in Candida albicans isolates from an HIV-infected patient. Antimicrob Agents Chemother 1997;41:1482–7.
31. Sanglard D. Emerging threats in antifungal-resistant fungal pathogens. Front Med 2016;3:11.
32. Townsend JJ, Wolinsky JS, Baringer JR, et al. Acquired toxoplasmosis. A neglected cause of treatable nervous system disease. Arch Neurol 1975;32: 335–43.
33. Lockhart SR, Etienne KA, Vallabhaneni S, et al. Simultaneous Emergence of Multidrug-Resistant Candida auris on 3 continents confirmed by whole genome sequencing and epidemiological analyses. Clin. Infect. Dis 2017;64:134–40.
34. Healey KR, Kordalewska M, Jimenez Ortigosa C, et al. Limited ERG11 mutations identified in isolates of candida auris directly contribute to reduced azole susceptibility. Antimicrob Agents Chemother 2018;62(10) [pii:e01427-18].
35. Chowdhary A, Prakash A, Sharma C, et al. A multicentre study of antifungal susceptibility patterns among 350 Candida auris isolates (2009-17) in India: role of the ERG11 and FKS1 genes in azole and echinocandin resistance. J Antimicrob Chemother 2018;73(4):891–9.
36. Perlin DS. Current perspectives on echinocandin class drugs. Future Microbiol 2011;6(4):441–57.
37. Johnson ME, Katiyar SK, Edlind TD. New Fks hot spot for acquired echinocandin resistance in Saccharomyces cerevisiae and its contribution to intrinsic resistance of Scedosporium species. Antimicrob Agents Chemother 2011; 55(8):3774–81.
38. Katiyar SK, Edlind TD. Role for Fks1 in the intrinsic echinocandin resistance of Fusarium solani as evidenced by hybrid expression in Saccharomyces cerevisiae. Antimicrob Agents Chemother 2009;53(5):1772–8.
39. Garcia-Effron G, Lee S, Park S, et al. Effect of Candida glabrata FKS1 and FKS2 mutations on echinocandin sensitivity and kinetics of 1,3-beta-D-glucan synthase: implication for the existing susceptibility breakpoint. Antimicrob Agents Chemother 2009;53(9):3690–9.
40. Perlin DS. Echinocandin resistance in Candida. Clin Infect Dis 2015;61(Suppl 6): S612–7.
41. Katiyar SK, Alastruey-Izquierdo A, Healey KR, et al. Fks1 and Fks2 are functionally redundant but differentially regulated in Candida glabrata: implications for echinocandin resistance. Antimicrob Agents Chemother 2012;56(12):6304–9.
42. Calo S, Shertz-Wall C, Lee SC, et al. Antifungal drug resistance evoked via RNAi-dependent epimutations. Nature 2014;513(7519):555–8.
43. Chang Z, Billmyre RB, Lee SC, et al. Broad antifungal resistance mediated by RNAi-dependent epimutation in the basal human fungal pathogen Mucor circinelloides. PLoS Genet 2019;15(2):e1007957.
44. Magobo RE, Corcoran C, Seetharam S, et al. Candida auris-associated candidemia, South Africa. Emerg Infect Dis 2014;20(7):1250–1.

45. Sears D, Schwartz BS. Candida auris: an emerging multidrug-resistant pathogen. Int J Infect Dis 2017;63:95–8.
46. Chowdhary A, Sharma C, Duggal S, et al. New clonal strain of Candida auris, Delhi, India. Emerg Infect Dis 2013;19(10):1670–3.
47. Calvo B, Melo AS, Perozo-Mena A, et al. First report of Candida auris in America: clinical and microbiological aspects of 18 episodes of candidemia. J Infect 2016;73(4):369–74.
48. Vallabhaneni S, Kallen A, Tsay S, et al. Investigation of the first seven reported cases of Candida auris, a Globally Emerging Invasive, Multidrug-Resistant Fungus-United States, May 2013-August 2016. Am J Transplant 2017;17(1):296–9.
49. Chowdhary A, Anil Kumar V, Sharma C, et al. Multidrug-resistant endemic clonal strain of Candida auris in India. Eur J Clin Microbiol Infect Dis 2014;33(6): 919–26.
50. Forsberg K, Woodworth K, Walters M, et al. Candida auris: the recent emergence of a multidrug-resistant fungal pathogen. Med Mycol 2019;57(1):1–12.
51. Lam M, Jou PC, Lattif AA, et al. Photodynamic therapy with Pc 4 induces apoptosis of Candida albicans. Photochem Photobiol 2011;87(4):904–9.
52. Lamoth F, Kontoyiannis DP. The Candida auris alert: facts and perspectives. J Infect Dis 2018;217(4):516–20.
53. Eyre DW, Sheppard AE, Madder H, et al. A Candida auris outbreak and its control in an intensive care setting. N Engl J Med 2018;379(14):1322–31.
54. Welsh RM, Bentz ML, Shams A, et al. Survival, persistence, and isolation of the emerging multidrug-resistant pathogenic yeast Candida auris on a plastic health care surface. J Clin Microbiol 2017;55(10):2996–3005.
55. Adams E, Quinn M, Tsay S, et al. Candida auris in Healthcare Facilities, New York, USA, 2013-2017. Emerg Infect Dis 2018;24(10):1816–24.
56. Kean R, McKloud E, Townsend EM, et al. The comparative efficacy of antiseptics against Candida auris biofilms. Int J Antimicrob Agents 2018;52(5):673–7.
57. Larkin E, Hager C, Chandra J, et al. The Emerging Pathogen Candida auris: growth phenotype, virulence factors, activity of antifungals, and effect of SCY-078, a novel glucan synthesis inhibitor, on growth morphology and biofilm formation. Antimicrob Agents Chemother 2017;61(5) [pii:e02396-16].
58. Sherry L, Ramage G, Kean R, et al. Biofilm-forming capability of highly virulent, multidrug-resistant Candida auris. Emerg Infect Dis 2017;23(2):328–31.
59. Short B, Brown J, Delaney C, et al. Candida auris exhibits resilient biofilm characteristics in vitro: implications for environmental persistence. J Hosp Infect 2019;103(1):92–6.
60. Johnson CJ, Davis JM, Huttenlocher A, et al. Emerging fungal pathogen candida auris evades neutrophil attack. mBio 2018;9(4) [pii:e01403-18].
61. Hager CL, Larkin EL, Long L, et al. In vitro and in vivo evaluation of the antifungal activity of APX001A/APX001 against Candida auris. Antimicrob Agents Chemother 2018;62(3) [pii:e02319-17].
62. Hager CL, Larkin EL, Long LA, et al. Evaluation of the efficacy of rezafungin, a novel echinocandin, in the treatment of disseminated Candida auris infection using an immunocompromised mouse model. J Antimicrob Chemother 2018; 73(8):2085–8.
63. Nett JE. Candida auris: an emerging pathogen "incognito"? PLoS Pathog 2019; 15(4):e1007638.
64. van der Linden JW CS, Kampinga GA, Arends JP, et al. Aspergillosis due to voriconazole highly resistant Aspergillus fumigatus and recovery of genetically related resistant isolates from domiciles. Clin Infect Dis 2013;57:513–20.

65. Verweij PE, Snelders E, Kema GH, et al. Azole resistance in Aspergillus fumigatus : a side-effect of environmental fungicide use? Lancet Infect Dis 2009;9(12):789–95.
66. Lestrade PP, Bentvelsen RG, Schauwvlieghe A, et al. Voriconazole resistance and mortality in invasive aspergillosis: a multicenter retrospective cohort study. Clin Infect Dis 2019;68(9):1463–71.
67. Snelders E, van der Lee HA, Kuijpers J, et al. Emergence of azole resistance in Aspergillus fumigatus and spread of a single resistance mechanism. PLoS Med 2008;5(11):e219.
68. Patterson TF, Thompson GR 3rd, Denning DW, et al. Practice guidelines for the diagnosis and management of aspergillosis: 2016 update by the Infectious Diseases Society of America. Clin Infect Dis 2016;63(4):e1–60.
69. Chen Y, Farrer RA, Giamberardino C, et al. Microevolution of serial clinical isolates of cryptococcus neoformans var. grubii and C. gattii. MBio 2017;8(2).
70. Aller AI, Martin-Manzuelos E, Lozano F, et al. Correlation of fluconazole MICs with clinical outcome in cryptococcal infection. Antimicrob Agents Chemother 2000;44:1544–8.
71. Dannaoui E, Abdul M, Arpin M, et al. Results obtained with various antifungal susceptibility testing methods do not predict early treatment outcome in patients with cryptococcosis. Antimicrob Agents Chemother 2008;50:2464–70.
72. Perfect JR, Dismukes WE, Pappas PG, et al. Clinical practice guidelines for the management of cryptococcal disease: 2010 Update by the Infectious Diseases Society of America. Clin Infect Dis 2010;50:291–322.
73. Sionov E, Chang YC, Garraffo HM, et al. Identification of a Cryptococcus neoformans cytochrome P450 lanosterol 14alpha-demethylase (Erg11) residue critical for differential susceptibility between fluconazole/voriconazole and itraconazole/posaconazole. Antimicrob Agents Chemother 2012;56(3):1162–9.
74. Bongomin F, Oladele RO, Gago S, et al. A systematic review of fluconazole resistance in clinical isolates of Cryptococcus species. Mycoses 2018;61(5):290–7.
75. Perfect JR, Cox GM. Drug resistance in Cryptococcus neoformans. Drug Resist Updat 1999;2:259–69.
76. Block ER, Jennings AE, Bennett JE. 5-Fluorocytosine resistance in Cryptococcus neoformans. Antimicrob Agents Chemother 1973;3:649–56.
77. Vu K, Thompson GR 3rd, Roe CC, et al. Flucytosine resistance in Cryptococcus gattii is indirectly mediated by the FCY2-FCY1-FUR1 pathway. Med Mycol 2018;56(7):857–67.
78. Joseph-Horne T, Loefflin RST, Halloman DW, et al. Amphotericin B resistant isolates of Cryptococcus neoformans without alteration in sterol biosynthesis. J Med Vet Mycol 1996;34:223–5.
79. Kelly SL, Lamb DC, Taylor M, et al. Resistance to amphotericin B associated with defective sterol delta 8-7 isomerase in a Cryptococcus neoformans strain from an AIDS patient. FEMS Microbiol Lett 1994;122:39–42.
80. Rodero L, Mellado E, Rodriguez AC, et al. G484S amino acid substitution in lanosterol 14-alpha demethylase (ERG11) is related to fluconazole resistance in a recurrent Cryptococcus neoformans clinical isolate. Antimicrob Agents Chemother 2003;47(11):3653–6.
81. Chang M, Sionov E, Khanal Lamichhane A, et al. Roles of three cryptococcus neoformans and Cryptococcus gattii efflux pump-coding genes in response to drug treatment. Antimicrob Agents Chemother 2018;62(4) [pii:e01751-17].

82. Bastos RW, Freitas GJC, Carneiro HCS, et al. From the environment to the host: how non-azole agrochemical exposure affects the antifungal susceptibility and virulence of Cryptococcus gattii. Sci Total Environ 2019;681:516–23.
83. Chen SLA, Meyer W, Sorrell TC. Cryptococcus gattii. Clin Microbiol Rev 2014; 27:980–1024.
84. Rosenberg A, Ene IV, Bibi M, et al. Antifungal tolerance is a subpopulation effect distinct from resistance and is associated with persistent candidemia. Nat Commun 2018;9(1):2470.
85. Sionov ECY, Garraffo HM, Kwon-Chung KJ. Heteroresistance to fluconazole in *Cryptococcus neoformans* is intrinsic and associated with virulence. Antimicrob Agents Chemother 2009;53:2804–15.
86. Stone NR, Rhodes J, Fisher MC, et al. Dynamic ploidy changes drive fluconazole resistance in human cryptococcal meningitis. J Clin Invest 2019;129(3): 999–1014.
87. Mondon P, Petter R, Amalfitano G, et al. Heteroresistance to fluconazole and voriconazole in Cryptococcus neoformans. Antimicrob Agents Chemother 1999;43: 1856–61.
88. Yamazumi T, Pfaller MA, Messer SA, et al. Characterization of heteroresistance to fluconazole among clinical isolates of Cryptococcus neoformans. J Clin Microbiol 2003;41(1):267–72.
89. Sionov E, Lee H, Chang YC, et al. *Cryptococcus neoformans* overcomes stress of azole drugs by formation of disomy in specific multiple chromosomes. PLoS Pathog 2010;16(4):e1000848.
90. Sionov ECY, Kwon-Chung KJ. Azole heteroresistance in Cryptococcus neoformans: emergence of resistant clones with chromosomal disomy in the mouse brain during fluconazole treatment. Antimicrob Agents Chemother 2013;57: 5127–30.
91. Waag DM. Immune response to Coxiella burnetti infection. In: Marrie TJ, editor. Fever, Volume 1. Boca Raton (FL): CRC Press, Inc; 1990. p. 107–23.
92. Semighini CPAA, Perfect JR, Heitman J. Deletion of Cryptococcus neoformans AIF ortholog promotes chromosome aneuploidy and fluconazole-resistance in a metacaspase-independent manner. PLoS Pathog 2011;7:1002364.
93. Hope W, Stone NRH, Johnson A, et al. Fluconazole monotherapy is a suboptimal option for initial treatment of cryptococcal meningitis because of emergence of resistance. mBio 2019;10(6) [pii:e02575-19.
94. Nussbaum JC, Jackson A, Namarika D, et al. Combination flucytosine and high-dose fluconazole compared with fluconazole monotherapy for the treatment of cryptococcal meningitis: a randomized trial in Malawi. Clin Infect Dis 2010; 50(3):338–44.
95. Molloy SF, Kanyama C, Heyderman RS, et al. Antifungal combinations for treatment of Cryptococcal Meningitis in Africa. N Engl J Med 2018;378(11):1004–17.
96. Altamirano S, Fang D, Simmons C, et al. Fluconazole-induced ploidy change in Cryptococcus neoformans results from the uncoupling of cell growth and nuclear division. mSphere 2017;2(3) [pii:e00205-17].
97. Kanafani ZA, Perfect JR. Antimicrobial resistance: resistance to antifungal agents: mechanisms and clinical impact. Clin Infect Dis 2008;46(1):120–8.
98. Singh N, Perfect JR. Immune reconstitution syndrome associated with opportunistic mycoses. Lancet Infect Dis 2007;7(6):395–401.
99. Garey KWRM, Pai MP, Mingo DE, et al. Time to initiation of fluconazole therapy impacts mortality in patients with candidemia: a multi-institutional study. Clin Infect Dis 2006;43:25–31.

100. Morrell M, Fraser VJ, Kollef MH. Delaying the empiric treatment of candida bloodstream infection until positive blood culture results are obtained: a potential risk factor for hospital mortality. Antimicrob Agents Chemother 2005;49(9): 3640–5.
101. Bicanic T, Harrison T, Niepieklo A, et al. Symptomatic relapse of HIV-associated cryptococcal meningitis after initial fluconazole monotherapy: the role of fluconazole resistance and immune reconstitution. Clin Infect Dis 2006;43(8):1069–73.
102. Fraser JA, Giles SS, Wenink EC, et al. Same-sex mating and the origin of the Vancouver Island Cryptococcus gattii outbreak. Nature 2005;437(7063):1360–4.
103. Beale MA, Sabiiti W, Robertson EJ, et al. Genotypic diversity is associated with clinical outcome and phenotype in Cryptococcal Meningitis across Southern Africa. PLoS Negl Trop Dis 2015;9(6):e0003847.
104. Trifilio S, Pennick G, Pi J, et al. Monitoring plasma voriconazole levels may be necessary to avoid subtherapeutic levels in hematopoietic stem cell transplant recipients. Cancer 2007;109(8):1532–5.
105. Pascual A, Calandra T, Bolay S, et al. Voriconazole therapeutic drug monitoring in patients with invasive mycoses improves efficacy and safety outcomes. Clin Infect Dis 2008;46(2):201–11.
106. Mourad A, Stiber JA, Perfect JR, et al. Real-world implications of QT prolongation in patients receiving voriconazole and amiodarone. J Antimicrob Chemother 2019;74(1):228–33.
107. Lutsar I, Roffey S, Troke P. Voriconazole concentrations in the cerebrospinal fluid and brain tissue of guinea pigs and immunocompromised patients. Clin Infect Dis 2003;37(5):728–32.
108. Kuhn DM, George T, Chandra J, et al. Antifungal susceptibility of Candida biofilms: unique efficacy of amphotericin B lipid formulations and echinocandins. Antimicrob Agents Chemother 2002;46(6):1773–80.
109. Raad I, Hanna H, Boktour M, et al. Management of central venous catheters in patients with cancer and candidemia. Clin Infect Dis 2004;38(8):1119–27.
110. Mora-Duarte J, Betts R, Rotstein C, et al. Comparison of caspofungin and amphotericin B for invasive candidiasis. N Engl J Med 2002;347(25):2020–9.
111. Zarakas MA, Desai JV, Chamilos G, et al. Fungal Infections with Ibrutinib and Other Small-Molecule Kinase Inhibitors. Curr Fungal Infect Rep 2019;13(3): 86–98.
112. Johnson MD, MacDougall C, Ostrosky-Zeichner L, et al. Combination antifungal therapy. Antimicrob Agents Chemother 2004;48(3):693–715.
113. Livengood S, Drew R, Perfect J. Combination therpy for invasive fungal infections. Curr Fung Infect, in press.
114. Johnson MD, Perfect JR. Use of antifungal combination therapy: agents, order, and timing. Curr Fungal Infect Rep 2010;4(2):87–95.
115. Day J, Chau TT, Wolbers M. Combination antifungal therapy for Cryptococcal Meningitis. N Engl J Med 2013;368:1291–302.
116. Brouwer AE, Rajanuwong A, Chierakul W, et al. Combination antifungal therapies for HIV-associated cryptococcal meningitis: feasibility and power of quantitative CSF cultures to determine fungicidal activity. Lancet 2004;363:1764–7.
117. Rex JH, Pappas PG, Karchmer AW, et al. A randomized and blinded multicenter trial of high-dose fluconazole plus placebo versus fluconazole plus amphotericin B as therapy for candidemia and its consequences in nonneutropenic subjects. Clin Infect Dis 2003;36(10):1221–8.
118. Schaffner A, Frick PG. The effect of ketoconazole on amphotericin B in a model of disseminated aspergillosis. J Infect Dis 1985;151:902–20.

119. Marr KA, Schlamm HT, Herbrecht R, et al. Combination antifungal therapy for invasive aspergillosis: a randomized trial. Ann Intern Med 2015;162(2):81–9.
120. Panackal AA, Parisini E, Proschan M. Salvage combination antifungal therapy for acute invasive aspergillosis may improve outcomes: a systematic review and meta-analysis. Int J Infect Dis 2014;28:80–94.
121. Reed C, Bryant R, Ibrahim AS, et al. Combination polyene-caspofungin treatment of rhino-orbital-cerebral mucormycosis. Clin Infect Dis 2008;47(3):364–71.
122. Spellberg BIA, Chin-Hong PV, Kontoyiannis DP, et al. The Deferasirox-AmBisome therapy for Mucormycosis (DEFEAT Mucor) study: a randomized, double-blinded, placebo-controlled trial. J Antimicrob Chemother 2012;67: 715–22.
123. Pouliot M, Jeanmart S. Pan assay interference compounds (PAINS) and other promiscuous compounds in antifungal research. J Med Chem 2016;59(2): 497–503.
124. Juvvadi PR, Lee SC, Heitman J, et al. Calcineurin in fungal virulence and drug resistance: prospects for harnessing targeted inhibition of calcineurin for an antifungal therapeutic approach. Virulence 2017;8(2):186–97.
125. Cowen LE, Sing SD, Kohler JR, et al. Harnessing Hsp90 function as a powerful, broadly effective therapeutic strategy for fungal infectious disease. Proc Natl Acad Sci U S A 2009;(106):2818–23.
126. Hast MA, Nichols CB, Armstrong SM, et al. Structures of Cryptococcus neoformans protein farnesyltransferase reveal strategies for developing inhibitors that target fungal pathogens. J Biol Chem 2011;286(40):35149–62.
127. Mor V, Rella A, Farnoud AM, et al. Identification of a new class of antifungals targeting the synthesis of fungal Sphingolipids. MBio 2015;6(3):e00647.
128. Perfect JR, Tenor JL, Miao Y, et al. Trehalose pathway as an antifungal target. Virulence 2017;8(2):143–9.
129. Hata K, Horii T, Miyazaki M, et al. Efficacy of oral E1210, a new broad-spectrum antifungal with a novel mechanism of action, in murine models of candidiasis, aspergillosis, and fusariosis. Antimicrob Agents Chemother 2011;55(10): 4543–51.
130. Mitsuyama J, Nomura N, Hashimoto K, et al. In vitro and in vivo antifungal activities of T-2307, a novel arylamidine. Antimicrob Agents Chemother 2008;52(4): 1318–24.
131. Miesel L, Lin KY, Ong V. Rezafungin treatment in mouse models of invasive candidiasis and aspergillosis: Insights on the PK/PD pharmacometrics of rezafungin efficacy. Pharmacol Res Perspect 2019;7(6):e00546.
132. Lindsay J, Sandaradura I, Wong K, et al. Serum levels, safety and tolerability of new formulation SUBA-itraconazole prophylaxis in patients with haematological malignancy or undergoing allogeneic stem cell transplantation. J Antimicrob Chemother 2017;72(12):3414–9.
133. Delmas G, Park S, Chen ZW, et al. Efficacy of orally delivered cochleates containing amphotericin B in a murine model of aspergillosis. Antimicrob Agents Chemother 2002;46(8):2704–7.
134. Spec A, Pullman J, Thompson GR, et al. MSG-10: a Phase 2 study of oral ibrexafungerp (SCY-078) following initial echinocandin therapy in non-neutropenic patients with invasive candidiasis. J Antimicrob Chemother 2019;74(10): 3056–62.
135. Wiederhold NP, Shubitz LF, Najvar LK, et al. The novel fungal Cyp51 inhibitor VT-1598 is efficacious in experimental models of central nervous system

coccidioidomycosis caused by Coccidioides posadasii and Coccidioides immitis. Antimicrob Agents Chemother 2018;62(4) [pii:e02258-17].
136. Brand SR, Degenhardt TP, Person K, et al. A phase 2, randomized, double-blind, placebo-controlled, dose-ranging study to evaluate the efficacy and safety of orally administered VT-1161 in the treatment of recurrent vulvovaginal candidiasis. Am J Obstet Gynecol 2018;218(6):624.e1–9.
137. Tramsen L, Schmidt S, Boenig H, et al. Clinical-scale generation of multi-specific anti-fungal T cells targeting Candida, Aspergillus and mucormycetes. Cytotherapy 2013;15(3):344–51.
138. Ambati S, Ellis EC, Lin J, et al. Dectin-2-targeted antifungal liposomes exhibit enhanced efficacy. mSphere 2019;4(5) [pii:e00715-19].
139. Pachl J, Svoboda P, Jacobs F, et al. A randomized, blinded, multicenter trial of lipid-associated Amphotericin B alone versus in combination with an antibody-based inhibitor of heat shock protein 90 in patients with invasive candidiasis. Clin Infect Dis 2006;42(10):1404–13.
140. Bryan RA, Guimaraes AJ, Hopcraft S, et al. Toward developing a universal treatment for fungal disease using radioimmunotherapy targeting common fungal antigens. Mycopathologia 2012;173(5–6):463–71.
141. Edwards JE Jr, Schwartz MM, Schmidt CS, et al. A fungal immunotherapeutic vaccine (NDV-3A) for treatment of recurrent vulvovaginal candidiasis-A phase 2 randomized, double-blind, placebo-controlled trial. Clin Infect Dis 2018;66(12):1928–36.

UNITED STATES POSTAL SERVICE®

Statement of Ownership, Management, and Circulation (All Periodicals Publications Except Requester Publications)

1. Publication Title	2. Publication Number	3. Filing Date
INFECTIOUS DISEASE CLINICS OF NORTH AMERICA	001 – 556	9/18/2020
4. Issue Frequency	5. Number of Issues Published Annually	6. Annual Subscription Price
MAR, JUN, SEP, DEC	4	$340.00

7. Complete Mailing Address of Known Office of Publication (Not printer) (Street, city, county, state, and ZIP+4®)
ELSEVIER INC.
230 Park Avenue, Suite 800
New York, NY 10169

Contact Person: Malathi Samayan
Telephone (Include area code): 91-44-4299-4507

8. Complete Mailing Address of Headquarters or General Business Office of Publisher (Not printer)
ELSEVIER INC.
230 Park Avenue, Suite 800
New York, NY 10169

9. Full Names and Complete Mailing Addresses of Publisher, Editor, and Managing Editor (Do not leave blank)

Publisher (Name and complete mailing address)
DOLORES MELONI, ELSEVIER INC
1600 JOHN F. KENNEDY BLVD. SUITE 1800
PHILADELPHIA, PA 19103-2899

Editor (Name and complete mailing address)
KERRY HOLLAND, ELSEVIER INC.
1600 JOHN F KENNEDY BLVD. SUITE 1800
PHILADELPHIA, PA 19103-2899

Managing Editor (Name and complete mailing address)
PATRICK MANLEY, ELSEVIER INC.
1600 JOHN F KENNEDY BLVD. SUITE 1800
PHILADELPHIA, PA 19103-2899

10. Owner (Do not leave blank. If the publication is owned by a corporation, give the name and address of the corporation immediately followed by the names and addresses of all stockholders owning or holding 1 percent or more of the total amount of stock. If not owned by a corporation, give the names and addresses of the individual owners. If owned by a partnership or other unincorporated firm, give its name and address as well as those of each individual owner. If the publication is published by a nonprofit organization, give its name and address.)

Full Name	Complete Mailing Address
WHOLLY OWNED SUBSIDIARY OF REED/ELSEVIER, US HOLDINGS	1600 JOHN F KENNEDY BLVD. SUITE 1800 PHILADELPHIA, PA 19103-2899

11. Known Bondholders, Mortgagees, and Other Security Holders Owning or Holding 1 Percent or More of Total Amount of Bonds, Mortgages, or Other Securities. If none, check box → ☐ None

Full Name	Complete Mailing Address
N/A	

12. Tax Status (For completion by nonprofit organizations authorized to mail at nonprofit rates) (Check one)
The purpose, function, and nonprofit status of this organization and the exempt status for federal income tax purposes:
☒ Has Not Changed During Preceding 12 Months
☐ Has Changed During Preceding 12 Months (Publisher must submit explanation of change with this statement)

13. Publication Title		14. Issue Date for Circulation Data Below	
INFECTIOUS DISEASE CLINICS OF NORTH AMERICA		JUNE 2020	
15. Extent and Nature of Circulation		Average No. Copies Each Issue During Preceding 12 Months	No. Copies of Single Issue Published Nearest to Filing Date
a. Total Number of Copies (Net press run)		246	216
b. Paid Circulation (By Mail and Outside the Mail)	(1) Mailed Outside-County Paid Subscriptions Stated on PS Form 3541 (Include paid distribution above nominal rate, advertiser's proof copies, and exchange copies)	162	150
	(2) Mailed In-County Paid Subscriptions Stated on PS Form 3541 (Include paid distribution above nominal rate, advertiser's proof copies, and exchange copies)	0	0
	(3) Paid Distribution Outside the Mails Including Sales Through Dealers and Carriers, Street Vendors, Counter Sales, and Other Paid Distribution Outside USPS®	49	43
	(4) Paid Distribution by Other Classes of Mail Through the USPS (e.g., First-Class Mail®)	0	0
c. Total Paid Distribution (Sum of 15b (1), (2), (3), and (4))		211	193
d. Free or Nominal Rate Distribution (By Mail and Outside the Mail)	(1) Free or Nominal Rate Outside-County Copies included on PS Form 3541	19	8
	(2) Free or Nominal Rate In-County Copies Included on PS Form 3541	0	0
	(3) Free or Nominal Rate Copies Mailed at Other Classes Through the USPS (e.g., First-Class Mail)	0	0
	(4) Free or Nominal Rate Distribution Outside the Mail (Carriers or other means)	0	0
e. Total Free or Nominal Rate Distribution (Sum of 15d (1), (2), (3) and (4))		19	8
f. Total Distribution (Sum of 15c and 15e)		230	201
g. Copies not Distributed (See Instructions to Publishers #4 (page #3))		16	15
h. Total (Sum of 15f and g)		246	216
i. Percent Paid (15c divided by 15f times 100)		91.73%	96.01%

* If you are claiming electronic copies, go to line 16 on page 3. If you are not claiming electronic copies, skip to line 17 on page 3.

16. Electronic Copy Circulation	Average No. Copies Each Issue During Preceding 12 Months	No. Copies of Single Issue Published Nearest to Filing Date
a. Paid Electronic Copies		
b. Total Paid Print Copies (Line 15c) + Paid Electronic Copies (Line 16a)		
c. Total Print Distribution (Line 15f) + Paid Electronic Copies (Line 16a)		
d. Percent Paid (Both Print & Electronic Copies) (16b divided by 16c × 100)		

☒ **I certify that 50% of all my distributed copies (electronic and print) are paid above a nominal price.**

17. Publication of Statement of Ownership
☒ If the publication is a general publication, publication of this statement is required. Will be printed in the DECEMBER 2020 issue of this publication. ☐ Publication not required

18. Signature and Title of Editor, Publisher, Business Manager, or Owner
Malathi Samayan - Distribution Controller *Malathi Samayan* Date 9/18/2020

I certify that all information furnished on this form is true and complete. I understand that anyone who furnishes false or misleading information on this form or who omits material or information requested on the form may be subject to criminal sanctions (including fines and imprisonment) and/or civil sanctions (including civil penalties).

Printed and bound by CPI Group (UK) Ltd, Croydon, CR0 4YY

03/10/2024

01040478-0012